WORLD HEALTH ORGANIZATION

INTERNATIONAL AGENCY FOR RESEARCH ON CANCER

STATISTICAL METHODS

IN

CANCER RESEARCH

VOLUME II – THE DESIGN AND ANALYSIS OF COHORT STUDIES

BY

N.E. BRESLOW & N.E. DAY

TECHNICAL EDITOR FOR IARC

E. HESELTINE

IARC Scientific Publications No. 82

INTERNATIONAL AGENCY FOR RESEARCH ON CANCER
LYON

1987

The International Agency for Research on Cancer (IARC) was established in 1965 by the World Health Assembly, as an independently financed organization within the framework of the World Health Organization. The headquarters of the Agency are at Lyon, France.

The Agency conducts a programme of research concentrating particularly on the epidemiology of cancer and the study of potential carcinogens in the human environment. Its field studies are supplemented by biological and chemical research carried out in the Agency's laboratories in Lyon and, through collaborative research agreements, in national research institutions in many countries. The Agency also conducts a programme for the education and training of personnel for cancer research.

The publications of the Agency are intended to contribute to the dissemination of authoritative information on different aspects of cancer research.

Distributed for the International Agency for Research on Cancer
by Oxford University Press, Walton Street, Oxford OX2 6DP, UK

London   New York   Toronto
Delhi   Bombay   Calcutta   Madras   Karachi
Kuala Lumpur   Singapore   Hong Kong   Tokyo
Nairobi   Dar es Salaam   Cape Town
Melbourne   Auckland

Oxford is a trade mark of Oxford University Press

Distributed in the United States
by Oxford University Press, New York

ISBN 92 832 1182 0
ISSN 0300–5085

© International Agency for Research on Cancer 1987
150 cours Albert Thomas, 69372 Lyon Cedex 08, France

CONTENTS

FOREWORD

Epidemiological studies provide the only definitive information on the degree of cancer risk to man. Since malignant diseases are clearly of multifactorial origin, their investigation in man has become increasingly complex, and epidemiological and statistical studies on cancer require a correspondingly complex and rigorous methodology.

The past 15 years have seen rapid developments of the analytic tools available to epidemiologists. These advances now permit a more flexible and quantitative approach to the use of epidemiological data, and thus greatly enhance the utility of such data for the primary purpose of disease prevention. For society now expects that if preventive measures are to be introduced, then quantitative assessments of the expected benefit should be available. The first volume in this series focused on case-control studies, reflecting the concentration on this approach in the 1970s for the identification of cancer hazards. Attention has recently turned to the more basic line of attack provided by cohort studies, and the more general modelling of risk that can ensue. This second volume gives an authoritative account of the methods now available for the interpretation of the results from this type of study.

The two volumes together give a comprehensive development of the principles and concepts underlying the design and analysis of both types of study currently used in analytic cancer epidemiology, and a detailed treatment of the quantitative methods now available. The IARC hopes that this text will be of value to the epidemiological and statistical community for many years to come.

L. Tomatis, MD
Director
International Agency
for Research on Cancer

PREFACE

Long-term follow-up (cohort) studies of human populations, particularly of industrial workers, of patients treated with radiation and cytotoxic chemotherapy, and of victims of nuclear and other disasters, have provided the most convincing evidence of the link between exposure to specific environmental agents and cancer occurrence. Of the chemicals and industrial processes for which working groups convened by the IARC have decided that there is 'sufficient evidence' of human carcinogenicity, cohort studies provided the definitive evidence in the great majority of cases. In the studies carried out in the 1950s and 1960s, high risks were associated with specific exposures. Relatively simple statistical methods were sufficient to demonstrate the effect, and the finer quantitative features of the relationship were not emphasized. It was not uncommon for reports of occupational hazards to be based primarily on the computation of standardized death rates or mortality ratios (SMRs) for a few causes of death, with virtually no attention paid to internal comparisons among differentially exposed workers. Since then, the picture has changed. More attention is now paid to the quantification of risk and the use of more refined dose-response models. Interest has also turned to a wider range of exposures and the interplay between physiological measures of nutritional status, dietary factors and other variables of modes of life. Multivariate methods are then necessary, often making use of serial measurements on the same individuals.

Increasingly, modern concepts of statistical inference and modelling are being used to maximize the information obtainable from these major endeavours and to provide the most precise estimates possible of quantitative risk. Indeed, some cohort studies have stimulated the development of new statistical methods of particular relevance to this field.

The primary purpose of this monograph is to bring together in one place the statistical developments that have taken place during the past few years that are of relevance to the design and analysis of cohort studies, and to illustrate their application to several sets of data of importance in the field of cancer epidemiology. We hope to present these new statistical methods in such a way that epidemiologists and other research workers without extensive statistical training can appreciate the possibilities they offer and, in many cases, can apply them to their own work. In addition, by providing a thorough introduction to the design and execution of cohort studies, including a detailed description of six landmark investigations of this type, we hope to interest students of statistical science in this field so that they may turn their attention both to the proper application of current methods and to the further development of those methods.

In the preface to the first volume in this series we stressed the essential similarity of statistical methods applicable to the case-control and cohort approaches to epidemiological research, the flexibility of new methods for handling a variety of data configurations and the wide range of problems that could be approached from a common conceptual foundation. This pursuit of unity and flexibility continues to be our goal. We show how elementary methods that have long been used for analysis of cohort data relate to explicit statistical models, and how they may be extended so as to achieve greater understanding of the collected data. The SMR, for example, has been used virtually without change for over 200 years to make age-adjusted comparisons of regional and occupational mortality. We show how this statistic may be derived as a maximum likelihood estimate in a well-defined statistical model, and how an extension of that model leads to a regression analysis of the SMR as a function of one or more risk factors. This approach shows us that the well-known 'lack of comparability' of SMRs is due to the problem of statistical confounding and may be alleviated by a proper analysis. Further extensions of the basic model permit variations in the SMR to be estimated as a nonparametric function of time for purposes of exploratory analyses of data.

Experience with the first volume taught us that one of its most important features, made possible through the generosity of our collaborators, was the provision of appendices containing several condensed, but nonetheless bona-fide, sets of data. These were used in worked examples that readers could follow to test their understanding of the material (and, occasionally, to find our mistakes). The present volume contains appendices that give grouped data from a study of respiratory cancer among smelter workers in Montana, USA, and both grouped and individual data records on 679 Welsh nickel refiners who had high rates of lung and nasal sinus cancer. Summary data from several other studies that appear in tables scattered throughout the monograph may also be useful for this purpose.

A major source of dissatisfaction with the first volume was its lack of a subject index. We have attempted to remedy the situation by including a combined index to both volumes.

N.E. Breslow and N.E. Day

ACKNOWLEDGEMENTS

Planning of this volume on cohort studies began shortly after the appearance of the first volume on case-control studies in 1980. Since then, many people have contributed to its development. Thirteen epidemiologists and statisticians participated in an IARC workshop on the statistical aspects of cohort studies that was held in Lyon on 23–27 May 1983 (see List of Participants). Initial drafts of several chapters were circulated and reviewed during that meeting, and the discussion was valuable for orientating subsequent developments. As those chapters were completed, they were sent to selected individuals for further comment. Persons who generously contributed their time in this regard include E. Bjelke, D. Clayton, T. Fletcher, E. Johnson, J. Kaldor, E. Läärä and P. Smith. We appreciate the significant efforts of these reviewers.

Data from two cohort studies are listed in the appendices and are utilized throughout the monograph in illustrative analyses that demonstrate the relationships between various statistical methods. We are indebted to Professor Sir Richard Doll and Professor J. Peto for permission to reproduce a working version of the recently updated data on Welsh nickel refiners in Appendices VI, VII and VIII. Likewise, we appreciate the generosity of Dr J. Fraumeni, Dr A. Lee-Feldstein and Dr J. Lubin in providing access to the latest follow-up data from their study of Montana smelter workers, portions of which are reproduced in Appendix V. We believe that the availability of these data sets to readers who wish to verify our results, or who wish to test their own ideas for statistical analysis on the basis of bona-fide and well-documented sets of epidemiological data, is extremely important in achieving the goals towards which the monograph is directed.

Several people assisted with the computer programming, data management and statistical analyses required for the illustrative examples, tables and figures. NEB would like to thank particularly Dr B. Langholz, who contributed to this effort over a period of several years, Mr P. Marek for computer programming and Mr J. Cologne who assisted with many of the final preparations. NED would like to acknowledge Ms D. Magnin and Dr J. Kaldor.

Primary secretarial support for this project was provided by Jean Hawkins who was responsible for the typing of innumerable drafts and the transfer of material among several word-processing systems. She also provided valuable assistance with editing, reference checking, and a myriad of necessary details. We should like to thank also Mrs A. Rivoire, Mrs E. Nasco and Mrs M. Kaad for their contributions. The figures were carefully prepared by Mr Jacques Déchaux. We thank Mrs E. Heseltine and her staff for editing and shepherding the manuscript through the final stages of publication.

This project would not have been possible without the generous financial support of the US National Cancer Institute. During the initial years of preparation, NEB held a Preventive Oncology Academic Award, and in later years a research grant awarded by the National Cancer Institute. First drafts of several chapters were written during the 1982–1983 academic year while he was on sabbatical leave from the University of Washington at the German Cancer Research Center in Heidelberg. He would like to thank Dr H. Neurath and Dr G. Wagner, as well as the Alexander von Humboldt Foundation, for arranging this visit and his colleagues in Seattle, particularly Dr V. Farewell and Dr P. Feigl, for continuation of work in progress during his absence.

LIST OF PARTICIPANTS AT IARC WORKSHOP
25–27 May 1983

Professor E. Bjelke
Institute of Hygiene and Social Medicine
University of Bergen
5016 Haukeland Sykehus, Norway

Professor N.E. Breslow
Department of Biostatistics, SC-32
University of Washington
Seattle, WA 98195, USA

Dr T. Hirayama
Chief, Epidemiology Division
National Cancer Center Research Institute
Tokyo, Japan

Dr B. Langholz
German Cancer Research Center
Im Neuenheimer Feld 280
6900 Heidelberg 1, Federal Republic of Germany

Dr O. Møller Jensen
Director, Danish Cancer Registry
2100 Copenhagen Ø, Denmark

Professor J. Peto
Division of Epidemiology
Institute of Cancer Research
Sutton, Surrey, UK

Dr P.G. Smith
Department of Medical Statistics
London School of Hygiene and Tropical Medicine
London WC1E 7HT, UK

Dr D.C. Thomas
Department of Family and Preventive Medicine
University of Southern California
Los Angeles, CA 90033, USA

Dr A. Whittemore
Department of Family, Community and Preventive Medicine
Stanford University School of Medicine
Stanford, CA 94305, USA

IARC participants:

Dr N.E. Day
Dr J. Estève
Dr J. Wahrendorf
Dr A.M. Walker

1. THE ROLE OF COHORT STUDIES IN CANCER EPIDEMIOLOGY

CHAPTER 1

THE ROLE OF COHORT STUDIES IN CANCER EPIDEMIOLOGY

Longitudinal studies are of fundamental importance in human biology. In the study of physical growth, of mental and hormonal development, and in the process of ageing, the longitudinal approach has played a central role. The essential feature of such investigation is that changes over time are followed at the individual level. Most chronic diseases are the result of a process extending over decades, and many of the events occurring in this period play a substantial role. The longitudinal surveillance and recording of these events is therefore a natural model of study to obtain a complete picture of disease causation. Fortunately, for the study of a large number of chronic diseases, most of the relevant information on exposure can be summarized in a few relatively simple measures, so that continuous monitoring is not required. But the regular assessment of exposure variables may well be necessary, and in the epidemiology of cardiovascular disease, with its emphasis on physiological and biochemical explanatory measures, this approach has been the one of choice.

The essence of longitudinal studies in epidemiology is the identification of a group of individuals about whom certain exposure information is collected; the group is then followed forward in time to ascertain the occurrence of the diseases of interest, so that for each individual prior exposure information can be related to subsequent disease experience. Since the first requirement of such studies is the identification of the individuals forming the study group – or cohort – longitudinal studies in cancer epidemiology are usually referred to as *cohort* studies. (This use of the word 'cohort' first appeared in the literature in a demographic setting in 1944, according to the Oxford English Dictionary. It had apparently been introduced informally in 1935, as described by Wall & William, 1970.)

There are two ways in which the follow-up over time may be conducted. First, one may assemble the cohort in the present, and follow the individuals prospectively into the future. This type of study is often referred to as a *prospective cohort* study. It has the advantage that one may collect exactly the information thought to be required, and the disadvantage that many years may elapse before sufficient cases of disease have developed for analysis.

Second, one may identify a group with certain exposure characteristics, by means of historical records, at a certain defined time in the past, and then reconstruct the disease experience of the group between the defined time in the past and the present. This type of study has been called a *historical cohort* study. The advantage is that results are potentially available immediately; the disadvantage is that the information available on the cohort may not be completely satisfactory, since it would almost certainly have been collected for other purposes. Much may be missing, and it may not correspond closely to the question of interest. The term 'retrospective cohort study' is also commonly used, but is slightly misleading, since the essential viewpoint in most such studies is forward in time, although starting in the past. The term 'historical cohort study' is preferable logically. In both types of study, the individuals comprising the cohort are identified, and information on their exposure obtained, before their disease experience is ascertained.

Cohort studies, by recording disease occurrence in a defined group, provide measures of incidence, or mortality rates, and it is these rates that provide the basic measures of disease risk. By allowing one to measure the basic risk associated with different levels and types of exposure, cohort studies provide the foundation of cancer epidemiology. It so happens, however, that a frequently convenient way of expressing the excess risk in one group compared to another is in terms of the ratio of the rates in the two groups, and to estimate the ratio of the rates one can use just a sample of the overall cohort. Since it is often easier and cheaper to obtain information on a sample rather than on the entire cohort, the case-control study has become widely adopted in cancer epidemiology as an alternative to the cohort study.

In fact, as commonly used, the case-control approach departs more radically from a cohort study than simply by sampling. In many case-control studies, the individuals with the disease in question and some comparison group are ascertained first, and their exposure experiences for some defined period of time in the past obtained retrospectively. The results are used to derive rate ratios. A cohort study faces forwards in time, starting with the defined population and its exposure status, and observing the subsequent disease experience, whereas a retrospective case-control study faces backwards in time, starting with the disease status and reconstructing the exposure history from which it emerged. Graphically, the distinction can be expressed as shown in Figure 1.1

Notwithstanding these differences, however, the rate ratios estimated in a case-control study should refer to rates in some defined population. As argued in Volume 1 of this series, the inferences one draws from the results of a case-control study depend logically on the interpretation one can give to it as having arisen by sampling from some underlying cohort. The less clear the definition of the underlying population, the less confidence can be put in the results of the case-control study. Thus, although the case-control and cohort approaches appear clearly distinct, they share the same logical framework of inference. An increasing number of studies have components of both approaches in their design. In these hybrid designs, the cohort component would usually identify the group and ascertain the disease experiences in the follow-up period; the exposure experience would then be obtained using the case-control approach. In this way, one ensures strict definition of the study cohort, but the effort and resources devoted to obtaining accurate exposure data can be concentrated on the most informative individuals. We discuss later at some length (§1.4i) the interplay between the cohort and the case-control approach.

Common to both cohort and case-control studies is the extended period of

Fig. 1.1   Differences between cohort and case-control studies

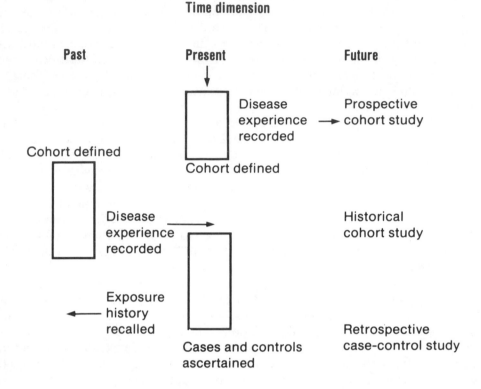

observation, relating to disease experience in the former and to exposure experience in the latter, and sometimes both in either case, and the fact that the individual is the unit of observation. These two features contrast with those of studies in which populations are compared by using cross-sectional data on both exposure and disease occurrence – so-called 'population correlation' or 'ecological' studies. This type of study would normally be given little weight in assessing the basic causality of a relationship, and, in the series of *IARC Monographs on the Evaluation of the Carcinogenic Risk of Chemicals to Humans,* a prerequisite for evidence to be deemed sufficient to establish carcinogenicity in humans is that it derive from individual-based studies. Correlation studies may be useful in suggesting interesting areas of study, that is, for hypothesis generation. The distinctions, however, are not absolute. Population comparisons may be made on the basis of temporal changes or of the experience with respect to exposure and disease of different birth cohorts, rather than among populations defined geographically, and such comparisons are often given greater weight. A cohort study, on the other hand, may include little or no information on variations in exposure between individuals, it being known simply that the cohort as a whole was exposed – for example, had received Bacillus Calmette–Guérin (BCG) vaccination in the first year of life.

1.1 Historical role

In 1954, two papers were published that are landmarks in the historical development of cancer epidemiology. The first, called a 'preliminary report', described the rationale for, and the first results of, the prospective cohort study of British doctors (Doll & Hill, 1954), designed to investigate the relatonship of tobacco smoking to lung cancer. The second, a historical cohort study, reported on the risk of bladder cancer in the British chemical industry (Case *et al.*, 1954; Case & Pearson, 1954).

The prospective study of British doctors was initiated in 1951, when the results of a number of case-control studies had already been published demonstrating an association between lung cancer and cigarette smoking. (The design and execution of the study are described in detail in Appendix IA.) It is interesting to examine why, in view of the results of the case-control studies, a large scale, long-term study was felt necessary. The 1954 paper by Doll and Hill starts as follows:

'In the last five years a number of studies have been made of the smoking habits of patients with and without lung cancer. All these studies agree in showing that there are more heavy smokers and fewer nonsmokers among patients with lung cancer than among patients with other diseases. While, therefore, the various authors have all shown that there is an "association" between lung cancer and the amount of tobacco smoked, they have differed in their interpretation. Some have considered that the only reasonable explanation is that smoking is a factor in the production of the disease; others have not been prepared to deduce causation and have left the association unexplained.

'Further retrospective studies of that same kind would seem to us unlikely to advance our knowledge materially or to throw any new light upon the nature of the association. If, too, there were any undetected flaw in the evidence that such studies have produced, it would be exposed only by some entirely new approach. That approach we considered should be "prospective". It should determine the frequency with which the disease appeared, in the future, among groups of persons whose smoking habits were already known.'

In this initial report on the British doctors study, the authors stressed that the results of the prospective study were in close agreement (Table 1.1) with the results of their earlier case-control study (Doll & Hill, 1950), in terms of the ratios of the rates in the different smoking categories. The absolute level of the rates, however, appeared to be more than twice as high in the case-control study (confined to the subset of the study consisting of residents of Greater London) than in the cohort of doctors. It should be noted that the results of the case-control study were converted into absolute incidence rates for lung cancer and were not limited to a description of the effect of smoking in terms of the ratios of rates in the different smoking categories.

The results of 20 years or more of follow-up have been published in some detail (Doll & Peto, 1976, 1978; Doll *et al.*, 1980). A comparison of these results with those of the case-control study published in the early 1950s (Doll & Hill, 1950, 1952) highlights the relative merits of the two approaches. The case-control study was begun in April 1948, and the final results published in December 1952. A total of 4342 people were interviewed, of whom 1488 were lung cancer cases. Most of the analyses referred

Table 1.1 Comparison of the relation between risk of dying from lung cancer and the most recent number of cigarettes smoked per day, among men aged 45–74, obtained from a prospective cohort study and a retrospective case-control study

	Non-smokers	Smokers			All groups
		1–14 cig./day	15–24 cig./day	25+ cig./day	
Standardized rates: 'Backward' study[a] of patients' histories	0.11	1.56	2.20	4.00	1.97
'Forward' study[b] of mortality of doctors	0.00	0.50	0.97	1.45	0.73
Each rate as a % of the rate for all groups: 'Backward' study of patients' histories	6%	79%	112%	203%	100%
'forward' study of mortality of doctors	0%	68%	133%	199%	100%

[a] From Doll and Hill (1950)
[b] From Doll and Hill (1954)

to 1465 lung cancer cases and a series of 1465 individually matched controls. By contrast, the prospective study was begun in October 1951, the month the British doctors were first approached, and the most recent results for men, based on 20 years of follow-up, appeared in 1978, and for women, based on 22 years of follow-up, in 1980. During these years, 441 lung cancer deaths were registered among the 34 440 men, and 27 among the 6194 women, enrolled in the study. The advantages of the case-control study are clear: many more cases of lung cancer could be assembled in a much shorter time. In addition, the total number of persons interviewed in the case-control study was only one-tenth the number who completed the questionnaire in the prospective study. This reduction in numbers facilitates the asking of a broader range of questions, allowing one to obtain information on a wider range of potential risk factors. In the prospective study, the questionnaire was kept short and simple, in order, as the authors say, 'to encourage a high proportion of replies'.

What was achieved in return, then, for the high cost and length of the prospective study? Part of the answer is given by comparing Table 1.2a, from the prospective study, and Table 1.2b, from the case-control study. Attention has been limited to males; a similar comparison could be made for females. The results of the case-control study with regard to the health effects of cigarette smoking, relative to the average amount smoked per day, are summarized in Table 1.2b. For the prospective study, in addition to the 441 lung cancer deaths, there were 9631 other deaths, and the full range of the effect of cigarette smoking on mortality can be examined, either for each individual cause of death or for all causes combined. One can see that there is nearly a two-fold difference in the annual death rate between heavy smokers and nonsmokers.

Table 1.2a   Death rates between November 1951 and October 1971 by cause of death and by smoking habits when last asked: male British doctors[a]

Cause of death	No. of deaths	Annual death rate per 100 000 men, standardized for age							χ^2	
		Non-smokers	Current or ex-smokers	Ex-smokers	Current smokers, any tobacco	Current smokers, any tobacco (cig./day)			Others *versus* non-smokers[b]	Trend[b]
						1–14	15–24	≥25		
Cancer										
Lung	441	10	83	43	104	52	106	224	41.98	197.04
Oesophagus	65	3	12	5	16	12	13	30	3.94	14.94
Other respiratory sites	46	1	9	4	11	6	9	27	3.31	21.68
Stomach	163	23	28	21	32	28	38	32	—	—
Colon	195	27	34	34	34	35	33	31	—	—
Rectum	78	6	14	14	14	10	14	27	2.81	10.76
Pancreas	93	14	16	12	18	14	18	27	—	3.98
Prostate	186	39	30	31	30	28	31	38	—	—
Kidney	46	3	8	9	8	8	9	9	—	—
Bladder	80	9	14	11	16	16	16	12	—	—
Marrow and reticulo-endothelial system	152	33	24	26	24	27	22	19	—	(3.51)
Unknown site	64	12	11	9	12	10	13	14	—	—
Other site	151	25	26	29	24	19	24	35	—	—
Respiratory disease										
Respiratory tuberculosis	57	3	11	11	10	8	7	21	3.83	10.51
Asthma	40	4	7	12	5	5	7	0	—	—
Pneumonia	345	54	59	62	57	47	62	91	—	6.94
Chronic bronchitis and emphysema	254	3	48	44	50	38	50	88	25.58	47.23
Other respiratory disease	121	16	21	24	19	20	14	26	—	—
Pulmonary heart disease	50	0	9	7	11	9	10	19	4.72	8.37
Cardiac and vascular disease										
Rheumatic heart disease	77	14	13	12	13	14	16	5	—	—
Ischaemic heart disease	3191	413	554	533	565	501	598	677	22.59	53.56
Myocardial degeneration	615	67	108	98	116	111	111	160	9.58	13.92
Hypertension	239	37	41	41	41	33	43	58	—	4.67
Arteriosclerosis	117	21	20	17	21	17	21	46	—	4.85
Aortic aneurysm (non-syphilitic)	121	5	22	16	26	18	28	45	8.40	25.60
Venous thromboembolism	48	9	8	8	8	8	5	14	—	—
Cerebral thrombosis	616	86	106	105	107	92	123	131	—	0.54
Other cerebrovascular disease	692	107	118	122	115	112	114	128	—	—
Other cardiovascular disease	267	53	44	49	41	37	42	52	—	—

[a] From Doll and Peto (1976)
[b] Figures are given whenever the value was greater than 2.71 ($p < 0.1$); figures in parentheses indicate a decreasing trend from nonsmokers to heavy smokers; others indicate an increasing trend

Table 1.2a—*contd.*

Cause of death	No. of deaths	Annual death rate per 100 000 men, standardized for age							χ^2	
		Non-smokers	Current or ex-smokers	Ex-smokers	Current smokers, any tobacco	Current smokers, any tobacco (cig./day)			Others versus non-smokers[b]	Trend[b]
						1–14	15–24	≥25		
Other diseases										
Parkinsonism	51	14	8	13	5	8	1	4	—	(9.10)
Peptic ulcer	79	8	14	12	15	10	20	23	—	8.26
Cirrhosis of liver,										
alcoholism	80	7	14	10	16	10	10	40	—	22.53
Hernia	16	0	3	2	4	3	4	7	—	4.16
Other digestive disease	144	20	25	27	24	18	33	26	—	3.25
Nephritis	79	10	14	10	16	15	14	21	—	—
Other genitourinary										
disease	136	19	23	24	23	22	24	26	—	—
Other disease	391	59	67	73	64	65	58	73	—	—
Violence										
Suicide	173	21	31	27	32	30	28	46	—	6.26
Poisoning	74	9	13	6	16	16	14	26	—	6.86
Trauma	240	46	39	36	41	47	25	56	—	—
All causes	10 072	1317	1748	1652	1802	1581	1829	2452	68.47	244.16
(no. of deaths)		(490)	(9132)	(3114)	(6018)	(2707)	(1986)	(1325)		

Table 1.2b   Most recent amount of tobacco smoked regularly before the onset of the present illness: lung carcinoma patients and matched control patients with other diseases (males only)[a]

Disease group	Number of non-smokers	Number smoking daily:				
		1 cig.	5 cig.	15 cig.	25 cig.	50 cig.
1357 lung cancer patients	7	49	516	445	299	41
	0.5%	3.6%	38.0%	32.8%	22.0%	3.0%
1357 control patients	61	91	615	408	162	20
	4.5%	6.7%	45.3%	30.1%	11.9%	1.5%

[a] From Doll and Hill (1952)

For an exposure with a wide range of deleterious effects, there is no substitute for the broad picture given by Table 1.2a.

A second advantage to be gained from the extended duration of a prospective study is the opportunity it affords to obtain further information on the exposure of interest. In the British doctors study, four separate questionnaires were sent (in 1951, 1957, 1963 and 1971). The good compliance of the population under study is well indicated by the low proportion of non-responders to the second, third and fourth questionnaires

Table 1.3 Response to questionnaires

	Second questionnaire	Third questionnaire	Fourth questionnaire
Survey period	November 1957– October 1958	March– October 1966	July– October 1972
No. known to have died before end of survey period	3122	7301	10 634
No. presumably alive at end of survey period	31 318	27 139	23 806
No. who replied by end of survey (and % of men then alive)	30 810 (98.4)	26 163 (96.4)	23 299 (97.9)
Reasons for non-response:			
Too ill	31	65	21
Refused	36	63[a]	102[a]
Address not found	72	403	22
Unknown and other reasons	369	445	362

[a] Includes all men who had refused previously

(see Table 1.3); it was not sent to those who had refused to reply previously or who had been struck off the Medical Register. These additional questionnaires certainly improved the quality of the basic information that was being sought, namely, the average amount smoked in the few years preceding onset of disease, and also provide much useful information on the time sequence of events, particularly changing smoking habits. The relationship between the years since stopping smoking and the level of excess risk for lung cancer, both absolute and relative, has been more clearly defined from the prospective studies.

The British doctors prospective study was followed rapidly by a similar study undertaken by the American Cancer Society, started in 1952 (Hammond, 1966), and two years later, in 1954, by a study of United States veterans (Kahn, 1966). Other studies have followed since, notably a prospective study in Japan (Hirayama, 1975). The impact of these studies was much greater than their unambiguous demonstration of the health effects of tobacco smoking. They were the studies which, at least in the field of cancer, established chronic disease epidemiology as a rigorous scientific discipline.

The case-control studies, when they were first reported, appeared fraught with possible biases. The potential for error, so many claimed, was such that little credence could be put in the results. The large prospective studies begun in the early 1950s have shown that observational studies in humans can produce results that establish beyond reasonable doubt associations between exposure and disease. Furthermore, they demonstrated pragmatically that prospective cohort studies and retrospective case-control studies can, under favourable circumstances, give the same results. This demonstration, complementing the theoretical arguments developed at that time for the equivalence of the two study designs, at least in terms of estimating relative risks

Table 1.4   The number of death certificates expected if no special risk were operating and the number of cases and death certificates found for the various exposure classes[a]

Rank	Class	Group	Total no. of cases found	No. of cases on nominal roll			No of cases on nominal roll for whom death certificate mentions bladder tumour	Expected no. of such cases	% of expected no. derived from incomplete data	Significance of difference	P
				Total	Alive	Dead					
1	Aniline without	I	4	4[b]	2[b]	2[b]	1	0.30	35.8	None	>0.1
	magenta contact	II	0	0	0	0	0	0.23		None	>0.1
		III	0	0	0	0	0	0.01		None	>0.1
		All	4	4[b]	2[b]	2[b]	1	0.54		None	>0.1
2	Aniline with	I	8	5	3	2	2	0.30	15.6	Suspicious	0.025
	possible	II	1	1	0	1	1	0.05		None	>0.1
	magenta contact	III	0	0	0	0	0	0.00		None	>0.9
		All	9	6	3	3	3	0.35		Signicant	<0.02
3	All aniline	I	12	9[b]	5[b]	4[b]	3	0.60	20.3	Suspicious	0.025
		II	1	1	0	1	1	0.28		None	>0.01
		III	0	0	0	0	0	0.01		None	>0.1
		All	13	10[b]	5[b]	5[b]	4	0.89		Suspicious	0.025
4	Benzidine	I	38	34	21	13	10	0.54	3.7	Very high	<0.001
		II	0	0	0	0	0	0.17		None	>0.1
		III	0	0	0	0	0	0.01		None	>0.1
		All	38	34	21	13	10	0.72		Very high	<0.001
5	α-Naphthylamine	I	28	19	13	6	6	0.66	3.2	High	0.005
		II	0	0	0	0	0	0.04		None	>0.1
		III	0	0	0	0	0	0.00		None	>0.9
		All	28	19	13	6	6	0.70		High	<0.005
6	β-Naphthylamine	I	59	55	28	27	26	0.30	4.1	Very high	<0.001
		II	0	0	0	0	0	0.00		None	>0.9
		III	0	0	0	0	0	0.00		None	>0.9
		All	59	55	28	27	26	0.30		Very high	<0.001
7	Mixed exposures	I	162	135	50	85	75	1.15	13.5	Very high	<0.001
		II	9	7	0	7	5	0.32		High	<0.005
		III	2	2	1	1	1	0.006		Significant	<0.005
		All	173	144	51	93	81	1.48		Very high	<0.001
8	All classes,	I	287	243	112	131	117	2.65	7.3	Very high	<0.001
	excluding	II	9	7	0	7	5	0.53		High	<0.005
	aniline	III	2	2	1	1	1	0.02		Suspicious	0.025
		All	298	252	113	139	123	3.20		Very high	<0.001
9	All classes	I	299	252	117	135	120	3.25	9.3	Very high	<0.001
		II	10	8	0	8	6	0.81		High	<0.005
		III	2	2	1	1	1	0.03		Suspicious	0.025
		All	311	262	118	144	127	4.09		Very high	<0.001

[a] From Case et al. (1954)
[b] Also manufacturer of auramine

(Cornfield, 1951), has led to the case-control study becoming the major methodological tool in cancer epidemiology.

The bladder cancer study of the British chemical industry (Case *et al.*, 1954) also played a seminal role in the evolution of cancer epidemiology and is the prototype of historical cohort studies. Its purpose was to determine 'whether the manufacture or use of aniline, benzidine, β-naphthylamine or α-naphthylamine could be shown to produce tumours of the urinary bladder in men so engaged'. It had been suspected since the last century that the production of aniline-based dyestuffs might produce bladder cancers among the men employed. There was lack of unanimity concerning the agent or agents responsible, however, and little information on the level of the excess risk.

In the early 1950s, Case and his co-workers constructed a list, or nominal roll as they termed it, of all those who had ever been employed in the chemical industry in the United Kingdom for at least six months since 1920, worked for one of the 21 firms which cooperated in the study, and for whom exposure to one of these compounds listed above had been documented. Age and the dates between which exposure to these substances occurred were recorded. A search was made retrospectively for all bladder cancer cases occurring among men who had been employed, in or after 1921 until 1 February 1952, in the chemical industry. Of the 455 cases identified, 127 were on the nominal roll, had died, and had bladder cancer mentioned on the death certificate. Since bladder cancer death rates based on death certificates mentioning bladder cancer were known between 1921 and 1952, the nominal roll could be used to calculate expected numbers, strictly comparable to the 127 observed bladder cancer deaths, using calendar time- and age-specific rates. The results of these calculations are given in Table 1.4. Accepting the authors' use of the terms 'aniline', 'benzidine' and so on to mean these substances as encountered in industrial practice, rather than to mean the pure chemicals, Table 1.4 gives clear, quantitative evidence of the carcinogenicity to humans of β-naphthylamine, α-naphthylamine and benzidine. Aniline exposure, as it occurred in the British chemical industry in the first half of this century, presents a risk to the human bladder of a lower order of magnitude than the risk associated with β-naphthylamine, if it presents a risk at all. It is interesting to note that, 28 years later, in 1982 (IARC, 1982a), this study was still considered the soundest evidence on which to base an evaluation of the carcinogenicity of aniline to humans.

No real alternative existed to the strategy adopted by Case, since an answer to the question was urgently required. A prospective study was therefore out of the question, and, furthermore, exposure had already been substantially reduced so that present levels were no longer indicative of past exposure. Since only a very small proportion of all bladder cancer cases in the general population of England and Wales were related to the chemical industry, a general case-control study of bladder cancer would not have been informative. Reconstruction of the past for a cohort of individuals with recorded exposure to the compounds of interest was the only feasible approach. In the 30 years since Case's study was reported, this methodology has become the approach of choice in many situations.

1.2 Present significance and specific strengths of cohort studies

In the next two sections, we discuss the relative merits and drawbacks of cohort and case-control studies. Although, as we have seen, the distinction is not always clear cut, and the two may merge into each other, what we have in mind in the following discussion is a comparison of two approaches: one in which a group of individuals is defined, their exposure determined and their subsequent disease experience ascertained; the other in which cases of a specific disease are identified together with a suitable comparison group, and information on exposure before disease onset obtained retrospectively. Described in this way, it would seem natural that the latter might appeal if the focus is on causation of a specific disease, and the former if interest is on the health consequences of a given exposure.

Certainly, cohort studies have played a major role in the last 30 years in identifying specific environmental agents or other factors as carcinogenic hazards. We give in Table 1.5 the factors that are currently recognized as causally related to cancer risk in man, together with the type of evidence on which causality has been established. Case reports have been excluded. The intention has been to categorize the first epidemiological study that could be regarded as conclusive, although the choice is necessarily subjective, at least on occasion. For some associations, such as that between sexual activity and cervical cancer, the first epidemiological study establishing the link is not readily identifiable. A series of studies over the years has refined the nature of the association. For others, the effect is so strong that a case series, complemented by theoretical calculation of the size of the expected number, has been sufficient to establish the existence of an excess. The induction of lymphomas following immuno-suppression of recipients of renal grafts using azathioprine is an example, but the excess of other malignancies emerged only from a formal cohort study. An immediately evident feature of Table 1.5 is that the cohort study has been the method used to incriminate the great majority of factors so far identified as carcinogenic hazards. In addition to their value in establishing qualitatively that a carcinogenic hazard exists, cohort studies have been of importance in establishing quantitative estimates of increased risk. In Table 1.6 we list the few agents given in Table 1.5 for which substantial quantitative information is available on dose-response or the temporal evolution of risk. In later chapters, particularly Chapter 6, we discuss the quantification of excess risk and its temporal evolution in considerable detail, but one can see from Table 1.6 that much of the information currently available, particularly on the temporal development of risk, has come from cohort studies.

Tables 1.5 and 1.6 outline the significance that cohort studies have had historically in cancer epidemiology. These tables might give the impression that cohort studies are mainly of value when studying specific exposures, often rare and of little relevance to the great majority of cancers. Certainly, for the factors identified as cancer risks to which exposure is widespread, case-control studies have often been the study method used. The present significance of cohort studies, however, is wider than that suggested by Table 1.5.

Although, in many situations, the relatively low cost of retrospective case-control studies and the speed with which they can be conducted make them the design of choice, there are clearly occasions in which such an approach is inadequate, and a study design is required that is directed more towards the continuous recording of events in the years before disease, or which focuses on a broad spectrum of disease. This approach is the essence of a longitudinal or cohort study, the strengths of which

Table 1.5 Established human carcinogenic agents and circumstances

Agent	Site affected	Type of exposure	Main type of evidence[a]
Aflatoxin	Liver	Food	Geographic[1]
Alcoholic drinks	Mouth Larynx Oesophagus Pharynx	Lifestyle	Case-control[2,3,4,5]
4-Aminobiphenyl	Bladder	Occupational	Cohort[6]
Analgesic mixtures containing phenacetin	Renal pelvis	Medicinal	Case-control[7]
Arsenic and arsenic compounds	Skin	Medicinal, occupational, drinking-water	? Case series Geographical[8]
	Lung	Occupational	Cohort[9]
Asbestos	Lung Pleura Peritoneum	Occupational and geographic	Cohort[10,11] (in an informal sense)
Auramine manufacture	Bladder	Occupational	Cohort[12]
Azathioprine	Lymphomas Squamous skin tumours Liver	Medicinal	Cohort[13,14] (after earlier reports of a very high incidence of lymphomas)
Benzene	Leukaemia	Occupational	Cohort[15]
Benzidine	Bladder	Occupational	Cohort[16]
Betel-quid and tobacco chewing	Oral cavity Oesophagus	Lifestyle	Case-control[17]
Bis-chloromethyl ether	Lung	Occupational	Cohort[18,19]
Boot and shoe (leather goods) manufacture	Nasal sinus	Occupational	Based on cases, but interpreted mainly as a case-control study[20]
Busulphan (myleran)	Leukaemia	Medicinal	Cohort[21]
Chlorambucil	Leukaemia	Medicinal	Cohort[22]
Chlornaphazine	Bladder	Medicinal	Cohort[23]
Chromium and certain chromium compounds	Lung	Occupational	Cohort[24]
Conjugated oestrogens	Endometrium	Medicinal	Case-control[25,26]
Cyclophosphamide	Bladder	Medicinal	Cohort[13,14]
	Leukaemia	Medicinal	Case-control within a cohort[27]
Diethylstilboestrol	Vagina	Medicinal	Case-control[28]
Furniture manufacture	Nasal sinus	Occupational	Cohort[29]
Ionizing radiation	Leukaemia	Occupational, medicinal	Cohort[30,31]
	Most other sites	Warfare	Cohort[32] (see references to Appendix IB)
Isopropyl alcohol manufacture	Nasal sinus	Occupation	Cohort[33]
Melphalan	Leukaemia	Medicinal	Cohort[34]
Methoxsalen with UV-A (PUVA)	Skin	Medicinal	Cohort[35] Case-control within a cohort[35]

Table 1.5 (*contd*)

Agent	Site affected	Type of exposure	Main type of evidence[a]
Mustard gas	Lung, larynx	Occupational	Cohort[36]
β-Naphthylamine	Bladder	Occupational	Cohort[16]
Nickel refining	Nasal sinus ⎫ Lung ⎭	Occupational	Cohort[37,38]
Obesity	Endometrium ⎫ Gallbladder ⎭	Lifestyle	Case-control[39] Cohort[40]
Sexual promiscuity	Cervix	Lifestyle	Case-control[41]
Soots, tars and oils	Scrotum ⎫ Skin ⎬ Lung ⎭	Occupational	Numerous industrial cohorts
Tobacco smoking	Many sites	Lifestyle	Both case-control and cohort (see § 1.1)
Treosulphan	Leukaemia	Medicinal	Cohort[42]
Ultraviolet light	Skin	Lifestyle (occupational)	Geographic and other[b,43]
Vinyl chloride	Liver (angiosarcoma) (lung, brain)	Occupational	Based on cases[44] but interpreted as a cohort study[45]
Hepatitis B virus	Liver	Lifestyle	Cohort (see Appendix IC)
Reproductive history, age at first birth, age at menarche, age at menopause, parity	Breast Ovary	Lifestyle	Case-control[46] Case-control[47]
Chlonarchis siensis	Liver (cholangio-carcinoma)	Lifestyle	Geographic[48]
Schistosoma haematobium	Bladder	Lifestyle	Geographic[49]
Epstein-Barr virus	Burkitt's lymphoma	Lifestyle	Cohort[50]

[a] References: [1] Peers, F.G. & Linsell, C.A. (1973) Dietary aflatoxin and liver cancer. A population based study in Kenya. *Br. J. Cancer*, **27**, 473–484; [2] Wynder, E.L., Bross, I.D.J. & Feldman, R.M. (1957) A study of the etiological factors in cancer of the mouth. *Cancer*, **10**, 1300–1323; [3] Wynder, E.L., Bross, I.J. & Day, E. (1956) A study of environmental factors in cancer of the larynx. *Cancer*, **9**, 86–110; [4] Wynder, E.L. & Bross, I.J. (1961) A study of etiological factors in cancer of the esophagus. *Cancer*, **14**, 389–413; [5] Vogler, W.R., Lloyd, J.W. & Milmore, B.K. (1962) A retrospective study of etiological factors in cancer of the mouth, pharynx and larynx. *Cancer*, **15**, 246–258; [6] Melick, W.F., Naryka, J.J. & Kelly, R.E. (1971) Bladder cancer due to exposure to para-aminobiphenyl: a 17-year follow-up. *J. Urol.*, **106**, 220–226; [7] McCredie, M., Ford, J.M., Taylor, J.S. & Stewart, J.H. (1982) Cancer of the renal pelvis in New South Wales. Relationship to analgesic consumption and smoking. *Cancer*, **49**, 2617–2625; [8] Tseng, W.P., Chu, H.M., How, S.W., Fong, J.M., Lin, C.S. & Yeh, S. (1968) Prevalence of skin cancer in an endemic area of chronic arsenicism in Taiwan. *J. natl Cancer Inst.*, **40**, 453–463; [9] Lee, A.M. & Fraumeni, J.F., Jr (1969) Arsenic and respiratory cancer in man: an occupational study. *J. natl Cancer Inst.*, **42**, 1045–1052; [10] Doll, R. (1955) Mortality from lung cancer in abestos workers. *Br. J. ind. Med.*, **12**, 81–86; [11] Wagner, J.C., Sleggs, C.A. & Marchand, P. (1960) Diffuse pleural mesothelioma and asbestos exposure in the North-western Cape Province. *Br. J. ind. Med.*, **17**, 260–271; [12] Case, R.A.M. & Pearson, J.T. (1954) Tumours of the urinary bladder in workmen engaged in the manufacture and use of certain dyestuff intermediates in the British chemical industry. Part II. Further considerations of the role of aniline and of the manufacture of auramine and magenta (fuchsine) as possible causative agents. *Br. J. ind. Med.*, **11**, 213–216; [13] Kinlen, L.J., Sheil, A.G.R. & Peto, J. (1979) Collaborative United Kingdom–Australasian study of cancer in patients treated with immunosuppressive drugs. *Br. med. J.*, **iv**, 1461–1466; [14] Kinlen, L.J., Peto, J., Doll, R. & Sheil, A.G.R. (1981) Cancer in patients treated with immunosuppressive drugs. *Br. med. J.*, **i**, 474; [15] Infante, P.F., Rinsky, R.A., Wagoner, J.K. & Young, R.J. (1977) Leukaemia in benzene workers. *Lancet*, **ii**, 868–869; [16] Case, R.A.M., Hosker, M.E., McDonald, D.B. & Pearson, J.T. (1954) Tumours of the urinary bladder in workmen engaged in the manufacture and use of certain dyestuff intermediates in the British chemical industry. Part I. The role of aniline, benzidine, alpha-naphthylamine and beta-naphthylamine. *Br. J. ind. Med.*, **11**, 75–104; [17] Sanghvi, L.D., Rao, K.C.M. & Khanolkar, V.R. (1955) Smoking and chewing of tobacco in relation to cancer of the upper alimentary tract. *Br. med. J.*, **i**, 1111–1114; [18] Figueroa, W.G., Raszkowski, R. & Weiss, W.

Table 1.5   (contd)

(1973) Lung cancer in chloromethyl methyl ether workers. New Engl. J. Med., 288, 1096–1097; [19] Thiess, A.M., Hey, W. & Zeller, H. (1973) Zur Toxikologie von Dichlordimethyläther – Verdacht auf kanzerogene Wirkung auch beim Menschen. Zbl. Arbeitsmed., 23, 97–102; [20] Acheson, E.D., Cowdell, R.H. & Jolles, B. (1970) Nasal cancer in the Northamptonshire boot and shoe industry. Br. med. J., i, 385–393; [21] Stott, H., Fox, W., Girling, D.J., Stephens, R.J. & Galton, D.A.G. (1977) Acute leukaemia after busulfan. Br. med. J., ii, 1513–1517; [22] Reimer, R.R., Hoover, R., Fraumeni, J.F., Jr & Young, R.C. (1977) Acute leukemia after alkylating-agent therapy of ovarian cancer. New Engl. J. Med., 297, 177–181; [23] Thiede, T., Chievitz, E. & Christensen, B.C. (1964) Chlornaphazine as a bladder carcinogen. Acta med. scand., 175, 721–725; [24] Bidstrup, P.L. & Case, R.A.M. (1956) Carcinoma of the lung in workmen in the bichromates-producing industry in Great Britain. Br. J. ind. Med., 13, 260–264; [25] Smith, C.D., Prentice, R., Thompson, D.J. & Herrmann, W.L. (1975) Association of exogeneous estrogen and endometrial carcinoma. New Engl. J. Med., 293, 1164–1167; [26] Ziel, H.K. & Finkle, W.D. (1975) Increased risk of endometrial carcinoma among users of conjugated estrogens. New Engl. J. Med., 293, 1167–1170; [27] Mehnert, W.H., Haas, J.F., Kaldor, J., Day, N.E., Kittelmann, B., Stanaczek, W. & Möhner, M. (1986) A case-control study of leukaemia as a second primary malignency following ovarian and breast neoplasms. In: Schmähl, D. & Kaldor, J.M., eds, Carcinogenicity of Alkylating Cytostatic Drugs (IARC Scientific Publications No. 78), Lyon, International Agency for Research on Cancer, pp. 203–221; [28] Herbst, A.L., Ulfelder, H. & Poskanzer, D.C. (1971) Adenocarcinoma of the vagina. Association of maternal stilbestrol therapy with tumor appearance in young women. New Engl. J. Med., 284, 878–881; [29] Rang, E.H. & Acheson, E.D. (1981) Cancer in furniture workers. Int. J. Epidemiol., 10, 253–261; [30] Dublin, L. & Spiegelmann, M. (1947) The longevity and mortality of American physicians 1938–42. J. Am. med. Assoc., 134, 1211–1220; [31] Court Brown, W.M. & Abbatt, J.D. (1955) The incidence of leukaemia in ankylosing spondylitis treated with X-rays. Lancet, i, 1283–1287; [32] Lange, R.D., Moloney, W.C. & Yamawaki, T. (1954) Leukaemia in atomic bomb survivors. Blood, 9, 574–580; [33] Hueper, W.C. (1966) Occupational and environmental cancers of the respiratory system. Recent Results Cancer Res., 3, 105–107; [34] Law, I.P. & Blom, J. (1977) Second malignancies in patients with multiple myeloma. Oncology, 34, 20–24; [35] Stern, R.S., Zierler, S. & Parrish, J.A. (1980) Skin carcinoma in patients with psoriasis treated with topical tar and artificial ultraviolet radiation. Lancet, i, 732–735; [36] Wada, S., Nishimoto, Y., Miyanishi, M., Kambe, S. & Miller, R.W. (1968) Mustard gas as a cause of respiratory neoplasia in man. Lancet, i, 1161–1163; [37] Doll, R. (1958) Cancer of the lung and nose in nickel workers. Br. J. ind. Med., 51, 217–223; [38] Doll, R., Morgan, L.G. & Speizer, F.E. (1970) Cancers of the lung and nasal sinuses in nickel workers. Br. J. Cancer, 24, 623–632; [39] Damon, A. (1960) Host factors in cancer of the breast and uterine cervix and corpus. J. natl Cancer Inst., 24, 483–516; [40] Friedman, G.D., Kannel, W.B. & Dawber, T.R. (1966) The epidemiology of gallbladder disease: observations in the Framingham study. J. chron. Dis., 19, 273–292; [41] Wynder, E.L., Cornfield, J., Schroff, P.D. et al. (1954) A study of environmental factors in carcinoma of the cervix. Am. J. Obstet Gynecol., 68, 1016–1047; [42] Pedersen-Bjergaard, J., Nissen, N.I., Sørensen, H.M., Hou-Jensen, K., Larsen, M.S., Ernst, P., Ersbøl, J., Knudtzon, S. & Rose, C. (1980) Acute non-lymphocytic leukemia in patients with ovarian carcinoma following long-term treatment with treosulphan (=dihydroxybusulfan). Cancer, 45, 19–29; [43] Scotto, J., Fears, T.R. & Fraumeni, J.F., Jr (1982) Solar radiation. In: Schottenfeld, D. & Fraumeni, J.F., Jr, eds, Cancer Epidemiology and Prevention, Philadelphia, W.B. Saunders Co., pp. 255–276; [44] Creech, J.L., Jr & Johnson, M.N. (1974) Angiosarcoma of the liver in the manufacture of polyvinyl chloride. J. occup. Med., 16, 150–151; [45] Waxweiler, R.J., Stringer, W., Wagoner, J.K., Jones, J., Falk, H. & Carter, C. (1976) Neoplastic risk among workers exposed to vinyl chloride. Ann. N.Y. Acad. Sci., 271, 40–48; [46] MacMahon, B., Cole, P., Lin, T.M., Lowe, C.R., Mirra, A.P., Ravniher, B., Salber, E.J., Valaoras, V.G. & Yuasa, S. (1970) Age at first birth and cancer of the breast. A summary of an international study. Bull. World Health Organ., 43, 209–221; [47] Joly, D.J., Lilienfeld, A.M., Diamond, E.L. & Bross, I.D.J. (1974) An epidemiological study of the relationship of reproductive experience to cancer of the ovary. Am. J. Epidemiol., 99, 190–209; [48] Balarmaric, J. (1973) Intrahepatic bile duct carcinoma and C. sinensis inflection in Hong Kong. Cancer, 31, 468–473; [49] Ferguson, A.R. (1911) Associated bilharziosis and primary malignant disease of the urinary bladder with observations in a series of forty cases. J. Pathol. Bacteriol., 16, 76–94; [50] de-Thé, G.B., Geser., A., Day, N.E., Tukei, P.M., Williams, E.H., Beri, D.P. Smith, P.G., Dean, A.G., Bornkamm, G.W., Feorino, P. & Henle, W. (1978) Epidemiological evidence for causal relationship between Epstein-Barr virus and Burkitt's lymphoma from Ugandan prospective study. Nature, 274, 756–761

   [b] The evidence comes from a wide variety of sources, and no single study can be regarded as definitive. The reference is to a review

compared to case-control studies are described as follows:

(a) A wider picture is obtained of the health hazards associated with a given exposure. This point was stressed when discussing the early studies on the effects of cigarette smoking (see Tables 1.2a and 1.2b). The link with the disease under prime suspicion, lung cancer, was established by retrospective case-control studies, but identification of the full range of diseases for which smoking increases the risk came from the prospective studies. Perhaps the most comprehensive longitudinal study of an exposed population with cancer as a major endpoint of interest is the follow-up of the survivors of the atomic bomb explosions in Japan (see Appendix IB for a description of the study design). An excess of leukaemia had been identified before the main programme started, but it was expressly stated when the atomic bomb survivor studies were launched that the overall aim was to study all the long-term health effects of

Table 1.6 Agents for which quantitative information is available on risk and exposure

Agent	Site	Type of study providing the principal information	
		Quantitative information on level of exposure	Quantitative information on temporal development
Cigarette smoking	Lung	Case-control and cohort	Cohort
	Other sites	Case-control	Little available
Alcohol	Oesophagus	Case-control	Little available
Asbestos	Lung	Cohort	Cohort
	Mesothelioma	Cohort	Cohort
Ionizing radiation	Most sites	Cohort	Cohort
Conjugated oestrogens	Endometrium	Case-control	Case-control

ionizing radiation, and in particular to determine if there was any evidence for a general acceleration of ageing. The enormous value of the study in providing the most precise estimates of the radiogenic cancer risk that are currently available for the majority of sites (Committee on the Biological Effects of Ionizing Radiation, 1980) has tended to obscure the major, if negative, findings that no detectable increase in mortality rates for nonmalignant diseases has occurred, nor is there evidence for an acceleration of the ageing process. The full picture of the long-term health effects of a given exposure can be provided only by the cohort approach.

(b) Recall and selection bias can usually be eliminated. This was perhaps the principal reason for launching the major prospective studies of cigarette smoking. Recall bias, a bugbear of case-control studies, should not occur in cohort studies. It is sufficient, of course, that recall bias could have occurred, rather than that it demonstrably did, for the results of a study to be questioned. An illustrative example of the doubts that may surround information that is obtained retrospectively is the early report of an excess of cancer among children irradiated *in utero* for diagnostic purposes (Stewart *et al.*, 1958). This study was based on interviews of mothers of cases and of controls about their pregnancy history after diagnosis of cancer in the case child. It was initially discounted because of the possible recall bias on the part of the mother – a criticism almost impossible to refute from within the study. A cohort study involving all births between the years 1947 and 1954 in the principal Massachusetts maternity hospitals, undertaken to test the validity of the association, gave quantitatively similar results (MacMahon, 1962). Since the cohort approach of this latter study avoids recall bias, any bias in the results must derive from the selection of women who undergo diagnostic X-ray during pregnancy and not from problems of recall. More detailed examination of the association in terms of year of irradiation (Bithell & Stewart, 1975), and more recent studies of twins (Boice *et al.*, 1985), suggest that the association is real.

Bias is not the only way in which differences in recall between cases and controls can

Table 1.7 Effect of different precision of response between cases and controls, for a polytomous exposure variable

| | Levels of exposure | | | | | |
	0	1	2	3	4	Total
'True' distribution (in cases and controls)	0.05	0.3	0.3	0.3	0.05	1.00
Observed distribution[a] in cases	0.075	0.275	0.3	0.275	0.075	1.00
Observed distribution[b] in controls	0.10	0.25	0.3	0.25	0.10	1.00
Apparent odds ratio	1.0	1.47	1.33	1.47	1.0	
			1.37			

[a] Obtained by spreading 10% of the true distribution on each side of the correct data point
[b] Obtained by spreading 20% of the true distribution on each side of the correct data point

distort risk estimates derived from case-control studies, although it may be the major one. Distortion can also arise if the precision of the recall is different between cases and controls, again not a problem that should arise in a properly conducted cohort study. Consider a situation such as that illustrated in Table 1.7, in which the true distribution of a polytomous response is the same in cases and controls. Among both cases and controls, there is some unbiased random error in response, with a greater standard error among the controls. The effect is to generate a spurious risk differential. The picture of apparent low risk among a nonexposed group of low frequency, and lack of dose-response among the exposed is similar to that seen, for example, in several studies associating coffee drinking with bladder cancer (Hartge et al., 1983).

Selection bias in case-control studies is often almost impossible to evaluate. If population controls are used, a large proportion of those originally selected may refuse to participate; if hospital controls are used, the choice of which disease categories to include is difficult to resolve, particularly for complex exposures like diet. It is rare for the case series to approach 100% of those arising in a defined population; if the series is eventually matched to a cancer registry, the proportion of eligible cases actually included seldom approaches the coverage of 90% or more considered acceptable for cohort studies (see Table 1.10). For cohort studies with good follow-up, problems of selection bias should not arise.

Provided that the follow-up mechanisms do not favour particular exposure groups, which can be checked by examining the data, then comparison of the disease experience among different subgroups of the study cohort should be unbiased. The cohort itself, however, will usually be a selected subgroup of the general population, and the disease experiences of the cohort and that of the general population may well not be comparable. The best known example of this lack of comparability is the so-called 'healthy worker effect'. The employed population is generally healthier than the nonemployed population of the same age, and their death rates for many causes of

Fig. 1.2   Evolution of the 'healthy worker effect' following entry into the study:
Swedish building workers. The permission of Drs A. Englund and G.
Engholm to reproduce this figure is gratefully acknowledged. · —· Cancer
incidence (SIR); – – – cancer mortality (SMR); ——— total mortality
(SMR)

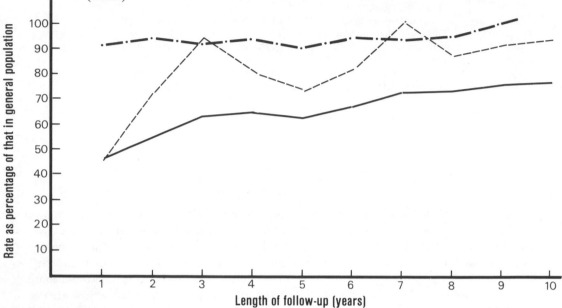

death are lower than the corresponding rates in the general population (Fox &
Goldblatt, 1982). Cancer death rates appear to suffer less from the healthy worker
effect than rates from most other causes, and cancer incidence rates probably are less
affected than cancer death rates (see Figure 1.2).

The cohort may also be a selected subgroup of those exposed to the agent of
interest. In both the Welsh nickel workers and Montana smelter workers studies
considered throughout this monograph (see Appendices ID and IE), exposure was
markedly higher before 1925 than in later periods. To qualify as a cohort member,
however, individuals had to have been employed at the respective plant at some date in
the 1930s or later. It may well be that employees not included, – for example, itinerant
workers given the dirtiest jobs or those retiring early for reasons of health – differ both
in their exposure and in their response from those included in the study. The cohort
would then represent a biased selection of all those employed. This bias does not of
course affect the inferences that are applied to the study cohort, but does affect the
generalizability of the conclusions to all those working at the plant.

(c) Effects are more efficiently studied of exposures that are both rare in the general
population and responsible for only a small proportion of any specific cancer. For many
of the agents listed in Table 1.5, the cohort approach was taken to study the possible
carcinogenic hazard because the exposure was rare. Only a very small proportion of

cases in the general population would have been associated with it, and a population-based case-control study would contain too few exposed cases to be informative. Cohort studies are sometimes claimed to be the approach of choice whenever an exposure is rare, but if a rare exposure is responsible for a substantial proportion of the cases of some cancer, presumably itself rare, then a case-control approach may well be more informative. Thus, the evidence relating adenocarcinomas of the vagina in young women to prenatal exposure to diethylstilboestrol, in general a rare exposure, comes essentially from case-control studies. In at least one prospective study of individuals exposed transplacentally to diethylstilboestrol no case of the disease was observed because, although the relative risk is very high, the baseline incidence from which the relative risk is calculated is extremely low. The associations of asbestos with mesothelioma and of vinyl chloride with angiosarcoma of the liver are also clearly demonstrated by a case-control approach, although quantitative aspects of the relationship may not be well estimated.

(d) Pre-disease information on biological parameters is available. Many physiological or biochemical measures, for example of nutritional status, will be modified by the disease itself, and observations taken on cases would be of doubtful value for etiological studies. As an illustrative example, in the early and mid-1970s, a series of case-control studies of hepatocellular carcinoma was performed investigating the differences in the prevalence of the carrier state of the hepatitis B virus surface antigen between the two groups. A much greater prevalence of the carrier state was seen among the cases in studies from a number of different countries (Szmuness, 1978). The etiological significance of this difference, however, was not accepted until it had been shown in a prospective study from Taiwan (Beasley et al., 1981) that the same differences in rates between carriers and noncarriers were observed even when the carrier state was ascertained years before the onset of disease. The findings of several prospective studies have now been published, confirming the Taiwan study, and the association is regarded as definitively established.

A second example is given by the present great interest in the role of micronutrients in cancer etiology. Since retrospective recall of diet gives only a weak indication of intake of specific micronutrients, attention has been focused on physiological measures of levels of vitamins and trace elements. For these measures to reflect etiology, rather than simply the presence of disease, the requisite biological samples have to be taken some time before onset of disease, thus necessitating a prospective cohort approach. Existing banks of biological materials can be of great value in this context, forming potentially the basis for historical cohort studies. As frequently happens with material being used for a purpose not envisaged when it was collected, the condition of the collection and storage may not have been optimal, may even have been inadequate, for the parameters of current interest. Care must also be taken to ensure that samples from cases are not manipulated, for example thawed and refrozen, more frequently than the samples taken from the rest of the cohort.

(e) Information obtained retrospectively may be essentially too inaccurate to be of use. Exposure to aflatoxin, say, might be estimated by dietary recall combined with tables of aflatoxin levels in common foodstuffs, but one would not expect such estimates to be accurate. The only way to obtain accurate measures of exposure is by direct observation of aflatoxin intake, either by assaying diet or measuring aflatoxin levels in body fluids. In another setting, quantitative estimates of exposure to benzene might be attempted by means of job histories linked to occupation-specific environmental measures, but better estimates of exposure are again clearly obtained by direct observation. The difficulty of interpreting past exposure measurements is well illustrated by the correspondence following the study of Infante *et al.* (1977) on benzene and leukaemia. The prospective study of gas workers in the United Kingdom, reported in 1965 and 1972 (Doll *et al.*, 1965, 1972), was initiated in 1953 because job histories could not be obtained retrospectively with acceptable accuracy. Assessment of exposure by biological monitoring has received increasing attention in recent years. Levels in the blood or in the urine of the compound itself or its metabolites can give measures of individual exposures, and this approach holds great promise for future prospective studies (Vainio, 1985).

(f) Repeated measurements can potentially be obtained. With an extended period of follow-up, serial measurements of the exposure may be possible. One consequence is that variables that have a time component are more accurately determined. A second consequence is that one can study the effect of changing levels of exposure. In breast cancer, for example, changes in weight may be of as much importance as weight just prior to diagnosis. Studying the effect of changing exposure levels provides one directly with estimates of the effect of intervention, although without the element of randomization. A third consequence is that misclassification rates or errors of measurement of exposures and of confounding variables can be assessed in unbiased fashion for the general population and for individuals destined to develop the disease of interest. These estimates can be used to infer the real rather than the apparent effect of exposure (Clayton & Kaldor, 1985). The use of prospective studies to generate repeat measurements of the variables of interest, and to use these repeat measurements to obtain estimates of the real disease-exposure relationship, is an area worth further elaboration.

(g) For some purposes, one requires not relative but absolute measures of risk. Cohort studies provide direct estimates of incidence rates, as opposed to the ratios of rates estimable from case-control studies. Both for public health decisions and for the study of the mechanisms of carcinogenesis, incidence rates, giving as they do absolute measures of risk, may sometimes be preferable.

1.3 Limitations of cohort studies

In spite of their advantages, a history of cancer epidemiology indicates that cohort studies have not been the major avenue of attack. Case-control studies have predominated. The limitations of cohort studies are summarized below.

(a) Prospective cohort studies imply a commitment over many years, and both individuals and granting agencies are loath to embark on a project that will not yield its main results for a decade or more. Furthermore, collecting accurate information on more than a short set of variables from the large number of individuals required for a cohort study may be very expensive. The use of case-control comparisons within a cohort (see §1.4*i* and Chapter 7) may reduce the workload involved in processing the data, but the costs of collecting the data still have to be taken into account.

(b) Historical cohort studies do not suffer from this extended commitment into the future, but they can obviously be performed only if a relevant cohort can be identified. For many exposures, the existence of such a cohort with accurate records of exposure dating back ten or more years cannot be guaranteed. Furthermore, even if a cohort which seems to approximate to the requirements of the study can be identified historically, information on other variables which may play an important confounding role is likely to be lacking. Thus, one can study diabetics as a group likely to consume greater than average quantities of artificial sweeteners, but the incidence of bladder cancer in the group is difficult to evaluate in the absence of information on smoking – less common among diabetics. The difficulty of evaluating the significance of moderate excesses of lung cancer among industrial cohorts for whom smoking histories are not recorded is well known.

(c) Most cancers are rare diseases. Even taking one of the most frequent cancers – breast cancer among women over 50 years of age from western countries – no more than one or two cancer cases could be expected per 1000 women per year. For most other cancers, the expected numbers would be considerably less. In fact, for rare cancers, cohort studies are unlikely to be of much value, unless the relative risk associated with the exposure under study is very large. Questions of power are considered in some detail in Chapter 7, but as a noteworthy illustration of the point, in the prospective study of British doctors, the association of smoking with bladder cancer, notwithstanding an observed increase in risk for current smokers of twofold, was not significant. Bladder cancer, although not one of the most common cancers in the United Kingdom, is also not one of the most rare, but nevertheless the number of cases was insufficient to demonstrate the effect convincingly. Given the relative ease with which a series of several hundred cases of cancer at many particular sites can be assembled, it is clear that on most occasions a comparison of the effort or cost per case included in the study will favour the case-control rather than the cohort approach. The justification for a cohort study has to be based, usually, on the superiority of the information it can yield.

(d) It is difficult to obtain estimates of attributable risk. On many occasions, there is interest not only in the degree of risk associated with a certain exposure, but also the importance of that risk in the general population. For a given cancer site, this can be expressed as the population attributable risk, a quantity which population-based case-control studies can provide in straightforward fashion. Many cohort studies, however, are based purposely on groups with a much higher prevalence of the relevant exposure than the general population and so cannot give estimates of the population attributable risk; when the results are extrapolated to the general population, bizarre conclusions can be drawn (as for example the unpublished but widely quoted report from the US National Institutes of Health on the proportion of cancers due to occupational exposures). Even cohorts such as the British doctors or US veterans differ sufficiently from the general population, in terms of economic level for example, to make extrapolation in terms of attributable risk hazardous.

The preceding discussion of the merits and drawbacks of a cohort study relative to a retrospective case-control study suggests that the two approaches have complementary attractions. The cohort approach provides a well-defined population from which cases can be identified in an unbiased manner, and for which some contemporary information on the exposure of interest will be available throughout the time period of interest. Time variables for this exposure may also be well recorded. The case-control approach concentrates effort on the informative individuals, that is the cases and a suitable set of controls, on whom extensive information on confounding variables may be obtainable. In an increasing number of situations, study designs are being used that incorporate the case-control approach within a cohort study, to take advantage of the merits of both approaches. These designs are discussed further in §1.4*i* and in detail in Chapters 5 and 7.

1.4   Implementation

The major concern in assembling a cohort for study is that the size and level of exposure of the cohort be sufficient to yield meaningful results. The two questions that arise are, first, is the study worth doing and, second, how should it be implemented. Chapter 7 considers the question of statistical power, a major element in assessing the potential informativeness of a study. In this section, we treat a range of issues which arise in the implementation of a study.

The design and execution of a cohort study will depend on the individual circumstances of the study, and on its aim. It is instructive to examine in detail the methods used in a number of studies, and for this purpose we give an extended account, in Appendices IA–IF, of the implementation of different types of cohort study – six in all. The studies vary widely in many respects. The study of atomic bonb survivors has been the largest single programme of research in chronic disease epidemiology. The Life-Span Study, on which the majority of the mortality results are based, forms both an infrastructure from which a broad range of activities has evolved and the main source of information on the cancer risks associated with radiation available at the present time (Committee on the Biological Effects of Ionizing Radiation, 1980). An enormous effort has gone into defining the cohort and estimating the radiation dose received by each member of the cohort, and to ensuring the completeness of follow-up and the validity of the death certificate information. All possibly fatal consequences of radiation exposure were included in the scope of the study.

By contrast, the hepatitis B prospective study was targeted closely on the association between the hepatitis B surface antigen carrier state and risk of primary liver cancer. A particular effort was made to confirm primary hepatocellular carcinoma as the cause of death, but otherwise the formation of the cohort and the follow-up procedures depended mainly on existing facilities.

Even though the scope and purpose of different studies may vary widely, however, there are a number of issues in the design and execution that require attention, irrespective of whether the study is prospective or historical. These questions include the following:

(a) Who should be included?
(b) What dates should be taken for each individual as the date of their entry into the study, and their date of exit from the study?
(c) What follow-up mechanisms or systems are to be used, and to what extent will demands of confidentiality impinge on the completeness of follow-up data?
(d) What endpoints will be used for assessing disease occurrence, and how are disease categories to be coded?
(e) What information should be obtained on exposure, and how often during the period of follow-up can it, and will it, be assessed?
(f) What information is available on other exposures, which are either of intrinsic interest or of importance as potential confounding factors?
(g) What comparisons will be made to assess the effect of exposure?
(h) What power will the study have to detect the levels of excess risk that might realistically be expected?
(i) Can a case-control approach be introduced into any component of the study, to improve feasibility or reduce costs, without reducing the information content?

(a) and (b) Who should be included, and how are dates of entry and exit defined?

The main requirement is that inclusion rules be clear and unambiguous. For each individual, the date on which observation begins must be well defined; after that date the individual contributes person-years of observation and is at risk to contribute events of interest. Table 1.8 summarizes the definition of the study cohort for the six studies described in detail in Appendices IA–IF. For each study, it is clear who is a cohort member, and from what date cohort membership starts. If should be stressed that an individual does not enter the cohort, and contribute person-years at risk, until all entry criteria have been satisfied. Thus, in the South Wales nickel workers study, an individual is included and starts to contribute person-years of exposure at the date on which his second appearance on a pay sheet occurs, not on the date of his first appearance on a pay sheet.

The date of exit from the study is the last date on which an individual could contribute person-years at risk. In every study, a date has to be specified as the end of the follow-up period for the current analysis. The vital status on that date should be ascertained for all cohort members and explicitly tabulated when reporting the study. In the Montana smelter workers study, the follow-up was originally to 31 December 1963, and later extended to 30 September 1977. Follow-up status in the original and the extended study is displayed in Tables 1.9a and 1.9b. For those whose vital status was known at the given date, the date of exit from the study is that date or the date of death – whichever is the earlier. Those whose vital status is not known at the end of follow-up will have been lost to follow-up, and the correct procedure is to terminate their follow-up on the last date their vital status is known.

It is important to note that date of entry into the study and date of first exposure are not necessarily the same, and will often be different. In the South Wales nickel workers

Table 1.8 Cohort definition in the studies described in Appendices IA–IF

Study	Source records used to define cohort	Inclusion criteria	Date of entry into cohort (i.e., into follow-up for calculation of person-years)
British doctors	UK medical register	Satisfactory reply to a mailed questionnaire, posted on 31 October 1951	1 November 1951
Atomic bomb survivors	National census data, 1 October 1950	Japanese citizens, present in city at time of bomb, resident in city at census date, place of family registration in or near city (later relaxed)[a]. All individuals within 2500 m of bomb hypocentre ATB, plus a sample of those more distant than 2500 m	1 October 1950
Taiwan hepatitis study	Taiwan government employees	Presented themselves at Government Employees' Clinic Centre for a routine free health examination, and agreed to provide an extra sample of blood	Date of visit to Clinic
South Wales nickel refinery	Company employment records (weekly pay sheets) for first week of April, 1934, 1939, 1944, 1949	Included[b] on at least two of the four pay sheets used	Date of the second pay sheet on which individual appears
Montana smelter workers	Company employment records	Employed for at least one year before 31 December 1956	At end of 1 year's employment or 1 January 1938 if employed for more than 1 year before that date
North American asbestos workers	Union membership records, 1966	All union members in 1966, alive on 1 January 1967, for asbestos study; asbestos and smoking study limited to 11 656 individuals who completed and returned a questionnaire on smoking habits	1 January 1967

[a] When the original cohort was assembled, a 'reserve' group was included who satisfied all criteria except that their place of family registration was distant from either city. This 'reserve' group was added to the rest of the cohort during the follow-up period (Beebe et al., 1977)

[b] This criterion refers to the original cohort described in the first paper (Doll et al., 1970). The cohort was later extended

Table 1.9a   Status of study group, 31 December 1963[a]

Known to be living		5397
Employed by smelters	1471	
Pensioned	389	
Other[b]	3537	
Known to be deceased		1877
Vital status not known		773
Total study group		8047

[a] From Lee and Fraumeni (1969)
[b] Includes persons receiving benefits or making claims to Bureau of Old Age and Survivors Insurance after December 1964

Table 1.9b   Follow-up status of study group[a]

Follow-up status, 30 September 1977	Total study group, 1977	Follow-up status, 31 December 1963		
		Known to be living	Known to be deceased	Vital status not known
Known to be living	3707[b]	3342	0	365[c]
Known to be deceased	3522	1534	1877	111
Vital status not known	816	520	0	296
Total, 1963	8045[d]	5396	1877	772

[a] From Lee-Feldstein (1983)
[b] Includes 442 men still employed at the smelter on 30 September 1977
[c] Approximately half of the men reported lost to follow-up by Lee and Fraumeni (1969) were found to be alive on 30 September 1977
[d] Two persons in the original study group of 8047 were women; they have been deleted from the present study

study, at least five years had to elapse after first exposure before entry into the period of observation. For many in the cohort, employment began ten, 20 or even 30 years before follow-up began. Among the atomic bomb survivors, five years elapsed between exposure and the census that defined the cohort. In some studies, it is possible to ensure that follow-up begins as soon as exposure occurs, but this is not usually so. A distinction has been made, mainly of interest in the occupational setting, between so-called 'prevalence cohorts', consisting of all those employed on a particular date, and 'incidence cohorts', consisting of all those first employed between two dates. The possible problems of interpretation when using prevalence cohorts have been mentioned earlier.

(c) Follow-up mechanisms

Follow-up over time of the individuals enrolled in a cohort study is the essential feature of the study. The success with which the follow-up is achieved is probably the basic measure of the quality of the study. If a substantial proportion of the cohort is lost to follow-up, the validity of the study's conclusions is seriously called into question.

Table 1.10   Completeness of follow-up in a number of cohort studies

Study	Date of end of follow-up	Proportion with unknown vital status at that date
British doctors	Males: 1 November 1971 Females: 1 November 1973	103 (0.3%) from 34 440 61 (1.0%) from 6194 (Authors estimate that at most 'a dozen' out of some 10 000 deaths would have been missed)
Atomic bomb survivors	31 December 1978	The follow-up depends on the national family registration system. Only 9 (0.7%) of 1300 known deaths were not recorded by the system in a pilot investigation (Beebe *et al.*, 1962). Losses to the cohort from emigration were estimated to be less than 100 (0.1%) by the end of 1974 (Beebe *et al.*, 1977)
Taiwan hepatitis study		Passive surveillance: 74 (0.3%) from 22 707 Active surveillance: 74 (1.1%) from 6908
South Wales nickel refinery workers	31 December 1971	37 (3.8%) from 967
Montana smelter workers	30 September 1977	816 (10.1%) from 8045
North American asbestos workers	31 December 1976	100% follow-up, according to the investigators (Hammond *et al.*, 1979)

The loss to follow-up reported in the studies described in appendices IA–IF is shown in Table 1.10, and indicates the target to be achieved. It is worth repeating the point made in an earlier section that case-control studies, insofar as they can be interpreted in a cohort context, would rarely achieve comparable coverage. In situations where new or untried follow-up mechanisms are to be used, a pilot study of their efficacy is recommended, as performed in the atomic bomb survivors study (see Table 1.10).

The purposes of the follow-up process are threefold:

(i) to determine which cohort members are currently under observation, by recording deaths and losses due to migration, i.e., to determine the denominator information;

(ii) to determine the disease events that are the defined endpoints of the study, i.e., to determine the numerator information; and

(iii) to obtain further information on the cohort members.

(i) *Determination of denominator information*

The mechanisms to be used for follow-up vary from country to country, depending on the national systems of population registration and on local laws on confidentiality. If the cohort is defined in terms of an occupational or professional group, or membership of a health insurance plan, then these group records often provide an accurate mechanism for follow-up. In Scandinavian countries, each individual has a unique identifying number which is in common use, accurate records of death using this number extend back over decades, and population rosters exist listing all persons presently living in the country. In principle one can therefore ascertain from among cohort members who has died in the country, who is currently alive in the country and thus, by default, who has left the country at some time in the past. This last group can be investigated further to determine the date of exit from observation. In England and Wales, linkage to death records can usually be achieved easily and with little error, but verification that the individual is currently alive and living in England and Wales is in general cumbersome. In the British doctors study, attempts were made to contact each individual at the end of the follow-up period to ascertain vital status. A range of mechanisms is available in other countries, which is of varying utility for cohort studies. In some countries, the contents of a death certificate are confidential, and it is illegal to know the cause of death.

Since many cohorts under study are defined in terms of membership of a particular group (professional body, occupational pension plan, union, health insurance plan, college alumnae), then, provided individuals remain members of the group, supplementary information from group records may be available, particularly on present vital status. For some cohorts, records kept by the group may be superior to the national system. The British doctors study, the Taiwan hepatitis study and the American insulators study used group records to ascertain vital status, and, as can be seen in Table 1.10, the losses to follow-up were small.

An issue that needs special attention if group membership is related to employment is the question of retirement. Loss to follow-up among the retired, if it achieves appreciable proportions, can vitiate a study, particularly since retirement can be caused by ill-health. Increased mortality soon after retirement is a common observation. Efforts made to trace those who had retired received special attention in the report on the Taiwan hepatitis study (see Appendix IC).

On occasion, follow-up may be active in the sense that the investigators attempt to see each cohort member on a regular basis. Such an approach can clearly be expensive, and it has tended to be used mainly when the cohort is already under some form of clinical care. Thus, in an early study of women irradiated for cancer of the cervix, on the routine post-treatment visits made by the cervical cancer patient to her treatment clinic, further investigations were carried out as part of the study – notably, haematological studies, since leukaemia was the main endpoint of interest at that time (Hutchison, 1968). In the Taiwan study, hepatitis B surface antigen carriers and a negative group of equal size were followed actively, with an annual examination. This active follow-up was undertaken partly to verify the completeness of the passive follow-up mechanism, and partly for sequential determination of hepatitis B virus status.

On occasion, acquisition of information on death and migration for every member of the cohort may involve greater expense than the study can meet. If the endpoints of interest can be ascertained on all cohort members, for example from a cancer registry, then a less complete approach could be considered to enumerate the relevant denominator. Two possibilities offer themselves. First, one can carry out the follow-up, for the purposes of person-year calculations, on a sample of the entire cohort. If the cohort is large, reasonably accurate denominator information may be obtained by sampling only a small fraction of the total. Second, one might use an actuarial approach and calculate what could be called 'expected' expected numbers, based on population deaths and migration rates. Either approach might be considered in a pilot phase of the study, to determine whether a full study was of interest. Section 1.6 treats briefly the proportional mortality approach, where denominators are simply ignored.

(ii) *Identification of cancer cases among the cohort*

In many countries, use of cancer registries for ascertainment of cancer occurring in cohort members is limited by incomplete coverage on a national level. There is considerable risk that individuals will have moved to areas of the country not covered by cancer registration. In some countries, however, cancer registration is nationwide. Use of the cancer registry to ascertain the cancer cases occurring in the cohort then has a number of advantages over use of the usual alternative source of information, namely, death certificates.

First, recording of cancer in cancer registries is often more accurate than on death certificates. Greater care is taken to ensure that the registered diagnosis is correct and more information is given, particularly on the histology of the cancer.

Second, more cases should be observed, since many cancers do not lead to death. The cases will also be observed earlier, death occurring after diagnosis, often with a delay of several years.

Third, population rates will be available for a wider variety of cancers. Observed and expected numbers can be given, for example, for different histological types of lung cancer.

A fourth advantage, of relevance mainly in occupational studies, is that the healthy worker effect should be less for cancer incidence than for cancer mortality, and may in fact be almost negligible (as in Figure 1.1).

Notwithstanding the advantages of cancer registry material, a large proportion of cohort studies have no choice but to use death certification as the main source of information on cancer in the cohort. For all comparisons with national mortality rates, it is essential that the cause of death as given in the death certificate be used. Only in this way can unbiased comparisons be made.

(iii) *Further information on cohort members*

For analyses, however, in which subgroups of the cohort under study are compared, the diagnosis as given on the death certificate may benefit from refinement based on additional information. Centralized review of available histological or haematological material to ensure uniform classification of subtypes of disease, or simply to confirm death certificate diagnoses, can be a valuable exercise. The resulting reclassification might be expected to sharpen the analyses performed within the cohort. In the British doctors study, for example, confirmation was sought whenever lung cancer was given on the death certificate as the underlying or contributing cause of death.

In the study of North America insulators, it was considered likely that at least asbestos-related disease might have been misclassified. Further information, including histology sections and X-ray films, was obtained where possible on asbestos workers who had died, and a revised cause of death assigned whenever indicated. Table 1.11 shows the differences in the number of deaths due to different causes between the

Table 1.11 Number of deaths occurring from five through 35 years after onset of work in an amosite asbestos factory, 1941–1945. Cause of death coded in two different ways[a,b]

Underlying cause of death	DC	BE	BE–DC	Expected
All causes	1946	1946	—	1148.0
Cancer, all sites	845	912	+67	259.0
Lung	397	450	+53	81.7
Pleural mesothelioma	23	61	+38	—
Peritoneal mesothelioma	24	109	+85	—
Mesothelioma not specified above	54	0	−54	—
Larynx, buccal and pharynx	21	27	+6	7.5
Oesophagus	17	17	0	5.1
Kidney	15	16	+1	8.5
Colon-rectum	54	55	+1	8.5
Stomach	18	21	+3	30.5
Prostate	24	26	+2	12.5
Bladder	7	9	+2	6.7
Pancreas	46	21	−25	16.0
Other specified sites	110	83	−27	72.1
Primary site unknown	35	17	−18	
Noninfectious pulmonary diseases, total	177	204	+27	68.2
Asbestosis	76	160	+27	—
Cardiovascular disease	638	566	−72	660.1
Other and unspecified causes	286	264	−22	160.8
Subtotal, all causes except cardiovascular diseases	1308	1380	+72	487.9

[a] DC, cause of death according to death certificate information only; BE, cause of death according to best evidence available
[b] From Hammond *et al.* (1979)

death certification and the cause based on the best available evidence. The death certificates severely underestimate the number of deaths due to asbestosis, mesothelioma and, to a lesser extent, lung cancer. More accurate estimates of dose-response, and of changing risk with time, are clearly given by the diagnoses based on the best available evidence. It is of interest to note that pancreatic cancers were overdiagnosed on the death certificates, and the confusion was usually with mesothelioma. What appears as a greater than two-fold excess, highly significant statistically, disappears if the more accurate cause of death is used. (In this situation, one might legitimately compare the refined diagnosis with expectations based on death certificate diagnoses since the main source of error, mesothelioma, affects inappreciably the general population rates.)

In the Taiwan hepatitis study, clinical and pathology records were sought for all deaths that occurred in the cohort, and primary hepatocellular carcinoma accepted as the cause of death only if the evidence was unambiguous. This degree of confirmation was required since the aim of the study was precisely to define the risk of primary hepatocellular carcinoma among carriers and noncarriers.

(d) *Coding of disease*

For many cohort studies, the follow-up period may cover a period of several decades. During this time, the codes used both for death certification and for cancer registration have changed. Of the International Classification of Diseases (ICD), the 6th revision was introduced in 1950, the 7th in 1955, the 8th in 1968 and the 9th in 1978. The World Health Organization has asked member countries to code death certificates according to the current revision. Unfortunately, several disease categories are subdivided differently in different revisions, confusing the comparisons between time periods. The cancer section of the ICD has been disturbed in this way less than many other sections, and most investigations extending back to the 1950s or earlier have devised tables of equivalence between the different revisions. The equivalences given in *Cancer Incidence in Five Continents* (Waterhouse *et al.*, 1976) are reproduced in Appendix II.

(e) *Information on exposure, and how often it should be assessed*

The aims of the study should help to define the detail that is required for the information on exposure. In the studies described earlier by Case, exposure was described solely in qualitative terms, whether or not employment for more than six months had occurred in an occupation with recorded exposure to the compounds of interest (e.g., α- and β-naphthylamine, benzidine, aniline). The cohort was classified according to the compounds to which individuals had been exposed (see Table 1.4). No data were available to quantify the level of exposure. The data, however, were considered adequate for the purpose at hand, which was identification of the major bladder carcinogens in the chemical industry, and the results sufficed as a basis for legislation. Thirty years later, no more quantitative relationship between levels of exposure to the aromatic amines and bladder cancer risk in humans has been established.

In contrast, studies on the leukaemogenicity of benzene, although unequivocally demonstrating that benzene causes leukaemia in man (Infante *et al.*, 1977; IARC, 1982b), have been insufficient at present for societal purposes, i.e., for setting safety limits, because of uncertainty over the levels to which the cohorts had been exposed. Further studies on benzene would be of value only if quantitative exposure levels could be determined for each individual during his period of exposure.

However, although the degree of quantification possible under different circumstances varies, the more quantitative that one can make the relationship between exposure and risk, the more it will be of value, for three reasons. First, the credibility of the causality of the relationship will be enhanced; second, the greater will be the potential for meaningful public health action; and, third, the contribution to an understanding of carcinogenic mechansims will be increased. It should be stressed that quantifying exposure requires recording not only the level of exposure, but when it occurred, for how long and whether it stopped. These temporal aspects may well be more powerful determinants of risk (as discussed in Chapter 6) and are often better recorded than is the exposure level.

To obtain quantitative relationships between exposure and excess risk, information

Table 1.12   Information on exposures in the six studies described in Appendices 1A–1F

British doctors	Smoking history from questionnaires. Amount currently smoked and age at which smoking started and stopped (for ex-smokers). Questionnaires sent on four separate occasions
Atomic bomb survivors	Detailed information on individual dose for each member of the cohort
Taiwan hepatitis study	One determination of hepatitis B virus carrier status on entry to study
South Wales nickel refinery workers	Specific job held during each year of employment. Job posts categorized retrospectively by analysis of associated risk
Montana smelter workers	Time and place of employment for each job held within smelter. Environmental measures taken in the smelter enabled each work area to be categorized on a 1 to 10 scale for arsenic trioxide levels.
North American asbestos workers	No information on level of asbestos exposure. Start and length of employment. Smoking history obtained in 1966

on exposure at the individual level is of the greatest value. Although mean levels for the entire cohort are not valueless, since they do give some impression of what dose has produced a given excess risk, they do not reflect the fact that the study is individual-based, and cannot yield estimates of dose-response.

The extent and detail of the information on exposure should reflect the relationship between exposure and excess risk that the investigator might expect. Table 1.12 summarizes the exposure data collected in the six studies described in Appendices IA–IF. Quantitative models of carcinogenesis, considered in Chapter 6 in some detail, suggest some of the required information. First, in relation to time of exposure, for each individual one should know the dates at which exposure started and stopped and the subject's age when exposure started. It is not unrealistic to expect such information to be available if it is based on employment or medical records, or is derived from questionnaires. If the exposure information comes from biological markers, however, exposure status will be determined only for the time points when the relevant samples are taken. The design of the study will then be critically influenced by the hypotheses under test. For an example in which this issue is discussed in detail – a prospective study relating Burkitt's lymphoma to infection by the Epstein-Barr virus – see Geser and de-Thé (1972).

Second, in relation to level of exposure, quantitative information is rarely available throughout the period of exposure. Exceptions might be workers exposed to radioactivity, who are continuously monitored, or patients given chemotherapy, for whom details of treatment should be available. One has to decide which summary measures are most informative. For many exposures, average levels during the whole period of exposure may be sufficient. For asbestos and mesothelioma, however, the levels in the first few years of exposure are likely to be the most relevant and levels in the years immediately preceding disease onset almost irrelevant (Peto, J. et al., 1981). In contrast, for cigarette smoking and lung cancer, Doll and Hill (1950) found from the results of their initial case-control study that among continuing smokers the amount most recently smoked was almost as informative as the full smoking history over many years.

Asking about current practices, or measuring current levels, has the advantage that it yields more accurate data than asking about former practices, although its value is restricted to prospective studies. It can also take advantage of new techniques for measuring metabolite levels in the urine, or binding to macromolecules in the blood, which offer the potential of measuring more relevant aspects of an individual's exposure. For many occupational or environmental exposures, however, levels have fallen steadily over the last three decades. For the determination of the present excess risk, the most relevant exposure levels may well be those in operation two or three decades ago, simply because at that time they were much higher. Unfortunately, if quantitative values are available for exposure levels 30 years ago, the methods used in their determination may not be comparable with those used today, or may not even be interpretable with more stringent modern criteria. Asbestos measurements, for example, taken in the 1940s are difficult to calibrate with modern measurements.

On many occasions the specific carcinogen may not have been identified, as for example in nickel refining, leather and wood working, or arsenic exposure in non-ferrous metal smelters. In these circumstances, dose cannot be defined in an absolute sense. One may, however, be able to assign degrees of exposure. Such a procedure was used when studying the Montana smelters exposed to arsenic, and in the most recent publications on the study of the South Wales nickel workers (Peto, J. *et al.*, 1984; Kaldor *et al.*, 1986).

In the Montana study, measurements of atmospheric arsenic trioxide were used to categorize working areas as providing heavy, medium or light arsenic exposure (Lee & Fraumeni, 1969). Each individual could then be categorized in terms of the jobs he had held within the smelter since the start of his empolyment there. It was noted that arsenic trioxide measurements were not made throughout the period of exposure, and that levels may have varied, but the authors considered that the relative exposure levels in different work areas would have remained fairly constant. In the nickel study, categorization of work areas was done *post hoc,* a high risk being associated with working in only a few of the refinery work places.

The degree of exposure defined categorically in this manner can then be used as a nonquantitative ordered variable in the analysis, affording the possibility of demonstrating a positive dose-response relationship. It may often happen that the categorization of level of exposure that gives the clearest trend with increasing risk will incorporate aspects of duration of exposure.

In prospective studies, the opportunity exists to repeat measurements of exposure, so that the degree of measurement error or of intrinsic intra-individual variation can be estimated. These estimates can be used to assess the real exposure-disease relationship (Clayton & Kaldor, 1985), but the planning of data collection to provide genuine estimates of intra-individual variation has at present received little attention in the context of prospective epidemiological studies.

(f) Information on other exposures

The main weakness of many historical cohort studies is the absence of information on potentially confounding variables. The lack will increase the uncertainty of the interpretation placed on the results. Two possible approaches could be taken to improve the situation. First, for the relevant cases and a series of controls, one could mount an intensive effort to obtain the missing information. For a historical cohort study that has involved several decades of follow-up, many of the cases may be long since dead. One could not expect a high degree of accuracy from a surviving spouse or friend on, say, the smoking and drinking habits of someone who had died 15 or more years previously. Limiting this case-control accrual of information to cohort members alive within five years of the interview should improve the accuracy of the information, but may remove most of the cases. A second approach would be to take a sample of the surviving members of the cohort and obtain the necessary information from them. This information cannot, of course, be handled in the usual way for information on confounding variables, by stratification or incorporation in regression models, but it can be used to give an estimate of the degree of confounding associated with that variable. This estimate has to involve use of external information on the risk associated with the confounding variable. The confounding risk ratio would then be calculated as in Chapter 3 of Volume 1.

In prospective cohort studies, one would expect to obtain prospectively some information on potential major confounding variables.

For both historical and prospective cohort studies, it is important that the information obtained on confounding variables be reasonably accurate. Approximate information, such as one might feel appropriate for factors of secondary inportance, can be almost useless (Tzonou et al., 1986). An example is given in Table 1.13, for a dichotomous exposure and a single dichotomous confounding variable, the latter being observed with error. The level of confounding that remains after the effect of the misclassified confounding variable has been taken into account is tabulated for a range of situations. Misclassification rates of 30%, not unknown in epidemiology, allow the removal of very little of the confounding effect; rates of 10%, which would often be considered relatively precise epidemiological measures, leave nearly half the confounding effect in operation. It is clear that one should attempt to obtain information prospectively on the entire cohort only if it is both economic and feasible to collect accurate information. Otherwise, the resources are probably better allocated to obtaining the information accurately on a case-control basis, concurrently if possible. An alternative approach, being developed, is to obtain repeat joint measures of the exposure and the confounder, and use the estimates of the joint error distribution to estimate the real relationship (Clayton & Kaldor, 1987).

(g) The need for the construction of special comparison groups

In most studies, the comparisons of interest that will be made are either among subgroups of the cohort or with the general population. On occasion, however, comparisons with an external group or among subgroups within the cohort will be insufficient. A separate control group will then have to be constructed. Such a situation is seen in the study of insulators, in which the emphasis is on the combined effect of smoking and asbestos exposure. To assess the effect of asbestos exposure among smokers and nonsmokers separately, one requires mortality rates among smokers and

Table 1.13 Bias in the estimation of the summary odds ratio if the confounding variable, C, is misclassified but the exposure variable, E, is not. The body of the table shows Δ_E, the ratio of the measured odds ratio to the true odds ratio (R_E)

P	p_1	p_2	$R_C = 2$				$R_C = 10$			
			$\delta = \gamma =$ 0.1	0.2	0.3	W	$\delta = \gamma =$ 0.1	0.2	0.3	W
0.1	0.6	0.4	1.05	1.09	1.12	1.14	1.15	1.26	1.34	1.39
	0.7	0.3	1.11	1.20	1.26	1.31	1.34	1.61	1.81	1.97
	0.8	0.2	1.20	1.34	1.43	1.50	1.62	2.16	2.58	2.93
	0.9	0.1	1.36	1.55	1.66	1.73	2.29	3.35	4.14	4.79
0.5	0.6	0.4	1.05	1.09	1.12	1.14	1.17	1.27	1.34	1.39
	0.7	0.3	1.12	1.20	1.26	1.31	1.40	1.67	1.84	1.97
	0.8	0.2	1.22	1.35	1.44	1.50	1.79	2.33	2.67	2.93
	0.9	0.1	1.41	1.58	1.67	1.73	2.74	3.76	4.36	4.79
0.9	0.6	0.4	1.05	1.09	1.12	1.14	1.18	1.28	1.35	1.39
	0.7	0.3	1.13	1.21	1.27	1.31	1.46	1.72	1.87	1.97
	0.8	0.2	1.23	1.37	1.45	1.50	2.00	2.49	2.75	2.93
	0.9	0.1	1.44	1.60	1.68	1.73	3.32	4.16	4.55	4.79

R_E = true odds ratio between exposure E and disease
P = (true) proportion of population exposed to E
R_C = true odds ratio between exposure C and disease
p_1 = proportion of those exposed to E who are also exposed to C
p_2 = proportion of those not exposed to E who are exposed to C
δ = proportion of those truly $C+$ classified as $C-$
γ = proportion of those truly $C-$ classified as $C+$
W = confounding risk ratio (for estimation of R_E) (= estimate of odds ratio ignoring C/true odds ratio)

nonsmokers without asbestos exposure. Since the entire group of insulators was considered to have been exposed to asbestos, this requirement necessitated the construction of an ad-hoc comparison group. The procedure is described in Appendix IF, where it can be seen that considerable care was taken to match the comparison group on socioeconomic and other factors. It is interesting to note that a nonexposed control group was also assembled in the atomic bomb survivor studies, consisting of people present in the two cities at the 1950 census but not at the time of the bomb. Fears were expressed at the outset that this group might not be comparable in a number of respects, and it emerged that their mortality rates differed from those of the study cohort in ways unrelated to exposure. They were not included in most of the major analyses.

(h) Power considerations

Before substantial resources are devoted to a study, the possible results the study could yield need to be investigated. In particular, the level of risk that has a high probability of being detected needs to be assessed. In another field, it is becoming increasingly recognized that small clinical trials are usually counterproductive. There is little probability that they can detect realistic differences in treatment; the only significant differences they can show will almost certainly overestimate the real effect. They might be considered biased against the correct result. The same considerations apply to small epidemiological studies. Studies that have low power of detecting realistic levels of excess risk should not be performed, unless their results can be merged with those from other studies.

Chapter 7 discusses in some detail power calculations for both cohort studies and case-control studies.

(i) *The possible role of a case-control approach within a cohort*

The essential feature of a cohort study is that each cohort member is followed from entry into the study to death or to the date at which follow-up ends. There are a number of different approaches, however, to the way in which the information on the relevant exposure variables is collected. Gathering the full information on all cohort members may on occasion be a waste of resources and so prevent more useful activities taking place. Typically, the final comparison will be based on a relatively small group of cases and a much larger group of controls. One can therefore take only a subsample of the controls without affecting appreciably the precision of the comparison. Omitting cases, of course, will lead directly to a loss in precision. The questions to face in the design, therefore, are whether and how one can limit the number of individuals for whom full information is obtained without jeopardizing either the validity or the precision of the study. The problem of precision, and of how the sampling might actually be performed, is discussed in detail in Chapters 5 and 7, where different sampling schemes are considered. The sample might consist, for example, of sets of controls, each set individually matched to a particular case, or it might consist of an unstructured subcohort (one in ten of all individuals, say). Designs in which a subcohort is chosen at the start of the study to constitute the control group are discussed by Prentice (1986). Here we consider the question of validity. The main options open to an investigator, set out in Table 1.14, are, first, to wait until the deaths (or other events) of interest have occurred, and then to obtain the information from only a sample of the rest of the cohort; second, to obtain the information on the entire cohort but process it only on a sample; thirdly, to obtain and to process information on the entire cohort, but to use only a sample of the entire cohort together with all the deaths of interest for the statistical analysis.

When the investigator can choose his approach, as would be the case in a prospective study, the design should specify at the start of the study for each variable under investigation the time in the study when information or samples are to be obtained, and when assay or processing is to be performed. The aim should be to reduce the overall burden of data collection and laboratory assays to the minimum consistent with validity, so that attention can be focused on maximizing the quality of the information obtained.

In historical cohort studies the investigator would usually not have the choice. He or she would simply have to decide whether further information, such as smoking histories, was worth obtaining retrospectively, and there would seldom be much value

Table 1.14 Possible approaches to data acquisition

Alternative approaches to the acquisition and treatment of exposure variables	Implication, given information required on all deaths (from a given cause)	Examples and remarks
1. Information obtained only on a sample of the cohort	Information collected when death status is known. Retrospective data must be equivalent to prospective data, and strictly comparable between cases and controls. Neither death nor disease state should affect the variable being measured.	Suitable for genetic markers, or when information from other sources is available independent of the study. No variable in which recall bias may operate should be ascertained in this manner, nor any metabolic or immunological marker affected by the disease in question.
2. Information (or biological specimens) collected on all the cohort, but processed (or assayed) only on a sample	Processing or assays performed only when death status is known. Long-term storage of unassayed samples required	Method of choice when the assay or processing makes heavy demands on resources (e.g., processing seven-day dietary diaries, assaying most metabolic and immunological markers). Essential to demonstrate that storage does not invalidate assay, and that records can be stored safely
3. All information available on entire cohort, but statistical analysis uses only a sample	None	A useful approach to exploratory data analysis (see Chapter 5)

in obtaining it on the whole cohort. He might also decide that further information was required to clarify the results for just one, or a few, causes of death. For example, in a study of Danish brewery workers, known to drink large quantities of beer, Jensen (1979) found an excess of oesophageal cancer (and of course many other diseases). An important question in the epidemiology of oesophageal cancer is whether the exposure of importance is alcohol itself or a particular type of alcoholic drink. In this situation, was it the beer that caused the excess, or were the oesophageal cancer cases heavy consumers of other types of alcohol as well? A subsequent case-control study showed that the association was mainly with beer, i.e., that in this cohort of brewery workers, heavy beer drinking was sufficient to lead to an excess of oesophageal cancer (Adelhardt et al., 1985).

1.5   Interpretation

The initial aim of most epidemiological studies is to determine, to the extent possible with the available data, whether some exposure represents a carcinogenic hazard. The previous section attempted to define what data should be collected for this purpose; this section considers how these data may be used. Criteria for assessing whether an observed association is likely to be causal were discussed at length in Chapter 3 of

Volume 1. Increasingly, however, the demand is not for qualitative evidence of carcinogenicity, but for quantification of the degree of risk. The analysis of the results of a cohort study should aim to extract the maximum quantitative information that the data can yield. The extent to which an analysis produces coherent quantitative descriptions of risk depends at least in part on the manner in which the exposure data are handled – what composite measures of exposure are used, for example.

It should be borne in mind that cohort studies are often the result of an unusual or even unique opportunity. Prospective studies are rarely undertaken, because of their cost and duration. Historical studies are often focused on one of the few cohorts that may exist for which there is clear evidence of exposure to the agent of interest. Either way, there may be few opportunities to repeat the study, unlike retrospective case-control studies, where, for most major sites, a large number of studies have been performed. There is thus an added onus on the investigator to exploit his material to the full.

The two major aspects of an observed excess risk that merit attention are indicators of a dose-response and the evolution of risk with time.

(a) Dose-response relationships

Both to identify the groups at highest risk and to demonstrate a dose-response, categorization of exposure is helpful, even if no reliable measure of exposure levels is available. Job categories, for example, can be classified as low, moderate or high exposure, as in the Montana smelter workers study (Chapters 4 and 5). The data themselves may indicate that some jobs comport a particularly high risk, as in the South Wales nickel workers (Chapters 4 and 6), although one must be wary of circular arguments. In some instances, little information may be available to classify either job categories or individuals. In this situation, length of employment may provide the best measure of degree of exposure. As mentioned earlier, time variables associated with exposure should be accurately recorded in a cohort study. Given the large effect that errors of measurement can have on estimates of the maximum degree of risk, and of the shape of a dose-response, the accuracy with which time variables are recorded may often make them more valuable than less accurate measures of level of exposure in distinguishing risk, even if the latter might appear *a priori* to be more relevant.

The exposure information available for the six studies summarized in Appendices IA–IF is shown in Table 1.12. When adequate dose information is available, one has to decide how to incorporate it most informatively into the analysis. In Chapter 4, straightforward methods of analysis are described in which categorization of an exposure history into a few levels is required. Chapters 5 and 6 discuss how continuous exposure levels can be treated in the analysis. In each chapter, the aim is the same: how can the data be best utilized to assess causality and to throw quantitative relationships into the clearest light.

(b) Time relationships

In describing the excess risk associated with an exposure, it is of interest to know not only the level of risk that can be expected, but also when that excess is likely to occur.

Among continuing cigarette smokers, lung cancer incidence rises with the fourth power of duration of smoking. Mesothelioma rates rise as the third or fourth power of time since first exposure to asbestos. Excess leukaemia mortality forms a wave with a peak at some five years after short-term exposure to radiation. These relationships, discussed in greater detail in Chapter 6, indicate that the temporal behaviour of excess cancer incidence following carcinogenic exposures exhibits well-defined patterns. These patterns may vary from site to site and between exposures, but the pattern of the change with time of an observed excess risk can be determinant in deciding whether an association is causal.

An example is given by a follow-up study of women treated by radiation for cancer of the cervix, in which a large (fourfold) excess of lung cancer was observed (Day & Boice, 1983). Luckily, a nonirradiated group was also included in the study, in whom a similar excess was seen, so that the excess was clearly independent of the irradiation. It is instructive to examine, however, the evolution after the radiation treatment of the excess lung cancer risk, displayed in Figure 1.3. The change in risk with time is unlike that seen for lung cancer in other studies of radiation, in which a genuine exposure-related excess was observed. The normal pattern is for the excess to appear only some ten years after exposure starts. When examined by age at irradiation (i.e., diagnosis of cervical cancer), the picture among those under 50 years of age at irradiation is even more extreme than that shown in Figure 1.3, and for women under age 40 at irradiation the initial excess was nearly 20-fold. Thus, even without the

Fig. 1.3   Observed to expected ratios of lung cancer by time since diagnosis of cervical cancer for patients with invasive cervical cancer treated with radiotherapy and patients with invasive cancer not treated with radiotherapy; 80% confidence intervals presented. From Day *et al.* (1983)

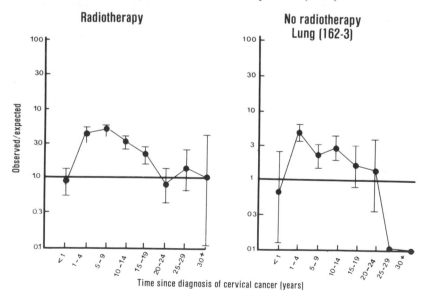

evidence from the nonirradiated group, the shape of the time-risk curve is such that one would feel confident that the observed excess risk is not causally related to the radiation. An alternative explanation, that the excess lung cancers observed are in fact misclassified metastases from the original cervical cancer, fits the observed changes with time and age closely. Smoking, an obvious confounder, is responsible for only a small part of the excess (Day *et al.*, 1983).

Apart from the evolution of risk with time since the start of exposure and with duration of exposure, the change in risk after exposure stops is also of importance. Not only does it aid interpretation, in that a decreasing excess risk after exposure stops would be further evidence of a causal relationship, but the effect of removing exposure is of major intrinsic interest. It is the main epidemiological guide to the effects of intervention measures, and to when public health measures may yield results. Part of the analysis of a cohort study should be orientated specifically at this aspect, and in the design of the study particular efforts should be made to include those formerly exposed.

(c) Problems in the interpretation of cohort studies

A number of issues arise in the interpretation of cohort studies, some of which are due to the longitudinal nature of the data acquisition, some of which are common to most analytical studies in which emphasis is put on quantification.

(i) Choice of comparison groups and the healthy worker effect

For studies in which subcohorts can be distinguished in terms of level or duration of exposure, most weight in the interpretation will usually be given to comparisons between subgroups within the cohort. Internal comparisons may not always be possible, however, and reliance may have to be put on comparisons with population rates external to the cohort. The question is then to decide which rates to use. Industrial cohorts usually live in urban areas; manual workers smoke more than professional and managerial groups; for a variety of reasons national rates may be inappropriate. Under these circumstances, one can attempt to use rates for a specific socioeconomic group, or for a locality if these are available. The issue of which rates to use to calculate expected numbers is well discussed in a report of the UK Medical Research Council (MRC Environmental Epidemiology Unit, 1984).

A common experience when studying cohorts of employed individuals is that the risk of dying in the first years after entry into the cohort, i.e., after identification as an employed individual, is less than that of the general population. Fox and Goldblatt (1982) have shown conversely, using UK census data, that mortality among the unemployed is particularly high. The reduction in mortality, the healthy worker effect, varies between disease categories and appears to be smaller for cancer than for other major groups. For cancer, the effect also appears to be smaller for cancer incidence than for cancer mortality, reflecting the fact that those with cancer are more likely to have left their job. The healthy worker effect tapers off as years pass since entry into the cohort, unfortunately confounding any real increase in risk with years since first exposure.

An analogue of the healthy worker effect may also occur when the cohort is made up of those who respond to invitations or mailed questionnaires. In the British doctors study, those who replied to the initial questionnaire had, in the first few years of follow-up, an overall mortality considerably less than that of all British doctors. As Doll and Hill put it: ' . . . there may be some general association between mortality and the tendency not to reply to such an enquiry, whether the tendency be due to a deliberate refusal (which is rare) or a mere neglect of things (which is frequent). In this respect it is perhaps not too fanciful to note that one non-replier died of smallpox and another of diabetic coma.' In the controlled trial of breast cancer screening in New York, among those invited to screening, the women who accepted had half the overall mortality of those who did not attend, even though they were at considerably higher risk for breast cancer (Shapiro *et al.*, 1982).

The healthy worker effect, since it produces lower mortality rates for many causes of death, may mask real effects. This masking is particularly difficult to interpret if comparisons are made with an external standard population. The more that comparisons are made between different exposure categories within the cohort, the less distortion to the overall interpretation will be caused by the healthy worker effect.

One aspect of the healthy worker effect requires special treatment since it is not eliminated by confining comparisons to those between subgroups of the cohort. Employment status often changes due to ill health. People may retire because they are chronically sick or, because of incapacity, move to lighter work or change jobs. Mortality is therefore likely to be particularly high in the year or two succeeding changes in employment, and conversely relative low in those not changing employment. Odd peaks and troughs may thus appear if risk is examined in relation to time since, or time before, change in job category. One means commonly used to alleviate this problem is to lag changes in status by a number of years – often two or three. In this way, the first year or two after retirement, and the deaths that occur within them, are treated as if the individual were still employed. The matter is discussed further in Chapter 3 (p. 87).

(ii) *Losses to follow-up*

The validity of a cohort study depends fundamentally on complete ascertainment of the events of interest (e.g., cancer deaths) and correct computation of the population at risk. Unless at the start of the study one can be confident that losses to follow-up can be limited to the levels seen in Table 1.10, a study should probably not be launched.

Individuals leave the population at risk either through death, or through migration to a country or region where the follow-up mechanisms of the study are not operative. If an individual has left the population at risk, i.e., the observable cohort, but this fact is unrecorded, then he will continue to contribute to the person–years at risk, but can no longer contribute to the events of interest. Mortality and incidence rates for each cause will be biased downwards. An evaluation of the extent to which follow-up losses have occurred is important, documentation of low loss rates adding to the credibility of the results. Thus, at the date chosen as the end of follow-up, the status should be ascertained of those still thought to be active members of the cohort and under observation. The proportion not found gives the proportion lost to follow-up. In some situations, this ascertainment may be laborious, and it might be undertaken on a sample, if selected in unbiased fashion.

(iii) *Biases due to errors of measurement*

One of the advantages of cohort studies over case-control studies is that information on exposure is obtained before disease status is ascertained. One can therefore have considerable confidence that errors in measurement are the same for individuals who become cases of the disease of interest, and the remainder of the cohort. The complexities possible in retrospective case-control studies because of differences in recall between cases and controls do not apply. Measurement error will bias estimates of relative risk and standardized mortality ratio (SMR); the extent of the bias is indicated in Table 1.15 for different rates of misclassification.

The shape of dose-response curves, and not just their overall level, will also be altered by error in measurement (Doll & Peto, 1978). A linear dose-response, for example, may be transformed into one concave upwards, concave downwards, or

Table 1.15   Bias in the estimation of the odds ratio associated with a dichotomous exposure variable in a case-control study if there is misclassification of exposure levels. The body of the table shows the ratio of the odds ratio estimated using misclassified data to the true odds ratio[a]

P	β	$R_E = 2$						$R_E = 10$					
		$\alpha = 0$	0.1	0.2	0.3	0.4	0.5	$\alpha = 0$	0.1	0.2	0.3	0.4	0.5
0.1	0.0	1.00	0.99	0.98	0.97	0.96	0.95	1.00	0.91	0.84	0.77	0.72	0.68
	0.1	0.76	0.74	0.72	0.69	0.67	0.64	0.57	0.50	0.43	0.37	0.32	0.28
	0.2	0.68	0.66	0.64	0.62	0.59	0.57	0.42	0.36	0.30	0.26	0.22	0.19
	0.3	0.64	0.62	0.60	0.58	0.56	0.54	0.34	0.28	0.24	0.20	0.17	0.14
	0.4	0.61	0.59	0.57	0.55	0.53	0.52	0.30	0.24	0.20	0.17	0.14	0.12
	0.5	0.59	0.57	0.55	0.53	0.52	0.50	0.20	0.21	0.17	0.14	0.12	0.10
0.5	0.0	1.00	0.92	0.86	0.81	0.78	0.75	1.00	0.55	0.40	0.32	0.28	0.25
	0.1	0.95	0.86	0.80	0.75	0.71	0.68	0.92	0.48	0.34	0.27	0.23	0.20
	0.2	0.92	0.82	0.75	0.70	0.66	0.62	0.85	0.42	0.29	0.23	0.19	0.17
	0.3	0.88	0.78	0.71	0.65	0.61	0.57	0.79	0.36	0.25	0.20	0.16	0.14
	0.4	0.86	0.74	0.67	0.61	0.57	0.53	0.74	0.32	0.22	0.17	0.14	0.12
	0.5	0.83	0.70	0.63	0.58	0.53	0.50	0.70	0.27	0.18	0.14	0.12	0.10
0.9	0.0	1.00	0.68	0.61	0.58	0.56	0.55	1.00	0.19	0.15	0.13	0.12	0.12
	0.1	0.99	0.66	0.60	0.57	0.55	0.54	0.99	0.18	0.14	0.13	0.12	0.12
	0.2	0.99	0.65	0.58	0.56	0.54	0.53	0.98	0.17	0.13	0.12	0.12	0.11
	0.3	0.98	0.63	0.57	0.54	0.53	0.52	0.97	0.16	0.13	0.12	0.11	0.11
	0.4	0.98	0.61	0.56	0.53	0.52	0.51	0.96	0.15	0.12	0.11	0.11	0.10
	0.5	0.97	0.59	0.54	0.52	0.51	0.50	0.95	0.14	0.12	0.11	0.10	0.10

[a] From Tzonou *et al.* (1986)

R_E = true odds ratio between exposure E and disease

P = (true) proportion of population exposed to E

α = proportion of those truly $E+$ classified as $E-$

β = proportion of those truly $E-$ classified as $E+$

Table 1.16 Effects of misclassification on the shape
of a linear dose-response curve – exposure grouped
into three categories

	Real exposure		
	Low	Medium	High
Misclassification matrix			
Observed Low	0.65	0.175	0
exposure Medium	0.35	0.65	0.35
High	0	0.175	0.65
Relative risk of real			
exposure	1.0	5.0	9.0
(a) Creation of a dose-response curvilinear *upwards*			
Real distribution of:			
Control population	76%	16%	8%
Case population	33%	34%	33%
Observed relative risk	1.0	2.2	6.3
(b) Creation of a dose-response curvilinear *downwards*			
Control population	33%	34%	33%
Case population	6.7%	33.3%	60%
Observed relative risk	1.0	4.4	4.4

linear with lower slope. What happens will depend on the distribution of the exposure in the cohort under study, and on the misclassification rates. Examples are given in Table 1.16.

Interpretation of the results will be sharpened if information is available on the misclassification rates, and, in this respect again, cohort studies, particularly prospective studies, have a clear advantage over case-control studies. Contact with the study cohort during the period of follow-up will permit assessment not only of the change in exposure variables during this period, but also estimation of the misclassification rates. These rates are then equally applicable to future cases and to the controls, and valid adjustments can be made to the observed relative risk and dose-response curves and also to the corresponding confidence intervals. Furthermore, correct use can be made of information on confounding variables (Clayton, 1985; Clayton & Kaldor, 1987). One should note, however, that repeating the same questionnaire may well not provide a second, independent observation; it may simply repeat the same errors. A more subtle approach will often be required. In case-control studies, repeat measurements are rarely available and, if at all, only on the controls. Their applicability to the cases will be questionable.

(iv) *Lack of information on confounding factors*

In an earlier section, we considered how information on confounding variables might be acquired. In many historical cohort studies, however, no opportunity will exist for further data collection, and one is left with the problem of interpreting the results, knowing that information on an important variable is missing. The way in which a

Table 1.17 Excess relative risk of lung cancer among cervical cancer cases

	Proportion in the population	Relative risk of lung cancer	Average relative risk for lung cancer
Cervical cancer patients	Smokers 71%	10	$(10 \times 0.71) + (1 \times 0.29) = 7.4$
	Nonsmokers 29%	1	
Women in the general population	Smokers 34%	10	$(10 \times 0.34) + (1 \times 0.66) = 4.1$
	Nonsmokers 66%	1	

quantitative assessment can be made of the effect such factors may have had can be illustrated by an example from the study of second cancers among patients diagnosed with an initial cancer of the cervix (see §1.5b) (Day et al., 1983). The study cohort contained 84 000 women diagnosed with in-situ lesions, among whom distant metastases would be infrequent. Among these women, lung cancer rates were increased more than two fold (SMR = 2.1). The question arises as to whether this excess could be due to smoking, known to be more frequent among cervical cancer patients from other studies. No information was available on the smoking history of the study cohort, since cancer registry records were the only source of information. One can, however, calculate approximately the excess risk likely to be due to smoking using data from other sources. In a study by Buckley et al. (1981), 71% of cervical cancer patients had never smoked compared to 34% of controls. Assuming that the relative risk of lung cancer among smokers compared to nonsmokers is tenfold, one can evaluate the excess relative risk of lung cancer among cervical cancer cases as outlined in Chapter 2 of Volume 1 and shown in Table 1.17. The predicted value of (7.4/4.1) = 1.8 is close to the observed value of 2.1 – certainly within the bounds of statistical error – and one would feel confident that smoking was a satisfactory explanation of the observed lung cancer excess. By contrast, among the 96 000 patients with invasive cervical cancer, in the first ten years of follow-up the excess risk of lung cancer was about fourfold (SMR = 3.9). This excess is clearly considerably too large to be explicable in terms of smoking.

Thus, use of concomitant information, even on populations distinct from the cohort under study, can remove much of the uncertainty due to unrecorded confounding factors.

(v) *Multiple comparisons*

In most cohort studies, an assessment will be made of a large number of disease categories as endpoints: there may be more than 30 sites of cancer for which observed and expected values are compared. Some of these comparisons can be anticipated to achieve nominal significance levels just by chance. The situation is often compounded by the inclusion in the study of more than one factor of interest, and in the analysis by using a variety of ways of examining each factor. Search for interaction effects, or looking at subgroups defined by several variables simultaneously, will increase further the possible comparisons.

The topic of multiple comparisons was considered in Volume 1, in the context of case-control studies, where there may be many exposure variables. In cohort studies, the multiplicity of the comparison refers more often to disease categories. Most cohort studies, however, are not launched in an intellectual vacuum. Animal experiments may suggest the site of action of the exposure; the route of administration may indicate which sites are most exposed; preliminary data, from official statistics or proportional mortality studies, may have drawn attention to a particular risk. There will therefore be one, or a few, sites at which any effect might be hypothesized to occur. Results for these sites should be interpreted differently from results for other cancers, which should probably be regarded as hypothesis generating, and the significance values modified accordingly, for example by multiplying by the number of such sites. For the former sites, a stricter interpretation in terms of hypothesis testing would be appropriate. Feinleib and Detels (1985) refer to the reporting of results, nominally significant but outside the original aim of the study, as 'post-hoc bias'.

(vi) *Identification of forerunners of disease, rather than causes*

We have stressed one powerful feature of cohort studies, that measures of physiological status can be made before the appearance of disease clouds the picture. Care must be taken, however, to ensure that the levels of a particular metabolic parameter have not been influenced by a preclinical disease state. An association that appears to be causal may be a reflection of an early state of disease. A number of reports in the late 1970s and early 1980s indicated that serum cholesterol levels were low in individuals who subsequently developed cancer. One interpretation was that low cholesterol levels predispose to cancer. An alternative was that in the year or two immediately preceding clinical onset, low cholesterol levels may be the result of early disease (Rose & Shipley, 1980). Opinion now favours the second of these explanations, since low levels are seen only immediately before clinical onset, and not five or more years before. A review is given by McMichael *et al.* (1984). A similar fate seems to have overtaken earlier reports of low retinol levels observed before cancer onset (see Wald *et al.*, 1980; Kark *et al.*, 1981). The lesson to be drawn is that the association must be examined in relation to the time between measurement of the parameter and disease onset. If the association weakens steadily as the time interval increases, serious doubt would be cast on its interpretation as causal. If the association remains strong as the interval increases, however, one would favour a causal explanation. This behaviour is seen, for example, in the association of hepatitis B and liver cancer (Beasley *et al.*, 1981) and the association of the Epstein–Barr virus and Burkitt's lymphoma (de-Thé *et al.*, 1978).

(vii) *Conclusions to be drawn from negative results*

Much emphasis is put on criteria for interpreting positive results, the extent to which they can be taken as indicating causality, and on the degree to which they provide quantitative measures of excess risk. For studies in which no excess risk is demonstrated, a complementary approach should be taken. The data should be examined for their adequacy in ruling out a positive effect and for the level of excess risk with which they are compatible, and also for whether alternative explanations are possible, i.e., whether bias or confounding may have produced an apparently negative result when a real effect existed. The evaluation of apparently negative evidence has been the topic of a recent publication (Wald & Doll, 1985). The following points are among those that should receive attention.

- What are the confidence limits for the excess risk? In Table 2.10, values are given for confidence intervals for the SMR. Clearly, even a moderately sized study, with, say, 50 events of interest, with an estimated SMR of exactly 1.0, cannot exclude increases in risk of the order of 30%.
- How do the dose levels observed in the present study compare with the levels to which other segments of the population are exposed?
- Had sufficient time elapsed between the start of exposure and the end of follow-up for a potential risk to have expressed itself fully? In this respect, it is useful to examine the excess risk seen ten years or more after first exposure, for which the confidence intervals will usually be considerably wider than for the cohort overall.
- Is there any reason to suspect that the cohort is at substantially lower risk than the general population? In a study of nuns in the United Kingdom, for example (Kinlen, 1982), one would expect particularly low rates for cancer of the oesophagus since they use neither alcohol nor tobacco. The observed excess (11 observed against 5.57 expected), which numerically would be of marginal interest in most circumstances, is therefore of particular note.
- What is the consistency with other studies?

1.6 Proportional mortality studies

An extreme example of loss to follow-up occurs when one has no accurate data on the composition of the cohort, but one has a set of death records. The proportion of deaths due to each cause arising from a particular cohort is known, but not the absolute mortality rates. One is then led to a study of proportional mortality rates, comparison being made either with the proportions seen in the general population or among subgroups in the study group. A similar situation arises in cancer registries, where one may have, for example, information on occupation, but obtained in a way not comparable to available census data. One then has a proportional incidence study.

Proportional studies have been used considerably in descriptive cancer epidemiology where, in the absence of corresponding census data, they may draw attention to unusual or contrasting patterns of cancer occurrence (Parkin, 1986). In analytical epidemiology, proportional mortality studies may be of considerable value in the initial stages of an investigation. They may indicate a fruitful orientation for later, more rigorous studies, and certainly provide a cheap and rapid way of taking an initial look at a set of data. Results of studies of proportional mortality rates suffer from a particular difficulty in interpretation, in that a proportionate excess can reflect either an excess in the absolute rate for that disease, or a deficit in the absolute rates for some of the other causes. It is unlikely, however, that large proportionate excess rates would be produced in this way. The approach is formally equivalent to a case-control study based on deaths, in which the cases have died from one cause of death and the controls are selected from deaths from all other causes. Seriously biased results can be obtained, as for example an apparent strongly protective effect for cigarette smoking against dying from mesothelioma (Blot *et al.*, 1980); but, provided one is aware of the dangers, useful results can be obtained.

One must be particularly careful in conducting proportional mortality studies to include all deaths, or at least the great majority. Differential exclusion of a particular cause of death not only decreases the proportional rate for that disease, but increases the proportional rate for all others. Initial reports of an excess risk based on high proportional rates from incomplete information may well be modified when more complete data are available, as happened with claims of an excess of leukaemia in Portsmouth (USA) shipyard workers (see Example 3.7). The problem is compounded by the fact that in a full cohort study the extent to which follow-up is incomplete can be explicitly stated (as in Table 1.9), whereas, in a proportional study, almost by definition, the degree of incompleteness is unknown. If it were known, it would imply that sufficient information on the cohort and the follow-up would be available for a full cohort analysis to be performed (i.e., calculation of rates rather than proportions).

2. RATES AND RATE STANDARDIZATION

CHAPTER 2

RATES AND RATE STANDARDIZATION

Analysis of data from a cohort study involves estimation of the rates of cancer and other diseases of interest which occur among cohort members during the study period. Cancer occurrence is most appropriately measured in terms of incidence rates, for example, as the number of newly diagnosed cases per 100 000 person-years of observation time. For a variety of practical reasons, however, most of the important cohort studies discussed in the preceding chapter used death from disease rather than its diagnosis as their principal endpoint. From the point of view of formal statistical analysis, it makes little difference what endpoint is selected, and we refer almost exclusively to 'deaths', 'mortality' and 'survival', leaving it to the reader to make the necessary substitution of terminology (e.g., 'cases', 'morbidity' and 'disease-free survival') as required for incidence data. However, since death is often preceded by a period of ill health, and the health status of the subject may influence his exposure to the agents under investigation, mortality data are subject to particular problems of interpretation, as discussed in §1.5c. Lagging of exposure variables is one means of partially accounting for modification of exposures during the interval between first appearance of disease symptoms and death.

Cancer rates vary widely according to sex, age, calendar time and a number of other demographic variables. We begin the chapter with a description of procedures used to estimate age- and time-specific disease rates from cohort data. The rates may also be specific for sex and race. Methods of estimation of incidence rates using cancer registry material were also discussed in Chapter 2 of Volume 1, which the reader may wish to consult for further elaboration of the concepts of rate and risk and a discussion of alternative methods available for their determination.

Analysis of cohort data typically involves a comparison of the rates observed in the study group with rates for the general population. This is a useful way of identifying diseases which occur at especially high or low frequency in the cohort, so that they may be studied further in relation to particular exposures. Since the age distribution of the cohort will generally be different from that of the population as a whole, and may also be evolving with time, such comparisons are best made on an age-time-specific basis. Thus, the second topic considered in this chapter is the combination of age-time-specific cohort rates so as to facilitate their comparison with standard or general population rates. Direct and indirect standardizations are presented as the two basic methods of summarizing a set of component rates. The corresponding comparative measures, known as the comparative mortality figure (CMF) and the standardized mortality ratio (SMR), are introduced and discussed in terms of the advantages and disadvantages they offer. We develop methods for evaluating the statistical significance of the observed differences in age-time-specific rates between study and standard populations, and for putting confidence intervals around the comparative measures.

A final section briefly describes some analogous procedures for age adjustment of proportional incidence and mortality measures that are used to evaluate disease frequencies when person-years denominators are not available.

2.1 Calculation of age- and calendar period-specific rates

The basic feature of cohort studies that distinguishes them from cross-sectional, case-control or other types of investigation is that, at least in principle, each subject is kept under continuous surveillance for a defined interval of time. If the study endpoint is death, we assume that each subject is 'at risk' of death during the entire interval from his entry into the study until his exit. This means that the study period should contain no interval during which the subject is known to be alive as a condition of cohort membership. If the cohort is defined to consist of all workers with at least five years of employment in a certain factory, therefore, the first five years of their employment history would be excluded from the observation period. A second critical assumption is that any death that actually occurs during the study period will be recorded. For cohorts defined on the basis of past records, this implies that adequate mechanisms exist for tracing individuals from their date of entry into the study until death or until the study's closing date. If no record exists of someone's whereabouts after a certain point in time, he should generally be considered as having left the study at that point. Obvious problems of selection bias exist if such losses are at all frequent, since the causes of and ages at death for 'lost-to-follow-up' subjects may well differ from those for persons who are successfully traced.

The basic method used to estimate age-time-specific mortality rates is to determine for each individual the amount of observation time contributed to a given age × calendar period category and to sum up those contributions for all cohort members so as to obtain the total number of person-years of observation in that category. These person-years form the denominators of rates the numerators of which are simply the numbers of deaths due to a given disease, likewise classified by age and calendar year of death. The process is illustrated in Figure 2.1, which shows schematically the course of one worker who was entered on study (point A) at age 43.71 in year 1956.03 and left 11.12 years later (F). He contributed observation time to five separate cells, boundary crossings being made at points B through E. The duration of time spent in each cell is easily determined, as shown in Table 2.1. In some applications, particularly when the observation period is relatively short, the calendar-year axis is ignored and the rates are determined by age interval alone. Computer programs for performing the calculations have been developed by Hill (1972), Monson (1974), Waxweiler *et al.* (1983), Gilbert and Buchanan (1984) and Coleman *et al.* (1986), among others.

Sometimes the exact dates of birth and of entry and exit from study, which are needed to draw Figure 2.1, will not be available. Then, approximate numbers of person-years may be calculated as shown in the right-hand column of Table 2.1, using

Fig. 2.1   Schema showing the follow-up of one person in a cohort study

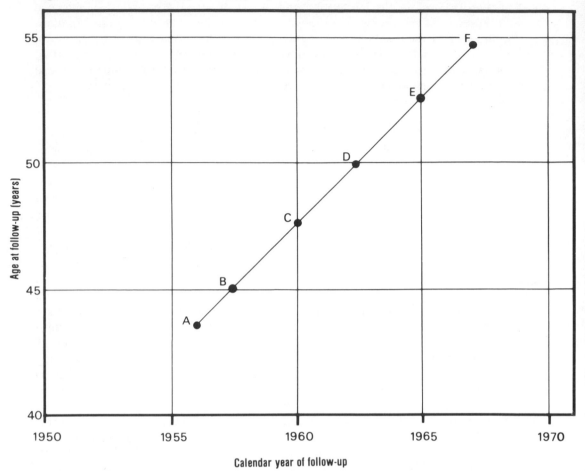

Table 2.1   Calculation of exact and approximate age- and year-specific person-years at risk

Point[a]	Coordinates (year, age)	Quinquinquennium		Person-years	
		Year	Age	Exact	Approximate
A	(1956.03, 43.71)	1955–1959	40–44	1.29	1.50
B	(1957.32, 45.00)	1955–1959	45–49	2.68	2.00
C	(1960.00, 47.68)	1960–1964	45–49	2.32	3.00
D	(1962.32, 50.00)	1960–1964	50–54	2.68	2.00
E	(1965.00, 52.68)	1965–1969	50–54	2.15	2.50
F	(1967.15, 54.83)				
Total				11.12	11.00

[a] See Figure 2.1

the three integer variables, age at entry, year of entry and year of exit. The approximation is based on the notion that a person aged 43 in 1956 will be 44 in 1957, 45 in 1958 and 54 in 1967. He contributes 0.5 years of observation time to the calendar year of entry (1956), 0.5 years to the year of exit (1967), and a full 1.0 year to each intervening year. There would be a single 0.25-year contribution for someone who enters and leaves the study in the same calendar year. The discrepancies between the exact and approximate figures tend to be averaged out when cumulated over individuals, so that the approximate method is sufficiently accurate for most practical purposes.

Cause-specific national death rates are typically published by five-year intervals of age and calendar year (Case & Pearson, 1957; Grove & Hetzel, 1968). Such 'quinquinquennia' are widely used in cancer epidemiology, and our example of the calculation of age- and calendar period-specific rates illustrates this standard breakdown. Analogous methods may be used if the age/time intervals are longer or shorter than five years.

Example 2.1

Appendix IE describes in some detail the design and execution of the Lee and Fraumeni (1969) study of Montana copper smelter workers, in which 8047 male subjects were entered into study on 1 January 1938 if they had worked for at least one year and were still employed on that date, or at the end of their first year of employment for those hired later. Table 2.2 shows the number of person-years in each quinquinquennium as determined by both exact and approximate methods for 8014 workers on whom full data were available. (Records had been lost for 33 of the original cohort.) These data include the follow-up through 1977 for workers who were still alive and under observation on 31 December 1963, the closing date of the original study (Lubin *et al.*, 1981).

The approximate method of calculation, based on integral ages and years, was modified to account for the fact that the 2517 men who entered the study at the beginning of 1938 were eligible for a full year's observation, whereas those who entered the study later were, on average, observed for only half of the first year. Likewise, nine months of observation during 1977 was counted for those still alive and being followed at the study's end (30 September 1977). Except for a few discrepancies along the boundaries of the table, this adjustment assures that the agreement between exact and approximate calculations is quite good.

Table 2.3 presents the numbers and rates of deaths from all causes classified by age and calendar period. The rates are based on sufficiently large numbers for most cells that they display a reasonable degree of numerical stability. For many specific causes of death, however, the numbers are smaller and a display of the age-period-specific rates in such a detailed manner is not helpful.

2.2 Summarizing a set of rates

Large tables of rates confront the investigator with a bewildering array of detail that is difficult to assimilate and utilize effectively. Even if attention is focused on a particular calendar period or column in Table 2.3, consideration of the rates in five-year age categories requires one to look at up to 18 separate numbers. There is a clear need for one or two summary measures that are easy to interpret yet retain most of the essential information in the age-specific data.

This section describes the calculation and interpretation of a commonly used summary measure, the directly standardized rate. We mention at the outset, however, that important information may be lost through use of this and other traditional approaches to data analysis. The remainder of the monograph emphasizes alternative

Table 2.2 Exact and approximate[a] person-years of observation in the Montana cohort, by age and calendar year

Age range (years)	Calendar period									Totals
	1938– 1939	1940– 1944	1945– 1949	1950– 1954	1955– 1959	1960– 1964	1965– 1969	1970– 1974	1975– 1977	
10–14	0.0	1.2	0.0	0.0	0.0	0.0	0.0	0.0	0.0	1.2
	0.0	1.5	0.0	0.0	0.0	0.0	0.0	0.0	0.0	1.5
15–19	42.6	208.1	387.7	173.8	59.8	0.0	0.0	0.0	0.0	871.9
	68.0	164.0	351.0	123.8	38.0	0.0	0.0	0.0	0.0	744.8
20–24	645.4	2157.6	2001.0	2361.4	1380.5	142.7	0.0	0.0	0.0	8 688.6
	679.0	2301.8	2012.0	2352.0	1349.5	118.5	0.0	0.0	0.0	8 812.8
25–29	690.3	2587.0	3143.6	3359.7	3038.4	1377.1	135.9	0.0	0.0	14 332.0
	682.5	2647.5	3290.8	3361.3	3039.5	1362.5	112.5	0.0	0.0	14 496.5
30–34	689.4	2378.9	3451.4	3941.6	3845.6	2950.1	1342.0	130.8	0.0	18 729.9
	693.0	2354.3	3508.0	4091.0	3844.8	2951.0	1327.5	108.0	0.0	18 877.5
35–39	607.9	2196.9	3091.0	3906.2	4313.5	3718.1	2883.8	1321.5	129.8	22 168.6
	598.5	2186.5	3076.8	3950.5	4456.5	3721.0	2885.0	1309.0	108.0	22 291.8
40–44	482.1	1829.2	2813.8	3603.3	4264.7	4164.2	3632.2	2815.4	941.9	24 546.9
	471.0	1784.5	2826.5	3573.0	4321.3	4296.5	3631.5	2815.5	945.5	24 665.3
45–49	451.4	1431.8	2298.9	3222.4	3851.7	4044.2	3967.8	3501.7	1812.1	24 581.9
	450.0	1426.5	2258.8	3227.8	3810.0	4108.0	4083.0	3505.5	1812.0	24 681.5
50–54	470.0	1230.1	1758.3	2598.0	3432.1	3613.6	3753.0	3728.5	2010.1	22 593.8
	465.0	1226.0	1747.0	2544.3	3437.0	3575.0	3810.0	3840.5	2018.0	22 663.3
55–59	424.5	1209.1	1389.6	1750.3	2560.2	3067.1	3263.4	3433.4	2101.5	19 199.0
	408.5	1206.0	1377.5	1737.5	2505.0	3062.5	3219.5	3486.0	2168.0	19 170.5
60–64	308.4	889.9	1221.2	1283.1	1574.6	2148.7	2535.5	2805.5	1790.9	14 557.9
	315.0	855.8	1217.0	1276.0	1561.0	2097.0	2527.0	2764.5	1799.0	14 412.3
65–69	248.4	667.2	762.9	1031.5	1054.8	1283.1	1699.4	2065.9	1338.7	10 152.1
	231.0	659.0	735.0	1014.0	1042.0	1270.5	1653.0	2056.5	1313.0	9 974.0
70–74	147.2	425.6	496.5	559.1	766.3	796.7	961.2	1325.3	951.2	6 429.1
	137.5	399.0	478.0	529.0	744.5	789.5	952.0	1285.5	941.5	6 256.5
75–79	49.2	215.3	259.5	287.7	324.6	493.6	526.8	647.3	499.9	3 303.8
	45.5	194.0	246.0	274.0	306.5	468.0	515.5	636.0	476.5	3 162.0
80–84	14.6	69.0	125.3	107.3	147.7	148.6	260.6	265.4	191.7	1 330.1
	11.0	63.5	111.0	97.5	140.0	132.5	245.5	253.5	187.0	1 241.5
85+	1.4	13.5	35.5	48.0	30.2	52.7	62.9	135.1	90.3	469.6
	1.0	10.0	31.5	41.0	26.5	47.5	53.5	127.0	81.5	419.5
Totals	5 272.7	17 510.5	23 236.3	28 233.4	30 644.7	28 000.3	25 024.5	22 175.7	11 858.2	191 956.3
	5 256.5	17 479.8	23 266.8	28 192.5	30 622.0	28 000.0	25 016.0	22 187.5	11 850.0	191 871.0

[a] Exact entries listed above approximate ones for each cell

methods of analysis that we believe are preferable for analytical epidemiology, namely the fitting of statistical models to the age- and period-specific rates in such a way that their essential structure is highlighted and purely 'random' fluctuations are identified as such.

(a) The directly standardized rate

Direct standardization appears to have been motivated originally by the idea of determining the crude disease rate that would be observed in the cohort if its age distribution were the same as that of the standard population. The directly standard-

Table 2.3 Number of deaths and death rates (per 1000 person-years)[a] from all causes in the Montana cohort, by age and calendar year

Age range (years)	Calendar period									Totals
	1938–1939	1940–1944	1945–1949	1950–1954	1955–1959	1960–1964	1965–1969	1970–1974	1975–1977	
15–19	0	2	0	0	0	0	0	0	0	2
	0.0	9.6	0.0	0.0	0.0	0.0	0.0	0.0	0.0	2.3
20–24	1	6	2	3	4	1	0	0	0	17
	1.5	2.8	1.0	1.3	2.9	7.0	0.0	0.0	0.0	2.0
25–29	2	11	2	4	7	2	1	0	0	29
	2.9	4.3	0.6	1.2	2.3	1.5	7.4	0.0	0.0	2.0
30–34	2	8	6	16	12	10	5	0	0	59
	2.9	3.4	1.7	4.1	3.1	3.4	3.7	0.0	0.0	3.2
35–39	0	10	14	23	16	14	7	2	0	86
	0.0	4.6	4.5	5.9	3.7	3.8	2.4	1.5	0.0	3.9
40–44	1	12	15	27	25	40	11	21	4	156
	2.1	6.6	5.3	7.5	5.9	9.6	3.0	7.5	4.2	6.4
45–49	1	13	21	26	40	40	43	28	15	227
	2.2	9.1	9.1	8.1	10.4	9.9	10.8	8.0	8.3	9.2
50–54	5	25	25	42	61	58	55	52	28	351
	10.6	20.3	14.2	16.2	17.8	16.1	14.7	13.9	13.9	15.5
55–59	1	28	26	48	78	86	82	76	37	462
	2.4	23.2	18.7	27.4	30.5	28.0	25.1	22.1	17.6	24.1
60–64	2	35	35	39	54	83	87	103	50	488
	6.5	39.3	28.7	30.4	34.3	38.6	34.3	36.7	27.0	33.5
65–69	11	29	35	51	56	68	71	83	53	457
	44.3	43.5	45.9	49.4	53.1	53.0	41.8	40.2	39.6	45.0
70–74	5	32	42	43	61	57	56	75	61	432
	34.0	75.2	84.6	76.9	79.6	71.5	58.3	56.6	64.1	67.2
75–79	3	16	30	34	37	55	57	63	46	341
	61.0	74.3	115.6	118.2	114.0	111.4	108.2	97.3	92.0	103.2
80–84	0	7	18	24	26	25	29	39	29	197
	0.0	101.4	143.6	223.7	176.1	168.3	111.3	147.0	151.3	148.1
85+	0	2	11	6	12	11	15	27	16	100
	0.0	147.7	309.5	125.0	397.7	208.7	238.7	199.8	177.2	213.0
Totals	34	236	282	386	489	550	519	569	339	3404
	6.4	13.5	12.1	13.7	16.0	19.6	20.7	25.7	28.6	17.7

Standardized rates (1950 US population aged 40–79 years):

12.8	26.5	26.0	27.9	29.5	29.4	25.0	24.4	22.4

[a] Numbers of deaths are listed above the corresponding rate

ized rate is obtained by applying the age-specific cohort rates to the standard age distribution. More formally, denote by d_j the number of deaths in the jth of J age groups, by n_j the person-years denominator, and by $\hat{\lambda}_j = d_j/n_j$ the corresponding rate. In statistical parlance $\hat{\lambda}_j$ is known as an estimate (hence the $\hat{\ }$) of the 'true' but unknown rate λ_j that would be observed if an infinite amount of data were available. If, in addition, w_j denotes the number (or proportion) of individuals in the standard population in the jth age group, the directly standardized rate is written

$$\hat{\Lambda} = \sum_{j=1}^{J} w_j \hat{\lambda}_j \qquad (2.1)$$

as a weighted sum (or average) of the age-specific rates. Λ denotes the corresponding 'true' quantity.

Table 2.4 shows several idealized populations used for direct standardization of cancer incidence rates (Waterhouse *et al.*, 1976). Since the weights sum to 100 000, the corresponding directly standardized rates calculated from (2.1) will have units of cases per 100 000 person-years. The African population is considerably younger than the European. The world population, which occupies an intermediate position, has long been used by Segi (1960) and associates to standardize cancer mortality data collected by the World Health Organization.

Table 2.5 shows the actual age distributions for 1 000 000 persons in the USA for the years 1950 and 1970. Note the effect of the post-war 'baby boom' on the two age structures. These figures are often used to standardize the mortality rates of US cohorts.

In order to promote comparability between series, we recommend that a published set of weights such as those shown in Table 2.4 or 2.5 be used for direct standardization, rather than an ad-hoc set constructed by the investigator. When world

Table 2.4   Standard populations used for the computation of age-standardized and truncated standardized incidence rates[a]

Age range (years)	African	World	European	Truncated
0–	2 000	2 400	1 600	—
1–4	8 000	9 600	6 400	—
5–9	10 000	10 000	7 000	—
10–14	10 000	9 000	7 000	—
15–19	10 000	9 000	7 000	—
20–24	10 000	8 000	7 000	—
25–29	10 000	8 000	7 000	—
30–34	10 000	6 000	7 000	—
35–39	10 000	6 000	7 000	6 000
40–44	5 000	6 000	7 000	6 000
45–49	5 000	6 000	7 000	6 000
50–54	3 000	5 000	7 000	5 000
55–59	2 000	4 000	6 000	4 000
60–64	2 000	4 000	5 000	4 000
65–69	1 000	3 000	4 000	—
70–74	1 000	2 000	3 000	—
75–79	500	1 000	2 000	—
80–84	300	500	1 000	—
85 and over	200	500	1 000	—
Total	100 000	100 000	100 000	31 000

[a] From Waterhouse *et al.* (1976)

Table 2.5 Standard million population[a] of the USA in 1950 and 1970

Age range (years)	Standard million population	
	1950	1970
0–4	107 258	84 416
5–9	85 591	98 204
10–14	73 785	102 304
15–19	70 450	93 845
20–24	76 191	80 561
25–29	81 237	66 320
30–34	76 425	56 249
35–39	74 629	54 656
40–44	67 712	58 958
45–49	60 190	59 622
50–54	54 893	54 643
55–59	48 011	49 077
60–64	40 210	42 403
65–69	33 199	34 406
70–74	22 641	26 789
75–79	14 725	18 871
80–84	7 025	11 241
85+	3 828	7 435
Total	1 000 000	1 000 000

[a] From US Bureau of Censuses (1972)

weights are used, one speaks of a rate that is 'standardized to the world population'. Alternatively, if the weights correspond to an actual age distribution, one would speak of a rate 'standardized to the population of the USA in 1950', for example, or of one standardized to 'the population of England and Wales in 1970'.

Example 2.2

The crude death rates shown in the penultimate row of Table 2.3 steadily increase as a consequence of the general ageing of the cohort over time. In order to summarize the age-specific rates for different calendar periods, we calculated directly standardized rates for each one, using the 1950 US population (Table 2.5) as the standard. However, only rates for ages 40–79 were included in the calculation since the other age groups lacked data for one or more calendar periods. This necessity of discarding relevant data is one of the disadvantages of direct standardization. The standardized rates first rise and decline, as is true for most of their age-specific components. The initial rise is probably due to the 'healthy worker' selection bias (see §1.5c) which would apply to a large number of workers in the first calendar period, since everyone followed from the beginning of 1938 was still employed at that time. The eventual fall in the age-specific or age-standardized rates conforms to the pattern observed in the general population.

Provided that the same standard age distribution is used in their construction, comparison of directly standardized rates between different groups is thought to eliminate the differences that are observed in the crude rates solely by virtue of one group having a different age structure from another. However, as the graphs of cross-sectional age-incidence curves in Figure 2.2 make clear, such comparisons may

Fig. 2.2 Relationship between incidence of cancer of the stomach and age in four areas: ▲, Iceland; ×, Miyagi, Japan; ○, Connecticut, USA; ●, Johannesburg & Kampala (African). From Doll and Cook (1967)

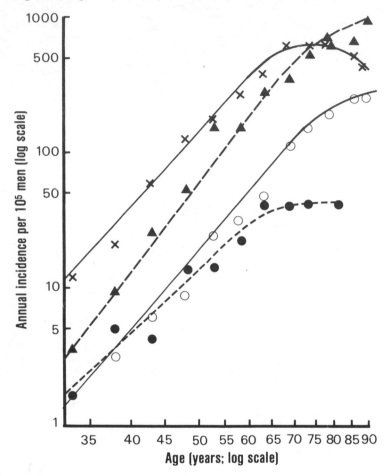

obscure important differences in the age-specific patterns. The apparent decline in stomach cancer incidence in older Japanese, in contrast to the rising age-incidence curve in Iceland, even among the elderly, means that the relative positions of the two countries as expressed in the age-standardized rate will depend to a large extent on the choice of the standard. If the standard population is heavily weighted towards the elderly, Iceland will have a relatively higher age standardized rate, while the reverse will be true if the standard population is younger. Doll and Cook (1967), from whose work the figure is taken, give several more examples of how the choice of the standard population affects the rank ordering of countries in terms of age-standardized incidence rates of specific cancers.

When incidence rates for cancers of epithelial tissues are plotted against age on a log–log scale, they are often remarkably close to straight lines, with slopes of 4 or 5. Doll (1971) and others have interpreted this basic feature of incidence data as support for the concept that such cancers are produced by a series of cellular events. If there is curvature in the log–log plot, as in Figure 2.2, it is generally in the downward direction (Cook *et al.*, 1969). Sometimes this is due to a 'birth cohort effect', i.e., a general increase in rates for successive generations due presumably to the introduction of new agents into the personal or ambient environment. In this case, the curves flatten out or otherwise assume similar shapes when arranged to present age-specific data for successive generations of individuals born in the same time interval (birth cohorts) rather than for separate calendar periods. In other situations, possibly including the data shown in Figure 2.2, the curvature may represent the failure to diagnose completely incident cases among the elderly. Largely for this reason, Doll and Cook (1967) suggested that the calculation of summary rates for epithelial tumours be restricted to people aged 35–64, and introduced for this purpose the truncated population shown in the fourth column of Table 2.4. They argued that the directly standardized rate based on this population was a good measure of the average level of incidence or mortality, that the ratio of rates for the 60–64 *versus* the 35–39-year age groups measured the steepness of the increase with age, and that the two measures taken together provided a basic summary of the age-specific data.

(b) The cumulative rate

Cumulative rates are defined by equation (2.1) if one takes for w_j the length of the jth age interval rather than the standard age proportion (see §2.3 of Volume 1). Essentially the same measure was introduced by Yule (1934), except that he calculated an average of the age-specific rates rather than their sum, and termed the result the 'equivalent average death rate'. Since the nonzero weights of the truncated population are almost constant across the five-year age groups, a rate that is standardized in this fashion will be very nearly proportional to the cumulative rate between 35 and 64 years.

The cumulative rate has several advantages as a method of reporting cancer incidence and mortality data (Day, 1976). First it dispenses with the rather arbitrary selection of the standard population, yet has the desired feature of summarizing the age-spectific data. Second, cumulative rates for different age ranges are additive. Thus, for example, the cumulative rate between 0 and 64 years is the sum of the cumulative rates for 0–34 and 35–64 years. Finally, the cumulative rate is easily converted into the cumulative risk by means of the formula $P = 1 - \exp(-\Lambda)$. This is the actuarial probability of disease development or death from the cause of interest, in the absence of other causes of death, for someone who is at risk throughout the designated age range. Since $1 - \exp(-\Lambda)$ is approximately equal to Λ for small Λ, moreover, the cumulative rate can be roughly interpreted as the cumulative risk (actuarial probability), provided that it is small, say less than 10%. See Table 2.6.

Example 2.3

Table 2.7 compares cumulative incidence rates between 0 and 74 years to directly standardized rates based on two different standard populations (Day, 1976). It illustrates clearly that, while cancer is a 'rare' disease

Table 2.6 Conversion of cumulative rates (100 Λ) into the corresponding cumulative risks (100(1 − $e^{-\Lambda}$))

100 Λ	0.1	0.5	1.0	5.0	7.0	10.00	15.00	20.00	30.00
100(1 − $e^{-\Lambda}$)	0.1	0.499	0.995	4.88	6.76	9.52	13.93	18.13	25.92

Table 2.7 Cumulative incidence rates, 0–74 years (percent), compared with rates standardized to the world population[a], and to the truncated rate[a], per 100 000 *per annum*

Population	Rate	Cancer site							
		Stomach	Lung	Breast	Cervix uteri	Leukaemia	Prostate	All sites[b]	
		Male	Male	Female	Female	Male	Male	Male	Female
Cali, Colombia	Cumulative (%)	7.34	2.14	3.08	8.35	0.38	2.71	29.11	29.78
	World population	57.5	17.5	27.3	75.6	5.2	23.2	(25.25)	(25.75)
	Truncated	87.7	29.0	62.6	183.6	5.6	2.15		
Alameda County, black	Cumulative (%)	2.69	5.85	4.15	3.18	1.05	7.54	30.80	20.81
	World population	24.4	43.8	38.6	30.5	8.3	65.3	(26.51)	(18.78)
	Truncated	33.0	88.9	75.0	75.4	8.9	55.6		
Birmingham, UK	Cumulative (%)	3.13	9.73	5.58	1.39	0.52	1.85	30.11	21.96
	World population	25.2	73.3	51.1	13.6	5.3	18.4	(26.00)	(19.50)
	Truncated	35.9	133.5	114.1	34.2	6.2	10.9		
Japan, Miyagi Prefecture	Cumulative (%)	11.97	2.16	1.06	2.28	0.36	0.35	24.22	16.30
	World population	95.3	15.6	11.0	20.6	4.4	3.2	(21.51)	(15.04)
	Truncated	164.1	22.6	27.5	52.8	4.7	2.0		

[a] From Doll *et al.* (1970)

[b] The figures given in parentheses are the exact cumulative probabilities $\hat{P} = 1 − \exp(−\hat{\Lambda})$ to compare with the cumulative incidence $\hat{\Lambda}$. See text and Table 2.6

when considered in terms of annual incidence, the total actuarial risk over a normal lifetime may be substantial. Japanese males, for example, have a cumulative actuarial risk for stomach cancer of 12%. Since the cumulative lifetime risk of many of the common cancers seen in laboratory animals is of the same order of magnitude (e.g., 5–40%), it is clear that expressing cancer incidence in such terms offers the possibility of more immediate extrapolation between epidemiology and laboratory investigations than does use of annual incidence rates (Peto, R. 1977).

(c) Standard error of the cumulative or directly standardized rate

When death rates are computed from national vital statistics, or incidence rates are determined from cancer registries that cover large populations, questions of statistical or sampling stability are generally of minor importance. Errors inherent in the process of data collection, in the coding of cause of death or cancer type, or in the estimation of the population denominators are usually of much greater magnitude and concern. Rates calculated for study cohorts of limited size, however, may be based on a relatively small number of cases. Then, a simple formula for the standard error is useful as a measure of the statistical precision with which the rate is determined.

The formula given here stems from the elementary statistical model for the sampling distribution of a rate that is developed in some detail in §4.2. For the moment it suffices to know that the sampling variability of the rate numerator is approximately $\text{Var}(d_j) = n_j\lambda_j$, which may be estimated by d_j itself, and that the person-years denominators n_j may be regarded as fixed constants. Thus, the standard error of the age-specific rate $\hat{\lambda}_j$, i.e., the square root of the estimated variance, is $\sqrt{d_j}/n_j$.

In order to determine the variance or standard error of the summary rate $\hat{\Lambda} = \sum w_j\hat{\lambda}_j$, we need to know the covariances between the observed numbers of deaths in the different age intervals. The covariances are zero if the observations are statistically independent. This is true when the rates are estimated from cross-sectional data, for then different individuals are at risk in different age intervals. In cohort studies, however, the same person may contribute observation time to several contiguous age groups. Then, the d_j are not statistically independent, since the death of an individual in one interval precludes his dying in the next. Nevertheless, the discussion in §4.2 suggests that even in this case the d_j may be regarded as being independent for purposes of making large-sample statistical inferences. Chiang (1961) argues that the d_j are uncorrelated (see also Keyfitz, 1966). It follows that the standard error is

$$\text{SE}(\hat{\Lambda}) = \left(\sum_{j=1}^{J} w_j^2 \, \text{Var}(\hat{\lambda}_j)\right)^{1/2} = \left(\sum_{j=1}^{J} w_j^2 d_j/n_j^2\right)^{1/2}. \tag{2.2}$$

Inspection of equation (2.2) emphasizes another potential weakness of direct standardization, namely that the a-priori weights w_j take no account of the precision with which the component rates are estimated. The data for a single age interval may make a major contribution to the sampling error if the corresponding rate is based on a small denominator yet is given a large weight.

Example 2.4

We illustrate the calculation of cumulative rates and their standard errors by applying equations (2.1) and (2.2) to data from the Montana cohort. Table 2.8 shows the number of respiratory cancer deaths that occurred among the smelter workers at ages 40–79 in four calendar periods. The population denominators differ slightly from the corresponding entries in Table 2.2, since they were calculated according to another approximate method that is described in §3.1. Note that the 40–79-year age range accounts for $276/288 = 96.5\%$ of the total deaths from this cancer. Since the age intervals are of equal length of ten years each, the formula for the standard error may be simplified to

$$\text{SE}(\hat{\Lambda}) = 10\sqrt{\sum_{j=1}^{J} d_j/n_j^2}.$$

Cumulative respiratory cancer mortality rates between ages 40–79 are 8.40, 14.07, 13.81 and 14.41% for the four calendar periods. These may be compared with cumulative rates of 2.19, 4.21, 6.58 and 8.92% for the US white male population for the periods 1940–1949, 1950–1959, 1960–1969 and 1970–1975 (Appendix III). Thus the Montana cohort has substantially higher rates in the early decades, but the effect is attenuated somewhat by the passage of time. Part of the explanation for the decline in both relative and excess risk is that the later calendar years contain more person-years of observation from workers first employed after 1925, when the smelting process was changed and airborne exposures were presumably reduced (Lee-Feldstein, 1983).

US mortality rates for respiratory cancer are higher than those of the three western states near the smelter, namely Montana, Idaho and Wyoming. Use of standard rates from these states alone therefore increases the discrepancy between the respiratory cancer rates for the cohort and those for the surrounding general

Table 2.8 Respiratory cancer deaths (d), person-years at risk (n, in thousands), and death rates ($\hat{\lambda}$, per 1000 person-years) in the Montana cohort. Calculation of the cumulative rate and its standard error

Age range (years)		Calendar period				Totals
		1938–1949	1950–1959	1960–1969	1970–1977	
40–49	d	5	5	7	4	21
	n	9.217	14.949	16.123	9.073	49.363
	$\hat{\lambda}$	0.542	0.334	0.434	0.441	0.425
50–59	d	11	24	28	17	80
	n	6.421	10.223	13.663	11.504	41.811
	$\hat{\lambda}$	1.713	2.348	2.049	1.478	1.913
60–69	d	14	24	44	35	117
	n	4.006	4.896	7.555	7.937	24.394
	$\hat{\lambda}$	3.495	4.902	5.824	4.410	4.796
70–79	d	4	12	15	27	58
	n	1.507	1.851	2.724	3.341	9.423
	$\hat{\lambda}$	2.654	6.483	5.506	8.081	6.155
Totals	d	34	65	94	83	276
	n	21.151	31.920	40.066	31.855	124.991
	$\hat{\lambda}$	1.608	2.036	2.346	2.606	2.208
Cumulative rate (%)		8.405	14.067	13.814	14.410	13.290
Standard error (%)		1.720	2.181	1.723	1.775	0.951

population. Regional rather than national death rates generally make a more appropriate standard, but they are often not available for the entire time period of interest or are based on such small populations as to be unstable.

Our next example confirms the basic point that age standardization techniques as discussed in this section can obscure important features of the data and should be used cautiously in analytical work.

Fig. 2.3   Thyroid cancer incidence rates, 1935–1975, for Connecticut, USA, age-adjusted to the 1950 US population: ○, females; ●, males; ×, both sexes. From Mendelsohn–Pottern *et al.* (1980)

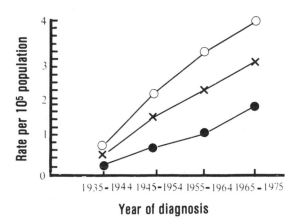

Example 2.5

Figure 2.3 shows age-adjusted incidence rates for thyroid cancer from the Connecticut Tumor Registry by sex and ten-year calendar period from 1935–1975 (Mendelsohn-Pottern *et al.*, 1980). They were calculated by direct standardization relative to the 1950 US population (Table 2.5). While they show a smoothly rising incidence over the 40-year period, they miss an important feature of the data for females. When the age-specific rates are plotted for each of the four periods (Figure 2.4), a clear bimodal age-incidence curve emerges for females after 1954, with a first peak between 25 and 44 years of age and a steady increase in rates from age 65 on. The first peak was less pronounced in males. It was discovered to be due to increases in rates for papillary and follicular carcinomas and was interpreted as probably due to increased childhood exposure to therapeutic radiation.

2.3 Comparative measures of incidence and mortality

A major goal of standardization, besides combining a set of age-/stratum-specific rates into a synoptic figure, is to provide a quantitative measure of the difference in rates between the study cohort and a standard population or other comparison group that is free from the effects of age or other confounding variables. Rather than taking the ratio or difference of the crude mortality rates for cohort *versus* standard as a measure of effect, one first divides the comparison groups into a number of strata that are reasonably homogeneous with respect to the confounding variables. The stratum-specific rates for both groups are calculated and their differences or ratios are summarized in a single comparative figure. Since ratios of age-specific cancer incidence rates are typically more nearly constant than are the rate differences (see §2.5 of Volume 1), a summary ratio is generally the more appropriate measure. However, caution must be exercised if, as in the last example, there are substantial variations between the comparison groups in the age-specific ratios. In such circumstances the investigator is better advised to choose some other measure of effect (such as a rate difference) that does remain constant, or else to model the variations in rate ratios or rate differences as a function of age and other stratification variables, rather than attempting to summarize them in a single number.

The choice of variables to be used as a basis for stratification or other statistical adjustment procedure raises several complicated issues (see §3.4 of Volume 1). One generally wants to adjust for variables that are causally related to disease, and the differential distribution of which among the comparison groups could therefore result in apparent differences in incidence or mortality that are secondary to the causal effects. This implies that some prior understanding or hypotheses about the causal nature of the disease process necessarily enters into the selection of stratification variables. Questions of the statistical significance, in the data under study, of their association with either the disease or the exposures are secondary if not irrelevant. Age is the paradigm case of a confounding variable since it is usually regarded as an independent cause, or at least as a surrogate for the accumulation of independent causes, of many cancers and other diseases.

(a) The comparative mortality figure (CMF)

A simple summary of the incidence or mortality rate ratios between the cohort and standard population that accounts for the possible confounding effects of age or other

Fig. 2.4 Age-specific thyroid cancer incidence rates, 1935–1975, for Connecticut, USA: ····, 1965–1975; ——, 1955–1964; ––––, 1945–1954; ———, 1935–1944. From Mendelsohn–Pottern *et al.* (1980)

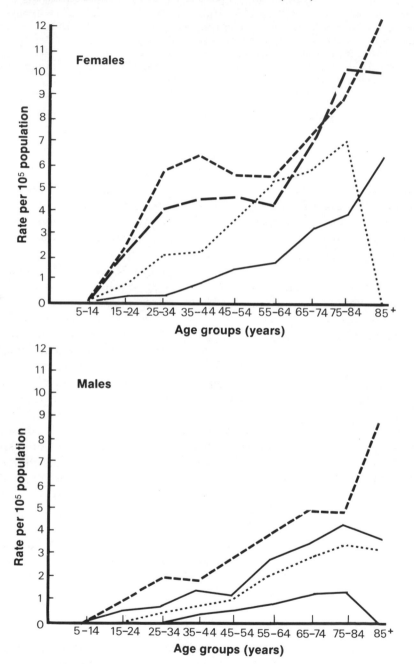

variables is obtained by dividing the directly standardized rate for the cohort by the standard population rate. Thus if λ_j^* denotes the standard death rate in stratum j, and w_j is the standard weight, the comparative mortality figure (CMF) is defined by

$$\text{CMF} = \frac{\sum_{j=1}^{J} w_j d_j / n_j}{\sum_{j=1}^{J} w_j \lambda_j^*}. \tag{2.3}$$

The ratio of CMFs calculated for two different cohorts using the same standard rates and weights is simply the ratio of the two directly standardized rates.

When we introduced the concept of direct standardization, the standard weights w_j were chosen to be equal to the person-years denominators n_j^* of the standard rates. With these weights one may write

$$\text{CMF} = \frac{\sum w_j d_j / n_j}{\sum w_j d_j^* / n_j^*} = \frac{\sum n_j^* d_j / n_j}{D^*}, \tag{2.4}$$

where d_j^* and n_j^* denote standard deaths and person-years in stratum j and $D^* = \sum d_j^*$ represents the total standard deaths. The second expression is easier for computation. An interpretation of the CMF in this case is as the ratio of the number of deaths that would be expected in the cohort if it had the same age structure as the standard population, using the stratum-specific cohort rates to calculate the expectation, divided by the number of deaths in the standard population. This version of the CMF may also be recognized as a weighted average of age-specific cohort to standard rate ratios $r_j = \hat{\lambda}_j / \lambda_j^*$,

$$\text{CMF} = \frac{\sum_{j=1}^{J} u_j r_j}{\sum_{j=1}^{J} u_j}, \tag{2.5}$$

where now the weights $u_j = n_j^* \lambda_j^* = d_j^*$ are equal to the number of deaths in each age group in the standard population.

A major disadvantage of the CMF is its instability when the component rates are based on small numbers of deaths. This is easily illustrated by means of a hypothetical example.

Example 2.6

Table 2.9, adapted from Mosteller and Tukey (1977, p. 237), presents fictitious data involving three age strata. The CMF is determined from equation (2.4) as

$$\text{CMF} = \frac{150\,000(10/10\,000) + 70\,000(9/3000) + 210(1/1)}{460} = 1.24.$$

However, if the single cohort member in the 85+ age stratum were to survive instead of die, the same calculation gives

$$\text{CMF} = \frac{150\,000(10/10\,000) + 70\,000(9/3000) + 210(0/1)}{460} = 0.78.$$

Thus, a change in only one of the 46 deaths has made a large difference in the comparative analysis.

Table 2.9 Fictitious data used to illustrate the instability
of the CMF[a]

Age stratum (years)	Cohort		Standard population	
	Deaths (d)	Person-years (n)	Deaths (d)	Person-years (n)
45–64	10	10 000	140	150 000
65–84	9	3 000	290	70 000
85+	1	1	30	210
Totals	20	13 001	460	220 210

[a] Adapted from Mosteller and Tukey (1977)

(b) Standard error of the CMF

Instead of examining its sensitivity to individual deaths, a more systematic way of measuring the statistical precision of the CMF is to calculate its standard error (SE). We assume that the standard population is very large relative to the cohort, so that sampling errors in the standard rates may be ignored. Then, the standard error of the CMF is obtained directly from the standard error of its numerator. From equations (2.2) and (2.3) we have

$$\text{SE(CMF)} = \frac{(\sum_{j=1}^{J} w_j^2 d_j / n_j^2)^{1/2}}{\sum_{j=1}^{J} w_j \lambda_j^*}. \tag{2.6}$$

Corrections to this equation are needed if the standard population is constructed as a pool of several cohorts that includes the one for which the CMF is being determined (Yule, 1934).

If the standard error is not regarded simply as a measure of statistical precision, but is to be used to construct test statistics or confidence intervals, it is preferable to make a transformation to the log scale. This helps to correct the skewness in the statistical distribution of the CMF itself and thus improves the normal approximation to the distribution of test statistics based on it. The standard error of the transformed CMF is

$$\text{SE(log CMF)} = \frac{\text{SE(CMF)}}{\text{CMF}} = \frac{(\sum_{j=1}^{J} w_j^2 d_j / n_j^2)^{1/2}}{\sum_{j=1}^{J} w_j d_j / n_j}. \tag{2.7}$$

A test of the null hypothesis CMF = 1 could be effected by referring log CMF/SE (log CMF) to tables of the normal distribution, but, in practice, such tests are better carried out directly in terms of the age-specific rates, as described in the next chapter.

Similar considerations apply to a comparison of the CMFs for two different cohorts, or equivalently to a comparison of the corresponding directly standardized rates. The standard error of the log ratio $\log(\text{CMF}_2/\text{CMF}_1) = \log \text{CMF}_2 - \log \text{CMF}_1$ is given by

$$\text{SE} \log \frac{\text{CMF}_2}{\text{CMF}_1} = \left\{ \frac{\sum_{j=1}^{J} w_j^2 d_{1j} / n_{1j}^2}{(\sum_{j=1}^{J} w_j d_{1j} / n_{1j})^2} + \frac{\sum_{j=1}^{J} w_j^2 d_{2j} / n_{2j}^2}{(\sum_{j=1}^{J} w_j d_{2j} / n_{2j})^2} \right\}^{1/2}.$$

(c) *The standardized mortality ratio* (*SMR*)

The standardized mortality ratio (SMR) has been in service at least since 1786 (Keiding, 1987). It was used by W.H. Farr in the 1855 annual report of the Registrar General of Great Britain to compare mortality in different occupational groups (Benjamin, 1968). It is also defined as a weighted average of the age-specific rate ratios (equation 2.5), where the weights $w_j = n_j \lambda_j^*$ are the expected number of deaths for the cohort in the jth age group, rather than the number of standard deaths as used for the CMF. Thus, the SMR compares the observed number of deaths in the cohort with an expected number obtained by applying the standard rates to the cohort age structure. In symbols,

$$\text{SMR} = \frac{\sum_{j=1}^{J} d_j}{\sum_{j=1}^{J} n_j \lambda_j^*} = \frac{D}{E^*}, \tag{2.8}$$

where $D = \sum d_j$ denotes the total observed number of deaths and E^* is the expected number.

In typical applications, the SMR is used to compare mortality from each of several causes of death in the cohort as a whole to that in the general population. Table 2.16, for example, shows the SMRs for four causes of death for the Montana smelter workers. Diseases identified as occurring in excess may then be studied in greater detail in relation to specific exposures. Of course, there is no guarantee that this process will identify those diseases or causes of death that are most closely associated with the exposures. Cause-specific rates for unexposed cohort members may be less than those in the general population, whereas rates for exposed members are higher, and the two effects may cancel each other out when averaged over the entire cohort. Nevertheless, use of the SMR as a device for screening a number of different causes of death seems firmly established. Other techniques to detect cancer sites or causes of death that are related to exposure, but without reference to an external standard population, are considered in Chapter 3.

One advantage of the SMR over the CMF is that age-specific numbers of deaths d_j are not required for its calculation. It suffices to know only the total D. This sometimes permits application of the SMR to published data for which the CMF could not be used. Details on numbers of deaths by cause, subgroup and age are often omitted from official publications for reasons of economy, whereas the subtotals by cause and subgroup and the person-years by subgroup and age are given. However, caution is required in such circumstances, because if the detailed data are missing there is no way of evaluating the hypothesis of constant rate ratios that is needed to justify fully the use of these summary measures (see below and also §4.6).

The SMR is also the preferred measure when analysing cross-sectional data according to birth cohort rather than calendar period. The reason is that the age intervals for which data are available differ for different generations, a feature that precludes calculation of comparable CMFs. Beral (1974) and Beral et al. (1978) have provided us with two particularly innovative examples that illustrate this type of application.

Example 2.7

Figure 2.5 shows SMRs for ovarian cancers calculated for successive generations of women from age-specific mortality rates. Data were available for women aged 30–74 years for the period 1931 to 1973 in the USA and for the same ages between 1931 and 1975 in the UK. Age-specific rates for the pooled calendar periods were used as a standard, and the SMRs consequently tend to cluster about 100. When the SMRs are plotted against average completed family size for the same generations, there is a near perfect negative correlation that suggests a possible protective effect of pregnancy or childbearing (Fig. 2.6).

In a similar analysis, Figure 2.7 shows plots of SMRs for cervical cancer in England and Wales by generation together with the rates of gonorrheal disease that prevailed at age 20 in those same generations. The similarity in the shapes of the two curves is striking.

Another advantage of the SMR, when viewed as a weighted average of the ratios of age-specific rates for cohort and standard population, is that the weights $w_j = n_j \lambda_j^*$ minimize the variance of the weighted average. Assuming that the true rate ratios are constant, the SMR is thus the minimum variance estimate of the common rate ratio. In practical terms, this means that it tends to be less sensitive to numerical instabilities in one or two of the age-specific rates, a property that is easy to demonstrate by returning to an earlier example.

Example 2.6 (contd)

The expected numbers of deaths for the cohort in Table 2.9 is

$$E^* = 10\,000(140/150\,000) + 3000(290/70\,000) + 1(30/210) = 21.90,$$

and thus the SMR is 20/21.9 = 0.91, indicating a slightly lower death rate among the cohort members as opposed to the general population. If the single exposed person in the 85+ age group had died instead of lived, we would have SMR = 19/21.90 = 0.87, a minor change compared to that observed earlier with the CMF.

Another means of demonstrating the greater numerical stability of the SMR is to

Fig. 2.5   Age-standardized mortality ratios for ovarian cancer in England and Wales (●) and the USA (○) for generations of women born at five-year intervals between 1861 and 1931. From Beral *et al.* (1978)

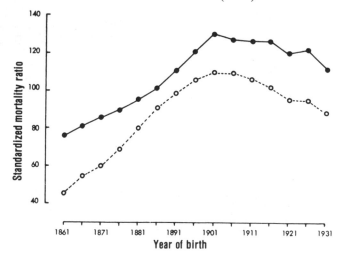

Fig. 2.6 Age-standardized mortality ratios for ovarian cancer plotted against the average completed family size (number of children) for different generations of women in England and Wales (●) and the USA (○). The mid-year of birth of each generation is shown in parentheses. From Beral *et al.* (1978)

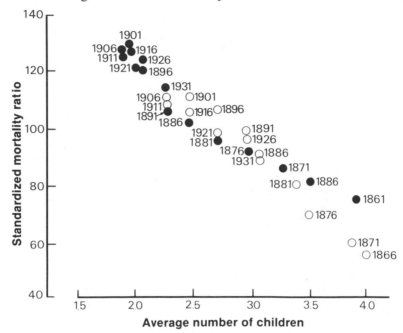

examine its standard error. Under the previous assumption that the numbers of deaths d_j in the different (age) strata are uncorrelated, whereas sampling errors associated with the standard population are negligible, we calculate

$$SE(SMR) = \left\{ \sum_{j=1}^{J} d_j \right\}^{1/2} \Big/ E^* = D^{1/2}/E^*,$$

or, more appropriately

$$SE(\log SMR) = SE(SMR)/SMR = 1/D^{1/2}. \tag{2.9}$$

Since the standard error of the SMR depends only on fluctuations in the total number rather than in the age-specific numbers of deaths, it is generally smaller than that of the CMF. As already noted, under the hypothesis of constant age-specific rate ratios, the SMR weights the ratios optimally, in inverse proportion to their statistical precision, whereas with the CMF the weights associated with unstable ratios may be much larger. The SMR is thus more appropriate when the sample is small and questions of statistical significance are at issue; we examine methods of making statistical inferences about this measure in more detail than we did for the CMF.

Fig. 2.7 Standardized mortality ratios (SMR) from cervical cancer by birth cohort
among women born between 1902 and 1947 in England and Wales and
incidence of gonorrhoea among women in England and Wales, 1925–1972.
From Beral (1974)

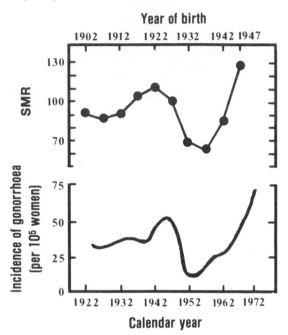

(d) Testing the significance of the observed SMR

The first question of interest relating to the SMR is simply whether the observed
cause-specific mortality in the study cohort can be explained adequately by the
standard rates and the play of chance. Conventional approaches (Monson, 1980) use
the simple continuity corrected chi-square statistic

$$\chi^2 = \frac{(|D - E^*| - 1/2)^2}{E^*} \tag{2.10}$$

in order to test whether the observed number of deaths is significantly different from
the number expected. This statistic is derived from the usual assumption that, under
the null hypothesis, the observed number of deaths D is approximately Poisson
distributed with mean and variance both equal to E^* (Armitage, 1971, section 4.3). It
is referred to tables of chi-square with one degree of freedom, or else its (signed)
square root χ is treated as an equivalent normal deviate. The 1/2 correction in the
numerator is intended to improve the correspondence between the percentiles of the
discrete Poisson distribution and the continuous normal one (see §4.3 of Volume 1).

When the number of deaths is small, the Poisson distribution is rather skewed, and the normal approximation implicit in the use of (2.10) will be inadequate. An 'exact' p value may be calculated using tail probabilities of the Poisson or (equivalently) chi-square distributions (Pearson & Hartley, 1966). However, these are tabled for only a limited range of values. Byar (see Rothman & Boice, 1979) suggested an extremely accurate approximation to the exact Poisson test, which is obtained by calculating the deviate

$$\chi = (9\bar{D})^{1/2}\left\{1 - \frac{1}{9\bar{D}} - \left(\frac{E^*}{\bar{D}}\right)^{1/3}\right\}, \tag{2.11}$$

where $\bar{D} = D$ if D exceeds E^*, and $\bar{D} = D + 1$ otherwise, and referring it to tables of the unit normal distribution (Rothman & Boice, 1979). Alternatively, and somewhat easier to remember, we may use the fact that the square-root transform is 'variance stabilizing' (Armitage, 1971), so that $D^{1/2}$ is approximately normal with mean $(E^*)^{1/2}$ and variance $1/4$ under the null hypothesis. This means treating

$$\chi = 2\{D^{1/2} - (E^*)^{1/2}\} \tag{2.12}$$

as a standard normal deviate.

(e) Confidence intervals for the SMR

A second statistical question of common interest is to determine a range of possible values for the true SMR that are reasonably consistent with the observed data. If the test of the null hypothesis gives the verdict 'not significant', it may be important to demonstrate that the study had sufficient precision to render large differences between cohort and standard rates implausible. Or, if the result is positive, one may wish to examine its consistency with that of other studies. Putting a confidence interval around the observed SMR can achieve these goals.

Exact confidence limits for the SMR are obtained by first finding lower (L) and upper (U) limits μ_L and μ_U for the mean $\mu = E(D)$ of the Poisson distributed observation D, and then calculating $SMR_L = \mu_L/E^*$ and $SMR_U = \mu_U/E^*$. Exploiting the general relationship between confidence limits and test statistics (§§4.2 and 4.3 of Volume 1), the limits on μ may be found by solution of equations involving Poisson probabilities. Table 2.10 presents exact 95% limits for a Poisson mean for selected values of D ranging from 1 to 1000 (Haenszel et al., 1962).

For other confidence levels and values of D not shown in Table 2.10, Byar's approximation is sufficiently accurate that one may avoid the iterative calculations needed for the exact results. Thus, for a $100(1 - \alpha)\%$ confidence interval, we have the approximate limits (Rothman & Boice, 1979)

$$\mu_L = D\left(1 - \frac{1}{9D} - \frac{Z_{\alpha/2}}{3D^{1/2}}\right)^3 \tag{2.13}$$

and

$$\mu_U = (D + 1)\left(1 - \frac{1}{9(D + 1)} + \frac{Z_{\alpha/2}}{3(D + 1)^{1/2}}\right)^3,$$

where $Z_{\alpha/2}$ denotes the $100(1 - \alpha/2)$ percentile of the unit normal distribution.

Table 2.10   Tabulated values of 95% confidence limit factors for estimating a Poisson-distributed variable[a]

Observed number on which estimate is based (n)	Lower limit factor (L)	Upper limit factor (U)	Observed number on which estimate is based (n)	Lower limit factor (L)	Upper limit factor (U)	Observed number on which estimate is based (n)	Lower limit factor (L)	Upper limit factor (U)
1	0.0253	5.57	21	0.619	1.53	120	0.833	1.200
2	0.121	3.61	22	0.627	1.51	140	0.844	1.184
3	0.206	2.92	23	0.634	1.50	160	0.854	1.171
4	0.272	2.56	24	0.641	1.48	180	0.862	1.160
5	0.324	2.33	25	0.647	1.48	200	0.868	1.151
6	0.367	2.18	26	0.653	1.47	250	0.882	1.134
7	0.401	2.06	27	0.659	1.46	300	0.892	1.121
8	0.431	1.97	28	0.665	1.45	350	0.899	1.112
9	0.458	1.90	29	0.670	1.44	400	0.906	1.104
10	0.480	1.84	30	0.675	1.43	450	0.911	1.098
11	0.499	1.79	35	0.697	1.39	500	0.915	1.093
12	0.517	1.75	40	0.714	1.36	600	0.922	1.084
13	0.532	1.71	45	0.729	1.34	700	0.928	1.078
14	0.546	1.68	50	0.742	1.32	800	0.932	1.072
15	0.560	1.65	60	0.770	1.30	900	0.936	1.068
16	0.572	1.62	70	0.785	1.27	1 000	0.939	1.064
17	0.583	1.60	80	0.798	1.25			
18	0.593	1.58	90	0.809	1.24			
19	0.602	1.56	100	0.818	1.22			
20	0.611	1.54						

[a] From Haenszel et al. (1962)

Somewhat less accurate but more easily remembered approximate limits for the SMR may be derived from analogues to the other statistics (2.10) and (2.12) used to test the null hypothesis. Specifically, denoting by θ the unknown value of the SMR, we solve the equation $(D - \theta E)^2/\theta E = Z^2_{\alpha/2}$ (ignoring the continuity correction) to find

$$\text{SMR}_L = \theta_L = \text{SMR}\left[1 + \frac{1}{2D}Z^2_{\alpha/2}\{1 - (1 + 4D/Z^2_{\alpha/2})^{1/2}\}\right] \qquad (2.14)$$

and

$$\text{SMR}_U = \theta_U = \text{SMR}\left[1 + \frac{1}{2D}Z^2_{\alpha/2}\{1 + (1 + 4D/Z^2_{\alpha/2})^{1/2}\}\right]$$

as the limits derived from the standard chi-square test. We have not used a continuity correction for this calculation, since to do so gives less accurate limits empirically. Alternatively, limits based on the square-root transform are obtained by solving the equation $2\{D^{1/2} - (\theta E)^{1/2}\} = Z_{\alpha/2}$, which gives

$$\text{SMR}_L = \text{SMR}\left(1 - \frac{Z_\alpha}{2D^{1/2}}\right)^2$$

and

$$\mathrm{SMR}_U = SMR\left(\frac{D+1}{D}\right)\left(1 + \frac{Z_\alpha}{2(D+1)^{1/2}}\right)^2. \tag{2.15}$$

The use of $D+1$ in the second equation is made on strictly empirical grounds in order to improve the approximation for small D (compare equation (2.13)).

The exact Poisson limits and all three sets of approximate confidence limits (2.13)–(2.15) can be expressed in the form $\mathrm{SMR}_L = \mathrm{SMR} \times M_L$ and $\mathrm{SMR}_U = \mathrm{SMR} \times M_U$, where M_L and M_U are multipliers determined by α and D. Table 2.11 compares the multipliers obtained by each method for several values of D, $\alpha = 0.05$ and $\alpha = 0.01$ (95% and 99% confidence). Byar's approximation is shown to be accurate even for quite small numbers of deaths. The square-root transform performs reasonably well as soon as D exceeds 10 or so. Especially as regards the lower bound, which is usually of prime interest, however, the approximation based on the simple chi-square statistic is not very satisfactory.

Table 2.11   Exact and approximate multipliers for computing confidence intervals for the SMR[a]

No. of deaths (D)	Exact limits		Byar's approximation (equation 2.13)		Square root (equation 2.15)		Chi-square (equation 2.14)	
	Lower	Upper	Lower	Upper	Lower	Upper	Lower	Upper
	95% intervals							
1	0.025	5.572	0.013	5.565	0.000	5.733	0.176	5.667
2	0.121	3.612	0.112	3.611	0.094	3.678	0.274	3.647
3	0.206	2.922	0.201	2.922	0.188	2.961	0.340	2.941
4	0.272	2.560	0.209	2.561	0.260	2.586	0.389	2.572
5	0.325	2.334	0.322	2.334	0.315	2.353	0.427	2.342
10	0.480	1.839	0.479	1.839	0.476	1.846	0.543	1.841
15	0.560	1.649	0.559	1.650	0.558	1.653	0.606	1.650
20	0.611	1.544	0.611	1.545	0.610	1.547	0.647	1.545
25	0.647	1.476	0.647	1.476	0.646	1.478	0.677	1.476
50	0.742	1.318	0.742	1.318	0.742	1.319	0.759	1.318
	99% intervals							
1	0.005	7.430	0.000	7.471	0.000	7.301	0.117	8.519
2	0.052	4.637	0.038	4.656	0.008	4.561	0.195	5.123
3	0.113	3.659	0.102	3.671	0.066	3.604	0.253	3.960
4	0.168	3.149	0.160	3.157	0.127	3.105	0.297	3.362
5	0.216	2.830	0.209	2.836	0.180	2.794	0.334	2.993
10	0.372	2.140	0.369	2.142	0.351	2.120	0.452	2.212
15	0.460	1.878	0.458	1.879	0.445	1.864	0.520	1.922
20	0.518	1.733	0.517	1.734	0.507	1.723	0.566	1.765
25	0.560	1.640	0.559	1.641	0.551	1.632	0.601	1.665
50	0.673	1.425	0.673	1.426	0.669	1.421	0.696	1.437

[a] Note: In order to obtain lower and upper limits for an SMR based on the indicated number of deaths, the computed SMR is multiplied by the values shown.

Example 2.8

Fifteen deaths from bladder cancer were recorded prior to 1964 among the Montana smelter workers, whereas only 8.33 were expected from US population rates: $SMR = 15/8.33 = 1.80$. The 95% confidence limits found from the exact multipliers corresponding to $D = 15$ in Table 2.10 are $SMR_L = 0.560 \times 1.80 = 1.01$ and $SMR_U = 1.649 \times 1.80 = 2.97$. Those based on Byar's formula are almost the same, and those for the square-root transform only very slightly wider (1.00, 2.98). However, the limits based on the chi-square test statistic (1.11, 2.97) have a lower limit which is seriously in error, as do those based on the standard error of $\log(SMR)$, namely $1.80 \times \exp(\pm 1.96/\sqrt{15}) = (1.09, 2.99)$.

Since the exact lower limit just excludes 1.0, we know that the exact two-sided significance level must be just under 0.05. Equation (2.11) gives $\chi = 1.98$ ($p = 0.048$), whereas with (2.12) we find $\chi = 1.97$ ($p = 0.049$). The conventional formula (2.10) yields $\chi = 2.14$ ($p = 0.033$) with continuity correction and $\chi = 2.31$ ($p = 0.021$) without. This reinforces our conclusion that the test statistics (2.11) and (2.12) should be used in preference to (2.10).

(f) SMR versus CMF: a tradeoff between bias and variance

Up until now we have emphasized the statistical advantages of the SMR over the CMF, but, unfortunately, this is not the entire story. The major weakness of the SMR is that ratios of SMRs for two comparison groups may not adequately represent the ensemble of ratios of their component age- or stratum-specific rates (Yule, 1934). In fact, as the schema shown in Table 2.12 makes clear, there is a precise analogy with the arithmetic of statistical confounding.

The ratios of SMRs for Cohort 1 *versus* Cohort 2 within each age group equal the odds ratio calculated from the corresponding 2×2 table, and likewise the overall SMR ratio is the odds ratio from the totals table. According to the general principle of statistical confounding (§3.4 of Volume 1), it follows that, even if the two age-specific odds ratios are equal, they may differ from the pooled odds ratio if both (i) the SMRs for each cohort vary from one age group to another and (ii) the age distributions of the two cohorts, and hence the distributions of expected numbers of deaths, are disparate. Since the age-specific ratios of SMRs equal the ratios of the corresponding rates (assuming that the standard rates are used in calculation of the expected numbers), it follows that the ratio of two SMRs determined by pooling observed and expected deaths across age groups may sometimes lie completely outside the range of the age-specific rate ratios.

The fictitious data in Table 2.13 provide a clear numerical illustration of this phenomenon. The overall SMR for each cohort is a weighted average of the two

Table 2.12 Confounding remaining after indirect standardization

	Age group 1		Age group 2		Total	
	Observed	Expected	Observed	Expected	Observed	Expected
Cohort 1	d_{11}	e_1^*	d_{12}	e_{12}^*	D_1	E_1^*
Cohort 2	d_{21}	e_{21}^*	d_{22}	e_{22}^*	D_2	E_2^*
SMR_1	$d_{11}e_{21}^*$		$d_{12}e_{22}^*$		$D_1E_2^*$	
SMR_2	$d_{21}e_{11}^*$		$d_{22}e_{12}^*$		$D_2E_1^*$	

d and D = number of deaths observed
e^* and E^* = number of deaths expected

Table 2.13 Example of a misleading ratio of SMRs[a]

Cohort		Age range (years)		
		20–44	45–64	Total (20–64)
I	d	100	1600	1700
	e^*	200	800	1000
	SMR_1 (%)	50	200	170
II	d	80	180	260
	e^*	120	60	180
	SMR_2 (%)	67	300	144
	SMR_1/SMR_2	75	67	118

[a] Adapted from Kilpatrick (1963)
d = number of deaths observed
e^* = number of deaths expected

age-specific d/e^* ratios, the weights being proportional to the expected number of deaths. Since Cohort 1 has more older people, the high d/e^* ratio for the 45–64-year age interval is weighted more heavily, whereas in Cohort 2 much more emphasis is given to the lower d/e^* ratio in the 25–44-year age interval. The overall result is a change of sign in the apparent effect, from an excess of deaths in Cohort 2 on an age-specific basis to an apparent excess in Cohort 1 when the data are pooled.

The CMF does not suffer from this problem. Ratios of two CMFs, being ratios of directly standardized rates, can be expressed as a weighted average of the age-specific rate ratios. If these are all equal to some constant value θ, therefore, the ratio of CMFs must also equal θ. However, this equality does not hold for the SMRs, unless, in addition, the age-specific rates for each comparison group are also in constant proportion with those for the standard population. This bias in the SMR has led many authors to conclude that the CMF is the preferred measure. Miettinen (1972) says of the SMR that 'estimates computed in this manner are internally standardized but not mutually comparable'. Kilpatrick (1963) notes that 'the ratio of two CMFs is a CMF but the ratio of two SMRs is not an SMR'.

In spite of these criticisms, the SMR and the CMF usually provide numerical results that are remarkably close in practice. In cases in which they differ, moreover, it is not necessarily true that the CMF is more nearly 'correct'. Table 2.14, compiled by the Office of Population Censuses and Surveys (1978), examines occupations of British men for which the CMF and SMR differ by 5 or more when each was expressed as a percentage. The large discrepancy between the two measures for trainee craftsmen in engineering trades is caused by undue weight in the CMF to the lack of deaths among men over 25 years of age, even though these men accounted for only 1% of the population. Since only one death in the 55–64-year age group would have increased the CMF from 1 to 35, this is another example of its extreme sensitivity to small numbers and serves as a reminder that we need to consider variance as well as bias in our choice of a summary statistic (see also Example 2.6).

The CMF may itself overemphasize biases in the basic data. As noted by the Office

Table 2.14 Occupation units for which the CMF and SMR differ[a]

Occupation unit		SMR (%)	CMF (%)		Age group (years)				
No.	Title				15–24	25–34	35–44	45–54	55–64
Major differences (10 or more)									
009	Workers below ground	112	138	Mortality ratio	139	112	61	46	184
				% Population	14	33	26	19	8
032	Trainee craftsmen (engineering trades)	26	1	Mortality ratio	27	0	0	0	0
				% Population	99	1	0	0	0
117	Pilots, navigators and flight engineers	86	151	Mortality ratio	190	82	26	80	195
				% Population	11	23	33	31	2
151	Fire brigade officers and men	99	117	Mortality ratio	102	83	63	66	145
				% Population	15	33	23	21	8
152	Police officers and men	109	213	Mortality ratio	76	68	66	72	299
				% Population	22	32	27	17	2
187	Chiropodists	74	101	Mortality ratio	805	145	94	79	67
				% Population	4	9	18	30	39
302	Metallurgists	96	107	Mortality ratio	—	85	64	114	117
				% Population	27	37	18	11	6
221	Armed forces (UK)	147	252	Mortality ratio	123	100	100	118	337
				% Population	43	31	17	7	1
222	Armed forces (foreign)	149	243	Mortality ratio	198	128	83	129	314
				% Population	41	33	21	4	1
Minor differences (5–9)									
61	Shoemakers and repairers	156	150	Mortality ratio	47	127	154	132	164
				% Population	10	14	20	23	33
114	Other labourers	201	209	Mortality ratio	292	369	285	113	81
				% Popoulation	23	15	16	20	26
134	Lorry drivers' mates van guards	120	128	Mortality ratio	97	118	115	153	123
				% Population	69	12	9	6	5
158	Domestic housekeepers	117	125	Mortality ratio	—	—	241	210	94
				% Population	—	5	16	29	50
163	Kitchen hands	113	123	Mortality ratio	172	253	225	147	91
				% Population	21	12	16	23	28
164	Maids, valets and related workers	121	129	Mortality ratio	198	200	190	151	105
				% Population	15	19	17	20	30
204	Chemists	89	95	Mortality ratio	104	53	66	96	100
				% Population	14	39	23	14	9
All men		100	100	Mortality ratio	100	100	100	100	100
				Population (15 – 64 = 100)	23.5	20.1	18.9	19.5	18.1

[a] From Office of Population Censuses & Surveys (1978)

of Population Censuses and Surveys for the data in Table 2.14:

'Pilots, policemen, firemen and members of the armed forces all recorded differences between the SMR and CMF of greater than 10. Although men in these units generally retired before 55 years of age and took up other work their main occupations instead of their last occupations were often recorded when the deaths were registered. The age-specific mortality ratio in the 55–64 age group was consequently inflated by this bias. The CMF placed considerable weight on the death rates in this age group since over 60 percent of the standard deaths occurred at this age. Since however for each of these occupation units the population in this age group was small, the SMR placed less weight on these high death rates, compensating for the bias introduced.'

Silcock (1959) determined analytically three conditions under which the CMF and SMR give substantially different results. Denote by $p_j = n_j/N$ and $p_j^* = n_j^*/N^*$ the age distributions of the comparison group and the standard population, both expressed as proportions, and by $\hat{\lambda}_j$ and λ_j^* the corresponding rates. Then the conditions are: (i) the differences $p_j - p_j^*$ must be non-negligible; (ii) the ratios $r_j = \hat{\lambda}_j/\lambda_j^*$ must vary substantially with age (j); and (iii) the differences in (i) and the ratios in (ii) must be correlated, such that positive differences tend to occur with high ratios and negative differences with low ratios, or *vice versa*. The 'data' in Table 2.13 confirm that these conditions hold in situations where the CMF and SMR differ.

(g) Summary ratios under heterogeneity of effect

Much of the preceding discussion of the relative merits of the CMF and SMR was conducted under the (sometimes only implicit) hypothesis that each measure was estimating the same quantity, namely the ratio of age-specific rates assumed constant from one age group to the next. The major exception was the fact just cited that the two measures could yield substantially different results only if the age-specific ratios varied in tandem with differences in the age distribution. Our basic viewpoint remains that summary measures should be avoided whenever there is substantial heterogeneity in the age-specific quantities being summarized.

Other authors have been more concerned with the issue of how to choose a summary measure in order to arrive at a scientifically meaningful result, even in the face of heterogeneity. Greenland (1982) notes that the CMF, viewed as a weighted average of ratios with weights equal to standard deaths (equation 2.5), represents the proportionate increase (or decrease) in the total disease rate that would be expected to occur in the standard population if its members had the same exposures as those in the cohort. Similarly, the SMR represents the proportionate increase in the cohort disease rate due to the exposures that occurred as a result of cohort membership. Following Miettinen (1976), he proposes yet another summary measure that uses the age distribution of the combined (cohort plus standard) population for calculation of the weights used to mutliply the age-specific ratios, namely: $u_j = (n_j + n_j^*)\lambda_j^*$.

Several other proposals are reviewed by Kilpatrick (1963) and Fleiss (1973). The relative mortality index (RMI) weights the ratios $r_j = \hat{\lambda}_j/\lambda_j^*$ by the age distribution of the cohort:

$$\text{RMI} = \frac{\sum_{j=1}^{J} n_j \hat{\lambda}_j/\lambda_j^*}{\sum_{j=1}^{J} n_j} = \frac{\sum_{j=1}^{J} d_j/\lambda_j^*}{\sum_{j=1}^{J} n_j}.$$

Liddell (1960) examines some properties of this measure, which he credits to Kerridge (1958) and Doering and Forbes (1939). Yerushalmy (1951) and Elveback (1966) use the length of the age interval to weight these same ratios, while Haenszel (1950) considers a ratio of directly standardized rates with weights equal to the number of years of working life (up to age 65) lost. Of course, if the ratios are constant, none of these schemes is optimal in the sense of minimum variance, as was true of the SMR, nor has any of them come into common use.

2.4 Proportional measures of incidence and mortality

Proportional mortality studies were mentioned in §1.6 as a timely and cost-effective way to provide a rough measure of the effect of cohort membership or of specific exposures on mortality caused by particular diseases. If the only data available concern incident cancer cases, information about their distribution by topographic site or histology can alert one to the possibility of unusual patterns of incidence that should be investigated using more orthodox methodologies. It is especially important in such studies to try to ascertain all deaths or cases that occur in a defined population during a defined period, or else to ensure that the probabilities of ascertainment do not depend on the cause of death or type of cancer. Otherwise one runs the risk of making misleading inferences due to selection bias. Even if such precautions are taken, major problems of interpretation remain due to the logical impossibility of making comparative statements about rates from 'numerator' data only

In this section we present the usual epidemiological methods for adjusting numerator or proportional mortality data so as to account for the differences in age distribution between the study group and the standard population. The same techniques may be used to control the effects of calendar year and other potentially confounding variables. We also show some empirical comparisons of the different results obtained from SMR and proportional mortality analyses when both are applied to the same set of data. A more theoretical evaluation of the behaviour of the proportional mortality measures is presented in §4.7, together with some suggestions for statistical modelling of this type of data.

(a) The proportional mortality ratio (PMR)

The basic idea of proportional mortality analysis is to compare the fraction of cohort deaths due to a specified cause with the corresponding fraction for the general population. Denote by d_j the number of deaths from the cause of interest observed in age interval j in the study group, and by d_j^* the corresponding number of standard deaths. Likewise denote by t_j and t_j^* the total numbers of age-specific deaths, regardless of cause. Then, with $D = \sum d_j$, $D^* = \sum d_j^*$, $T = \sum t_j$ and $T^* = \sum t_j^*$ indicating the totals of these quantities summed across age strata, the ratio $(D/T) \div (D^*/T^*)$ of the two proportions provides a crude measure of relative effect. Note that this can also be expressed as the ratio of the observed number of cause-specific deaths, D, to the number expected by applying the standard proportion to the total deaths, namely $T \times (D^*/T^*)$.

Since the death rates, and thus the proportions of deaths for different causes, depend on age in different ways, the age distribution of the comparison group can influence the overall proportion D/T. The conventional approach to adjusting for such age differences (Monson, 1980) is to calculate the expected numbers on an age-specific basis and then sum up. This yields a measure known as the proportional mortality ratio (PMR), namely:

$$\text{PMR} = \frac{D}{\sum_{j=1}^{J} t_j(d_j^*/t_j^*)}.$$ (2.16)

Under the null hypothesis that the age-specific proportions agree between cohort and standard population, the PMR will be approximately unity in large samples of data, regardless of differences in the age distributions. However, unless the disease is rare, the PMR does not estimate any well-defined or appropriate parameter under alternative hypotheses of interest (§4.7). For this reason, we do not recommend that statistical inference procedures be conducted on the PMR, but suggest instead that one use the parameter estimates, tests and confidence limits produced as a by-product of the model fitting described later. Nevertheless, we record here an equation for the standard error of log(PMR) that is based on the notion that the denominator is fixed whereas the numerator D is a sum of independent binomial variables:

$$\text{SE(log PMR)} = \frac{(\sum_{j=1}^{J} d_j(t_j - d_j)/t_j)^{1/2}}{D}.$$ (2.17)

The simpler equation (2.9) can be viewed as a conservative approximation to (2.17), to be used with the PMR as well as the SMR provided that the fraction of deaths due to the cause of interest is quite small.

(b) The PMR and the relative SMR

Several investigators have noted that, in practice, the PMR for a given cause of death is approximately equal to the SMR for that cause divided by the SMR for all causes combined. When there is no stratification by age or other factors one has:

$$\text{PMR} = \frac{D/T}{D^*/T^*} = \frac{D/N}{D^*/N^*} \div \frac{T/N}{T^*/N^*} = \frac{\text{SMR}}{\text{SMR(all)}},$$ (2.18)

where SMR(all) denotes the all-causes ratio (Decouflé et al., 1980). This equality does not hold, however, for the usual age-standardized PMRs and SMRs. Kupper et al. (1978), who refer to the ratio of cause-specific to all-causes SMR as the 'relative standardized mortality ratio' (RSMR), have attempted to establish confidence bounds within which the ratio of the two sides of the equation would be expected to lie with high probability. Unfortunately, their method relies on an assumption that cannot be verified from numerator data alone, namely that the age distribution of the deaths that would be expected to occur in the comparison group by applying the standard rates is roughly the same as the age distribution of the standard deaths. If this condition does not hold, the magnitude of the difference between the two sides of the equation could be larger than their calculations would suggest. Nevertheless, it is a frequent empirical finding that the PMR and RSMR tend to agree, probably because the age distributions in question are rarely all that different.

Table 2.15, adapted from Decouflé et al. (1980), illustrates the typical agreement

Table 2.15 Cause-specific mortality experience of non-white male foundry workers employed at a plant between 1938 and 1967[a]

Cause (ICD, 7th revision)	No. of observed deaths	SMR (%)	PMR (%)	RSMR (%)
All causes	172	55	100	100
Cancer (140–205)	35	88	153	160
Digestive (150–159)	14	92	161	167
Respiratory (160–165)	12	114	199	207
All other	9	65	111	118
Stroke (331, 332)	9	36	62	65
Circulatory disease (400–468)	54	53	93	96
Accidents, suicide, homicide	27	52	107	95
All other causes	47	48	92	87

[a] Adapted from Decouflé *et al.* (1980)
SMR = standardized mortality ratio
PMR = proportional mortality ratio
RSMR = relative standardized mortality ratio

found between PMRs and RSMRs for the same cause. In their example, the overall mortality of the workers was so low in comparison with that of the general population that there appeared to be a marked excess of respiratory cancers when numerator data alone were considered. If one believed that the selection bias that operates to make industrial workers healthier than the general population applied with equal force to all diseases, then it would be reasonable to conclude that the elevated PMR observed for respiratory cancer was indicative of an effect of exposure on that disease. However, a more plausible explanation in this case is that the elevated PMR results from the selection bias being less pronounced for cancer than it is for other diseases (Enterline, 1975). In view of the uncertainty surrounding these assumptions, use of the RSMR and PMR remains controversial (Wen *et al.*, 1983).

Our last example illustrates a number of the basic calculations introduced throughout the chapter using data from the Montana cohort.

Example 2.9

Table 2.16 presents the CMFs, SMRs, PMRs and RSMRs for four causes of death for the 8014 workers in the Montana cohort. The 1950 US standard population (Table 2.5) provided the weights used for direct standardization and calculation of the CMF. Expected numbers needed for determination of the SMRs were obtained by multiplying the exact person-years shown in each cell of Table 2.2 by the corresponding rates for US white males (Appendix III) and then summing. The denominators of the CMF statistics were obtained by applying the standard weights, a function of age alone, to the standard rates, which varied by both age and year. Thus, we have used equation (2.3) to calculate the CMF, rather than the simpler equation (2.4), which applies only when the weights are proportional to the denominators of the standard rates. The PMR was determined from equation (2.16); and the standard errors for the logarithms of the CMF, SMR and PMR (which equal the standard errors of the estimate expressed as a percentage of the estimate) were determined from equations (2.7), (2.9) and (2.17), respectively.

This working cohort was unusual in having an all-causes summary rate ratio (CMF or SMR) substantially above 100%. The PMRs and RMSRs show good agreement, as do the CMFs and SMRs. Note that the standard errors of log(PMR) are less than those for log(SMR). Part of the difference is due to the inherently smaller degree of variability in a proportion than in a rate. For example, had we used equation (2.9) to find the standard error of log(PMR) for circulatory diseases, the result would have been SE(log PMR) = 2.6% rather than 1.9%. Similarly, the log(SMRs) have smaller standard errors than do the log (CMFs). Besides

Table 2.16 Mortality ratios for the Montana cohort

	Cause of death			
	All causes	All cancers	Respiratory cancer	Circulatory disease
No. of observed deaths	3404	621	288	1535
No. of expected deaths	2761.0	485.4	137.1	1473.4
CMF($\times$100) $\pm$ SE(%)[a]	111.4 $\pm$ 2.5%	127.8 $\pm$ 5.0%	234.6 $\pm$ 7.0%	93.1 $\pm$ 3.1%
SMR($\times$100) $\pm$ SE(%)[a]	123.3 $\pm$ 1.7%	127.9 $\pm$ 4.0%	210.1 $\pm$ 5.9%	104.2 $\pm$ 2.6%
PMR(%) $\pm$ SE	100	102.9 $\pm$ 3.6%	166.4 $\pm$ 5.5%	84.5 $\pm$ 1.9%
RSMR(%)	100	103.7	170.4	84.5

[a] Standard errors are computed on a log scale, e.g., SE(log CMF) = 0.025, and we thus express the standard deviations of the estimate as a percentage of the estimated value

CMF = comparative mortality figure
SMR = standardized mortality ratio
PMR = proportional mortality ratio
RSMR = relative standardized mortality ratio

the excesses of respiratory cancer and circulatory disease (mostly diseases of the heart) shown in Table 2.15, there were more deaths observed from tuberculosis, cirrhosis of the liver and emphysema than would have been expected from the standard rates (Lee-Feldstein, 1983).

3. COMPARISONS AMONG EXPOSURE GROUPS

CHAPTER 3

COMPARISONS AMONG EXPOSURE GROUPS

The techniques of standardization introduced in the last chapter are typically used to determine whether the cause-specific mortality rates for the study cohort are comparable with those from some appropriate standard population. The observation of an elevated CMF or SMR for a particular cause of death may alert the investigator to the possibility that the cohort members are subject to exposures which increase their risk for that disease. However, a single elevated mortality ratio is usually not regarded in itself as sufficient evidence for a causal relationship, unless it is extremely large. A much better indication of causality is the demonstration of a trend in the mortality ratios with degree or duration of exposure.

In this chapter, we explore several elementary methods used by epidemiologists and biostatisticians to examine cohort data for evidence of differences in death rates between subgroups defined by exposures or other factors, and in particular for evidence of dose-response relationships. The most appropriate methods are adaptations of the classical Mantel–Haenszel analyses of grouped case-control data presented in Chapter 4 of Volume 1. These are covered in §3.6 below. Earlier sections consider methods based on the standardization techniques developed in the last chapter. These are of interest largely for historical reasons. Both the limitations and the potential of the various techniques are illustrated by their systematic application to the Montana smelter workers study. In addition, we cite several examples from the literature which point up notable innovations or pitfalls in the use of these statistical tools.

3.1 Allocation of person-years to time-dependent exposure categories

The first step in comparing death rates among different subgroups of the cohort is simply to estimate the rates for each of them separately using the techniques outlined in the previous chapter. This is quite straightforward when the subgroups are formed on the basis of information available at entry into the study – for example, when they are defined by age or calendar period at entry or by a classification of the initial work area according to measured levels of exposure. One simply treats each subgroup as a separate cohort and carries out the usual allocation of deaths and calculation of person-years by age and time for each one independently. Since a study member contributes person-years observation to only one subgroup, there is no ambiguity about the assignment of his observation time.

It is also of interest, however, to make comparisons among subgroups defined on the basis of variables that change values as the subject moves through the study. For example, subjects often continue to accumulate exposures of interest during the same period that they are being followed for evaluation of cause-specific mortality. Industrial workers may be entered on study while still relatively young and be followed through their working years and on into retirement. If the measured exposures are distributed continuously over the working lifetime, the subjects with the highest cumulative levels of exposure are frequently those who have lived the longest. This is even truer when a variable that reflects duration of exposure is being analysed for its relationship to the risk of disease. Special precautions are required to ensure that the allocation of person-years is made appropriately.

Several investigators have attempted to establish a dose-response trend in such circumstances by classifying each subject into a single subgroup on the basis of his total cumulative exposure or duration of employment at the end of the study. Mortality ratios computed separately for each subgroup are then compared. Unfortunately, results obtained in this manner are fallacious, since the early person-years of follow-up, when cumulative exposures are light, are being allocated to the same heavy exposure category as the later person-years. The death rates calculated in this fashion for the highest exposure categories are too low, since person-years during which no death could have occurred are included in the denominator. Rates for the lowest exposure categories are too high since it is only the individuals who die with short exposures who contribute to the denominator; the person-years of someone who might have died with short-term exposure, but in fact did not, are allocated elsewhere.

The correct assignment of each increment in person-years of follow-up is to that same exposure category to which a death would be assigned should it occur at that time. Subjects who change their exposure classification as they move through the study, as many in fact do, thus contribute to the person-years denominators of the rates for several exposure categories. Figure 3.1 illustrates schematically the proper, dynamic method of allocation as well as the improper, fixed method when duration of follow-up itself is used to define the subgroups being compared.

Table 3.1 presents an example of the magnitude of this dose-response fallacy in actual practice. In the original report of an early study of vinyl chloride workers (Duck *et al.*, 1975), the authors observed that the all-causes SMR declined from 110 for those employed for less than 15 years to 61 for those employed for 15 or more years and stated that no significant excess of mortality had occurred. However, the apparent decline in the SMRs was due entirely to the use of an improper methodology. After correcting the fixed person-years allocation used in the original analysis to an appropriate, dynamic one, the statistically significant negative trend in the SMRs disappeared. There was even an indication of a positive trend in the SMR for digestive cancer with duration of exposure (Duck & Carter, 1976; Wagoner *et al.*, 1976). Enterline (1976) discusses a similar error in the report of Mancuso and El-Attar (1967), who failed to detect a trend in respiratory cancer SMRs among asbestos workers who had been employed for increasing lengths of time.

We describe two algorithms for the correct assignment of person-years observation in the presence of time-dependent exposures categories, the use of which enables one

Fig. 3.1   Schematic diagram illustrating proper and improper methods of allocation of
person–years. ×, death from cause of interest; ○, withdrawal

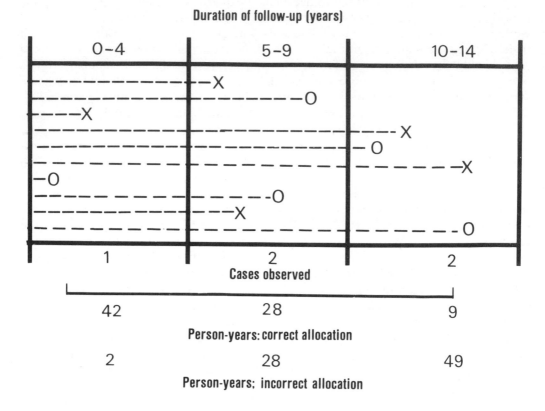

Duration of follow-up (years)

Table 3.1   Reanalysis of data by Duck *et al.* showing original *versus*
revised numbers of expected deaths and SMRs by duration of exposure
and cause of death[a]

Cause of death	Duration of exposure (years)	No. of observed deaths	No. of expected deaths		SMR	
			Original	Revised	Original	Revised
All causes	0–14	111	100.92	118.97	110	94
	15+	25	41.30	24.15	61	104
Total	0–14	27	25.55	29.93	106	90
cancers	15+	8	10.89	6.51	73	123
Digestive	0–14	7	7.77	9.10	90	77
system	15+	4	3.31	1.98	121	202
cancers						
Lung	0–14	13	10.73	12.57	121	103
cancer	15+	3	4.80	2.96	62	101

[a] From Duck *et al.* (1975); Duck & Carter (1976)

to avoid the dose-response fallacy caused by the overlapping of exposure and follow-up periods.

(a) Algorithms for exact allocation of person-years

In practice, there may be several time-dependent exposure variables of interest, and a simultaneous classification of deaths and person-years in a multidimensional table is required. For example, in addition to duration of time since start of employment, we usually need to keep track of age and calendar year, if only for purposes of standardization. Time since cessation of exposure adds a fourth dimension. Determination of the exact length of observation time that each individual contributes to each cell in the four-way table may seem initially to present a difficult problem.

Clayton (1982) describes a computing algorithm for making the appropriate allocation of person-years in such circumstances. It requires that one have available exact dates of entry into and exit from the various time-dependent classes. While not the most efficient method for all problems, this procedure has the advantage of simplicity and generality. Suppose, for example, that one wishes to determine the person-years observation time contributed by one subject to the cell defined by the age range 40–49, the calendar period from 1950–1954, and the interval from five to ten years since first exposure to some risk factor. Then Clayton's procedure is as follows:

(A) Choose the *latest* of the three dates: date of birth +40 years, 31 December 1949, and date of first exposure +five years.

(B) Choose the *earliest* of the four dates: date of birth +50 years, 31 December 1954, date of first exposure +ten years, and date of exit from study.

(C) If B precedes A, then the individual makes no contribution to this cell. Otherwise, the observation time contributed is the time interval from date A to date B.

The calculation must be repeated for each individual for each such cell in the multidimensional table (three dimensions in this example). It accommodates time-dependent variables defined in terms of cumulative length of exposure to particular agents, provided that one knows the exact dates at which cell boundaries are crossed. For example, one could add to the above specifications the requirement that the individual has received a cumulative exposure of between 5 and 10 units of radiation while employed in a nuclear industry. If periodic readings of radiation exposure were made, so that the dates of crossing the 5 and 10 unit boundaries could be estimated, these two dates would be added to those in parts (A) and (B) above.

An alternative, more efficient algorithm (Clayton, personal communication) is available when all of the axes of the multidimensional classification represent time variables that advance in pace with one another (age, calendar year, duration of time from initial exposure) rather than variables such as cumulative exposure or duration of (intermittent) employment, which advance at varying rates depending upon the entire history. This algorithm is presented in Appendix IV.

When using one of the standard programmes for cohort analysis it may be feasible to obtain the number of deaths and person-years in each age-time-exposure category by making separate passes through the data for each exposure category. One defines the dates of entry into and exit from the 'study' for each individual to correspond to the dates of entry into and exit from the particular exposure category. However, this approach is too cumbersome and inefficient to be practical when the number of separate exposure categories is very large.

(b) Approximate methods of allocating person-years

A drawback to Clayton's algorithms is that they require the exact dates at which an individual crosses from each time-dependent cell into another. In practice, exact dates may be available for some of the relevant variables but not others. For example, we may know a worker's birthdate and date of termination, but have available only the (integral) age and calendar year at which he entered the study or moved between jobs. Nevertheless, it may be possible in such cases to assign approximate dates to the relevant events so that a consistent ordering is maintained between the dates of entry, first exposure, termination and so on, and Clayton's method may then be used. It is important that the same procedure be applied also to the classification of deaths, so that one does not have person-years accumulating in cells where no deaths are possible, or *vice versa*.

An alternative approach to the problem of missing days and months in date variables is to use an approximate method of person-years allocation based on integral ages and calendar years. One such method was outlined in §2.1. For some of the examples in this monograph we have employed yet another approximation which divides each subject's observation period into annual intervals that are allocated in their entirety to a given time/exposure cell. Specifically, at the midpoint of each calendar year of follow-up, a determination is made as to the cell in which the subject should be classified at that moment. All of the observation time for that year, which may be less than a full year in case of entry into or exit from the study, is allocated to the one cell.

3.2 Grouped data from the Montana smelter workers study

One of the major themes of this monograph is the statistical analysis of grouped cohort data consisting of cause-specific deaths and person-years denominators classified by age, calendar period and relevant exposure variables, some of which may be time-dependent. In order to illustrate and compare the various analytical approaches, and to provide the reader with material that he can use to test his comprehension of the methodology, it is helpful to have available a data set that is reasonably typical of what one encounters in practice. Of course, one needs to balance the realism of the example against the need for simplicity if it is to be used as a pedagogic device.

For this purpose we used the approximate method of person-years allocation just mentioned to summarize the data from the Montana study into a three-way table with the dimensions age, calendar period and arsenic exposure. Cumulative exposure was measured in terms of the duration of time spent in certain areas of the smelter where airborne arsenic levels were thought to be higher than average. It thus represents a relatively crude way of separating workers (or, more precisely, their person-years of observation) according to the presumed degree of hazard. The largely descriptive analyses consist of estimating separate summary mortality measures for each exposure category and testing the statistical significance of the differences, especially for evidence of a trend with increasing exposure. Other, more refined approaches to dose-time-response analyses are discussed in Chapter 6.

The epidemiologists who conducted this study classified the 30 work areas within the plant into three levels of arsenic exposure (see Appendix IE). 'High' arsenic exposure areas comprised the arsenic kitchen, arsenic roaster and cottrell, whereas those with 'moderate' exposure levels were the convertor, reverbatory furnace, ore roaster and acid plant. All other areas were regarded as giving only 'light' exposures (Lee & Fraumeni, 1969). From the original data file containing the dates of entry into and exit from each work area for each worker, summary data consisting of the number of years worked in both high and moderate exposure areas were recorded by five-year calendar periods starting in 1910. By assuming that the exposure intensity was constant during each such period, we were able to determine the appropriate exposure duration category into which each individual should be classified at each point in time: (i) under 1.0 years moderate or high arsenic exposure; (ii) 1.0–4.9 years; (iii) 5.0–14.9 years; and (iv) 15 or more years.

The assignment of an exposure category to each calendar year was based on the duration of heavy/medium exposure experienced at a point two years earlier. Such adjustments to cumulative exposure variables are a crude way of coping with the bias that can arise from the fact that workers who have just entered a new cumulative exposure category are necessarily still employed and thus at lower risk of death, whereas those who change employment or retire for health reasons may have higher death rates (Gilbert, 1983). See the discussion in §1.5c of the selection biases, known collectively as the 'healthy worker effect', that are caused by the fact that health status has a major influence on hiring, job changes and termination. This adjustment would be less necessary if it were possible to use onset of disease as the endpoint, rather than death from disease, since onset presumably occurs closer to the time of any adverse health effect.

For the descriptive analyses reported in this chapter, the cohort was divided into two subcohorts, one consisting of the 1482 men employed prior to 1925 and the other of the remainder. The reason for this division was the fact that the selective flotation process introduced in 1924 apparently resulted in greatly reduced arsenic exposures (Lee-Feldstein, 1983). Substantially different dose-response trends are evident in the two groups. An alternative and possibly more appropriate means of coping with the change would be to classify the exposures as to the period during which they were actually received, namely before or after 1 January 1925. A man hired prior to 1925 could contribute to both sets of exposure duration variables, while someone employed later would contribute only to the post-1925 categories. However, this refinement is too complex for illustrative purposes.

We used four ten-year age groups of 40–49, 50–59, 60–69 and 70–79 years and four calendar periods, 1938–1949, 1950–1959, 1960–1969 and 1970–1977, in order to keep the data file to a reasonable size. In actual practice, five-year intervals of age by calendar year (quinquinquennia) would be considered more appropriate in order to take full account of their potentially confounding effects. In order to be able to

Table 3.2 Standard respiratory cancer death rates and standard weights used for comparative analyses of the Montana smelter workers data

Age range (years)	No. of deaths per 1000 person-years Calendar period				Standard weight (%)
	1938–1949	1950–1959	1960–1969	1970–1977	
40–49	0.14817	0.21896	0.28674	0.37391	37.4
50–59	0.47412	0.80277	1.05824	1.25469	30.1
60–69	0.73136	1.55946	2.33029	2.90461	21.5
70–79	0.73207	1.63585	2.85724	4.22945	11.0

calculate and compare SMRs for the various exposure classes, standard respiratory cancer death rates were determined for each of the 16 age/calendar cells by taking a weighted average of the death rates for the corresponding quinquinquennia (Appendix III), using weights proportional to the observed person–years. For calculation of directly standardized rates by exposure class, we chose weights to be proportional to the age distribution of the 1950 US population (Table 2.5). These weights thus depend only on age and not on calendar year. The standard rates and weights are both shown in Table 3.2.

Table 3.3 presents summary data on the numbers of respiratory cancer deaths and person-years allocated to each exposure category by this method, as well as the results of certain analyses described below. Deaths and person-years that occurred outside the age range 40–79 years are ignored. The entire set of data records, consisting of observed respiratory cancer deaths and person-years denominators for each combination of age, period and exposure, as well as other data, is listed in Appendix V. Note that age-year-exposure categories with no person-years of observation are omitted. The omissions are due largely to the fact that persons hired before 1925 could not contribute observations to the younger age groups during the later calendar intervals.

A major weakness of the Lee and Fraumeni study, which also affects all the analyses of the Montana data reported in this monograph, is the lack of smoking histories for the 8014 smelter workers. Welsh et al. (1982) subsequently ascertained smoking information by mail questionnaire or telephone interviews from a random sample of 1800 men, using proxy respondents for men who had died. They reported that the percentage of smokers was higher than for the USA as a whole, and this could well explain the high rates of respiratory cancer and ischaemic heart disease even in the 'low' exposure category. There was little difference in smoking habits among men in the arsenic categories, however, so that the dose-response relationships are unlikely to be confounded by smoking. However, the positive effects of certain other variables on respiratory cancer, notably foreign birthplace, could well be secondary to the effects of smoking. Unfortunately, the smoking data were not available and could not be considered in the illustrative analyses.

Table 3.3 Dose-response analysis of respiratory cancer deaths among Montana smelter workers, based on external standardization

	Cumulative years of moderate/heavy arsenic exposure (lagged two years)				
	0–0.9	1.0–4.9	5.0–14.9	15+	Total
Workers employed prior to 1925					
No. of observed deaths	51	17	13	34	115
Person-years (×1000)	19.017	2.683	2.600	3.871	28.171
Crude rate (per 1000 person-years)	2.681	6.337	5.000	8.783	4.082
Standardized rate (per 1000 person-years)	2.641	7.433	5.832	7.397	4.215
Standard population rate[a] (per 1000 person-years)	1.185	1.185	1.185	1.185	1.185
Expected deaths (E_k^*) (standard population)	21.47	2.95	2.76	4.44	31.62
CMF (%)	222.8	627.0	492.0	624.0	355.6
SMR (%)	237.5	577.1	471.7	765.0	363.7
Relative risk (ratio of SMRs)	1.0	2.43	1.99	3.22	
Adjusted expected ($\bar{E}_k^*$)	78.10	10.71	10.02	16.17	115.00

Test for homogeneity of SMR: $\chi_3^2 = 33.7$; test for trend: $\chi_1^2 = 30.5$

	0–0.9	1.0–4.9	5.0–14.9	15+	Total
Workers employed 1925 or later					
No. of observed deaths	100	38	15	8	161
Person-years (× 1000)	74.677	13.693	5.940	2.510	96.820
Crude rate (per 1000 person-years)	1.339	2.775	2.525	3.187	1.663
Standardized rate (per 1000 person-years)	1.557	2.409	2.482	3.949[b]	1.824
Standard population rate[a] (per 1000 person-years)	1.031	1.031	1.031	1.057[b]	1.031
Expected deaths (E_k^*) (standard population)	74.12	13.84	6.83	3.66	98.46
CMF (%)	155.1	233.7	240.8	373.6[b]	177.0
SMR (%)	134.9	274.6	219.6	218.4	163.5
Relative risk (ratio of SMRs)	1.0	2.04	1.63	1.62	
Adjusted expected ($\bar{E}_k^*$)	121.21	22.63	11.17	5.99	161.00

Test for homogeneity of SMR: $\chi_3^2 = 16.14$; test for trend: $\chi_1^2 = 8.74$

[a] See Example 3.1
[b] Based on 14 age × calendar periods for which data are available (see Appendix V) and therefore not comparable to the others. The other exposure categories have data for all 16 age × calendar periods.

3.3 Comparison of directly standardized rates

The goal of a comparative analysis is to describe the effects of the different levels of exposure on death rates from particular diseases. Ideally, this should be done at fixed levels of potentially confounding variables such as age and calendar year. However, the large number of comparisons and the instability of the component rates would then

Table 3.4 Notation used for two-way classification of
deaths and person-years

Stratum (j)		Exposure level (k)				
		1	2	... K	Total	
1	Deaths	d_{11}	d_{12}	... d_{1K}	D_1	
	Person-years	n_{11}	n_{12}	... n_{1K}	N_1	
2	Deaths	d_{21}	d_{22}	... d_{2K}	D_2	
	Person-years	n_{21}	n_{22}	... n_{2K}	N_2	
$\vdots$		$\vdots$	$\vdots$	$\vdots\vdots\vdots$	$\vdots$	
J	Deaths	d_{J1}	d_{J2}	... d_{JK}	D_J	
	Person-years	n_{J1}	n_{J2}	... n_{JK}	N_J	
Total	Deaths	O_1	O_2	... O_K	O_+	
	Person-years	n_{+1}	n_{+2}	... n_{+K}	$N_+ = n_{++}$	

make for a rather confusing picture. In our example, 16 separate evaluations depending on the particular age/year stratum would be required. One possible remedy is to base the evaluation on a summary measure such as the directly standardized rate.

Table 3.4 introduces some notation for the number of deaths and person-years of observation in each of J strata $(j = 1, \ldots, J)$ and K exposure categories $(k = 1, \ldots, K)$. Thus, the directly standardized rate for the kth exposure level may be written

$$\hat{\Lambda}_k = \sum_{j=1}^{J} w_j d_{jk}/n_{jk}, \tag{3.1}$$

where the weights are assumed to have been normalized so as to sum to one. These are divided by the standard population rate $\sum w_j \lambda_j^*$ in order to find the CMFs for each level. In the examples below, the standard weights depend only on age (Table 3.2).

Example 3.1

Table 3.3 illustrates the application of several elementary methods to the grouped data from the Montana study. Crude and directly standardized death rates are shown in the first few rows of each part of the table, the two parts corresponding to the pre- and post-1925 subcohorts created to illustrate the effect of date of hire. Stratum-specific death rates for each exposure group, calculated from the deaths and person-years in Appendix V, were multiplied by the standard weights (Table 3.2) and summed to give the directly standardized rate. The standard population rate used for comparison is simply the weighted average of the stratum-specific standard rates, the same weights being used for each calendar period. Both sets of standardized rates were divided by the total of the weights for those age × calendar periods that had some person-years of observation for the particular exposure category. In the second part of Table 3.3, note the limitation in the use of the standardized rate as a comparative measure caused by a lack of data for certain age × calendar periods for persons with the longest exposure. There is a substantial jump in the standardized rates as one progresses from the first to the second exposure category, but a less obvious trend thereafter.

In actual epidemiological practice, examination of dose-response trends in terms of directly standardized rates or CMFs seems largely and properly to be limited to studies in which there are substantial numbers of deaths in each exposure category. This ensures that the standardized rates are reasonably stable, so that evidence for a trend should be clear from a simple examination of the data. Although questions of statistical significance are generally not at issue, it is nonetheless prudent to report the standard

Table 3.5 Age-standardized death rates (all causes combined) and mortality ratios among male ex-smokers of 1–19 cigarettes per day, ages 50–74 years[a]

Smoking category	Number of men	Number of deaths	Standardized death rate (per 100 000 person-years)	CMF
Current smokers	118 373	9 117	2 359	172
Ex-smokers by years since last smoked				
Under 1	814	64	2 212	161
1–4	1 986	144	1 985	144
5–9	1 909	128	1 840	134
10+	4 578	255	1 397	102
Nonsmokers	62 332	3 512	1 374	100

[a] From Hammond (1966)

error of each summary rate (equation (2.7)) as a means of judging its stability. In case of uncertainty about the statistical significance of the observed results, the reciprocals of the corresponding variances could be employed as empirical weights in a formal regression analysis of the directly standardized rates on quantitative exposure variables. Such a regression analysis could also be helpful if the summary data were the only data available, for example, if they were obtained from published sources. However, statisticians have pointed out the need for caution in regression analyses of standard rates or other indices that have (age-specific) population denominators in both dependent and independent variables.

Example 3.2

The American Cancer Society study of one million men and women (Hammond, 1966) furnishes an example in which numbers of deaths are sufficiently large that direct standardization is appropriate. The effect of smoking on mortality was reported in terms of the ratios of the standardized death rates for various categories of smokers relative to the standardized rate for nonsmokers. Table 3.5, which concerns smokers of 1–19 cigarettes per day, indicates that cessation of smoking for increasing lengths of time results in a decline in the all-causes death rate compared to that for continuing smokers. Ten years after cessation of exposure, the death rate among ex-smokers is down nearly to the level among lifelong nonsmokers.

3.4 Comparison of standardized mortality ratios

If the data are not so extensive and questions of sampling variability are of greater concern, it is generally appropriate to use the SMR in place of the CMF as a measure of how the death rates in each exposure category compare with those of the standard population. Evidence for a dose-response trend may then be sought in terms of an increase or decrease in the SMRs with increasing exposure. Referring to Table 3.4, let us denote by $O_k = \sum_j d_{jk}$ the observed number of deaths in the kth exposure group. Keeping to the convention that quantities calculated from external standard rates are starred (*), the expected numbers of deaths may be written

$$E_k^* = \sum_j n_{jk} \lambda_j^* \tag{3.2}$$

and the standardized mortality ratios

$$\text{SMR}_k = O_k / E_k^* . \tag{3.3}$$

The grand totals of observed and expected deaths are denoted by $O_+ = \sum O_k$ and $E_+^* = \sum E_k^*$, respectively.

The overall SMR for the entire cohort is given by O_+/E_+^*, which was discussed in detail in Chapter 2. Here we are interested in comparisons among the different subcohorts, that is, among the different SMR_ks. When examining the SMR_ks for a trend with increasing exposure, it should be kept in mind that they are relative measures of effect calculated with reference to an external set of rates and that they may not be strictly comparable to one another. For reasons discussed at length in §2.3, ratios of the SMR_ks for different exposure categories may fail to summarize adequately the ratios of the stratum-specific rates. This occurs in precisely those circumstances when the SMR_ks themselves are not good summary measures, namely when the ratios of cohort to standard death rates vary widely from one stratum to another. For example, it might happen that heavier exposures had the effect of adding progressively greater amounts to the age-specific (background) rates that would be expected in the absence of exposure. However, if much higher background rates were expected with the heavier exposures, for instance, because persons with such exposures tended to be older, such an additive dose-response relationship could well be missed by a comparison of SMR_ks.

Example 3.3

Table 3.6 presents fictitious data that illustrate the phenomenon just described. The effect of increasing exposure is to increase the two age-specific death rates by 2 per 100 person-years (low exposure) or 4 per 100

Table 3.6   Fictitious data to illustrate a potential defect in the SMR

	Age range (years)			SMR (%)	CMF (%)
	35–44	45–54	Total		
Unexposed					
Rate (per 100)	3	10	3.7	176	100
Population	900	100	1000		
No. of observed deaths	27	10	37		
No. of expected deaths	9	12	21		
Lightly exposed					
Rate (per 100)	5	12	8.5	131	131
Population	500	500	1000		
No. of observed deaths	25	60	85		
No. of expected deaths	5	60	65		
Heavily exposed					
Rate (per 100)	7	14	13.3	121	161
Population	100	900	1000		
No. of observed deaths	7	126	133		
No. of expected deaths	1	108	109		
Standard population					
Rate	1	12	6.5		
Weight	0.5	0.5	1.0		

person-years (high exposure). These increases are reflected in increases in the CMFs, which are averages of the age-specific rates. However, due to the very skewed age distribution and the fact that the cohort to standard rate ratios vary markedly with age, the apparent trend as measured by the three SMR_ks is reversed. Compare Table 2.13.

Fortunately, the statistical confounding is not so serious in typical applications, and a dose-response analysis carried out in terms of SMR_ks often yields results that are quite similar to those obtained by other methods. The formal assumption required for an SMR analysis to be completely appropriate is that the stratum-specific death rates for each exposure class be proportional to the external standard rates, this being precisely the condition needed to assure comparability of the SMR_ks. This assumption may be investigated in practice by fitting an explicit model and comparing the observed and fitted number of deaths in each stratum-exposure cell, using the techniques described in the next chapter. Thus, the data themselves should give indications of situations in which inferences based on the SMR are liable to be seriously in error. When there appears to be heterogeneity of (multiplicative) dose-response effects between different age strata, it is better to use a different model to describe this heterogeneity rather than to summarize a number of disparate effects in a single SMR.

When the proportionality assumption holds, we may regard the total number of deaths, O_k, observed at the kth exposure level as having an approximate Poisson distribution with mean $\theta_k E_k^*$, where E_k^* represents the expected number of deaths and θ_k the unknown SMR for this level of exposure in relation to the standard rates (see §4.3). The ratios of SMR_ks, which we denote $\psi_k = \theta_k/\theta_1$, thus represent relative risks for each exposure level using the first level as baseline ($\psi_1 = 1$). These have precisely the same interpretation as do the relative risk parameters ψ_k estimated in case-control studies (§4.5 of Volume 1). They represent the ratios of age-specific rates for different exposure categories, assuming these to be constant over age-calendar year strata.

In this section we consider methods for estimating the individual relative risks, for determining their standard errors, for testing the statistical significance of each one individually, and for testing the global null hypothesis that the ψ_k equal unity (i.e., the SMR_ks are equal) for $k = 1, \ldots, K$ against alternatives of heterogeneity and trend. The tests involve a comparison of the observed numbers O_k with fitted values $\bar{E}_k^*$ calculated under the hypothesis that each θ_k is equal to some common value θ. These latter are easily obtained by distributing the total deaths O_+ among the K exposure levels in proportion to the expected numbers:

$$\bar{E}_k^* = O_+(E_k^*/E_+^*). \tag{3.4}$$

We refer to the $\bar{E}_k^*$ as 'adjusted expected values' to reflect the fact that they are equal to the E_k^* scaled by the overall SMR, O_+/E_+^*, so as to ensure that $\sum_k \bar{E}_k^* = \sum_k O_k$.

(a) Two dose levels: exposed versus unexposed

The simplest comparison is between two levels of exposure, say exposed ($k = 2$) versus unexposed ($k = 1$). Thus, we regard O_1 as a Poisson variable with mean $\theta_1 E_1^*$ and O_2 as Poisson with mean $\theta_2 E_2^*$. If we set $\theta = \theta_1$, $\psi = \psi_2 = \theta_2/\theta_1$ and $\theta\psi = \theta_2$, suppressing the subscripts for clarity, the parameter of interest is the relative risk ψ, θ

playing the role of a nuisance parameter that interferes with our inferences concerning ψ. According to standard principles of statistical inference (Cox & Hinkley, 1974), it is appropriate in such circumstances to consider a distribution for the observed data which depends only on the parameter of interest. This is quite easy here since the distribution of two Poisson variates conditional on their sum is binomial (Lehman, 1959). More precisely,

$$pr(O_2|O_+; \theta, \psi) = \binom{O_+}{O_2} \pi^{O_2}(1 - \pi)^{O_1}, \qquad (3.5)$$

where

$$\pi = \frac{\psi E_2^*}{E_1^* + \psi E_2^*}$$

or, equivalently,

$$\psi = \frac{\pi E_1^*}{(1 - \pi)E_2^*}. \qquad (3.6)$$

Statistical inferences about the relative risk ψ, whether exact or approximate, may therefore be carried out by making inferences about the binomial parameter π in (3.5) and then transforming *via* (3.6). They are formally identical to those used in the analysis of matched case-control pairs with dichotomous exposures (§5.2 of Volume 1). The relevant equations need merely be rewritten for use with cohort data.

Under the null hypothesis $\psi_0 = 1$ we have $\pi_0 = E_2^*/E_+^*$, and an exact test is obtained from the tail probability of the corresponding binomial distribution. For example, if $O_2 > E_2^*$, the one-sided significance level or p value is given by

$$p = \sum_{x=O_2}^{O_+} \binom{O_+}{O_2} \pi_0^x (1 - \pi_0)^{O_+-x}.$$

In practice, it will usually suffice to use the approximate chi-square statistic based on the observed deviation of O_2 from its expectation. This may be written

$$\chi^2 = \frac{\{|O_2 - E(O_2)| - \frac{1}{2}\}^2}{\mathrm{Var}(O_2)} = \frac{\{|O_1 - \bar{E}_1^*| - \frac{1}{2}\}^2}{\bar{E}_1^*} + \frac{\{|O_2 - \bar{E}_2^*| - \frac{1}{2}\}^2}{\bar{E}_2^*}, \qquad (3.7)$$

where we have used the fact that $\mathrm{Var}(O_2) = O_+\pi_0(1 - \pi_0) = \bar{E}_1^*\bar{E}_2^*/(\bar{E}_1^* + \bar{E}_2^*)$ and $O_1 - \bar{E}_1^* = -(O_2 - \bar{E}_2^*)$. The numerator(s) in (3.7) are reduced in absolute value by 1/2 before squaring for a continuity correction.

(b) Point and interval estimation of the relative risk

The maximum likelihood estimate of π is $\hat{\pi} = O_2/O_+$, from which it follows that the maximum likelihood estimate of ψ is

$$\hat{\psi} = \frac{\hat{\pi}\bar{E}_1^*}{(1 - \hat{\pi})\bar{E}_2^*} = \frac{O_2 E_1^*}{O_1 E_2^*}, \qquad (3.8)$$

the ratio of the two SMR_ks. Exact $100(1 - \alpha)\%$ confidence limits for π may be found from the charts of Pearson and Hartley (1966) or computed using the equations

$$\pi_L = \frac{O_2}{O_2 + (O_1 + 1)F_{\alpha/2}(2O_1 + 2, 2O_2)}$$

and (3.9)

$$\pi_U = \frac{(O_2 + 1)F_{\alpha/2}(2O_2 + 2, 2O_1)}{O_1 + (O_2 + 1)F_{\alpha/2}(2O_2 + 2, 2O_1)}$$

where $F_{\alpha/2}(v_1, v_2)$ denotes the upper $100_{\alpha/2}$ percentile of the F distribution with v_1 and v_2 degrees of freedom. The limits (3.9) are inserted into (3.6) to obtain confidence limits ψ_L and ψ_U for the relative risk. Alternatively, approximate limits based on the normal approximation to the binomial probabilities (Cornfield, 1956) are given as the solutions to the equations

$$E_1^*(O_2 - 1/2) - \psi_L E_2^*(O_1 + 1/2) = +Z_{\alpha/2}\{\psi_L E_1^* E_2^*(O_1 + O_2)\}^{1/2}$$

and (3.10)

$$E_1^*(O_2 + 1/2) - \psi_U E_2^*(O_1 - 1/2) = -Z_{\alpha/2}\{\psi_U E_1^* E_2^*(O_1 + O_2)\}^{1/2}.$$

These are quadratic equations in the unknown variable $\xi = \sqrt{\psi}$.

Example 3.4

Suppose $O_1 = 5$ and $O_2 = 14$ bladder cancer deaths are observed among unexposed and exposed members of an industrial cohort, respectively, whereas $E_1 = 7.3$ and $E_2 = 5.5$ were expected from vital statistics available for the region in which the plant was located. The overall SMR is $O_+/E_+ = 19/12.8 = 1.484$, and adjusted expected values are $\bar{E}_1^* = 7.3 \times 1.484 = 10.84$ and $\bar{E}_2^* = 5.5 \times 1.484 = 8.16$. Individual SMRs are $5/7.3 = 0.685$ and $14/5.5 = 2.545$ for unexposed and exposed so that $\hat{\psi} = 2.545/0.685 = 3.72$ is the point estimate of relative risk. The test (3.7) for the hypothesis $\psi = 1$ gives

$$\chi^2 = \frac{(5 - 10.84 + 0.5)^2}{8.16} + \frac{(14 - 8.16 - 0.5)^2}{10.84} = 6.13$$

with continuity correction ($p = 0.01$). Using equation (3.9) and the fact that $F_{0.025}(12, 28) = 2.45$ and $F_{0.025}(30, 10) = 3.31$, exact 95% confidence limits on the associated binominal probability are

$$\pi_L = \frac{14}{14 + 6(2.45)} = 0.488$$

and

$$\pi_U = \frac{15(3.31)}{5 + 15(3.31)} = 0.908,$$

from which we determine $\psi_L = 1.26$ and $\psi_U = 13.2$ as limits on the relative risk. The approximate limits are found as solutions to

$$98.55 - \psi_L 30.25 = 1.96\{\psi_L 762.85\}^{1/2}$$

and

$$105.85 - \psi_U 24.75 = -1.96\{\psi_U 762.85\}^{1/2},$$

these being $\psi_L = 1.25$ and $\psi_U = 11.8$, respectively.

(c) Testing for heterogeneity and trend in the SMRs

The same methods may be used to estimate the relative risks ψ_k for each level of exposure $k = 2, \ldots, K$ and to test the significance of each one individually. One merely substitutes O_k and $\bar{E}_k^*$ for O_2 and $\bar{E}_2^*$ in equations (3.7) through (3.10). However, since interpretation of a large number of separate comparisons is difficult, we also need a test of the hypothesis that all K ψ_k are simultaneously equal to unity. This is easy to derive using the framework already introduced (Kilpatrick, 1962, 1963). Conditional on the total observed deaths, O_+, the joint distribution of $O = (O_1, \ldots, O_K)$ under the null hypothesis is multinomial with cell occupancy probabilities $(\pi_1, \ldots, \pi_K)$ where $\pi_k = E_k^*/E_+^*$. A test of the global null hypothesis is thus achieved by comparing the O_k to the fitted values $\bar{E}_k^*$ using the standard criterion

$$\chi_{K-1}^2 = \sum_{k=1}^{K} \frac{(O_k - \bar{E}_k^*)^2}{\bar{E}_k^*}, \qquad (3.11)$$

which should be referred to tables of the chi-square distribution with $K - 1$ degrees of freedom.

One disadvantage of (3.11) is its relative lack of power against the specific alternative hypothesis of a trend in the SMR_ks with increasing exposure. Even if none of the pairwise comparisons of baseline and exposure groups nor the multi-degree of freedom statistic (3.11) yields a significant result, substantial evidence for a dose-response trend may nevertheless be generated if the estimated relative risks are in the hypothesized order. The Poisson trend statistic (Armitage, 1955; Tarone, 1982) was designed especially to detect such monotonic dose-response relationships. If x_k denotes a quantitative dose level associated with the kth exposure category, this single degree of freedom test is given by

$$\chi_1^2 = \frac{\{\sum_{k=1}^{K} x_k(O_k - \bar{E}_k^*)\}^2}{\sum_{k=1}^{K} x_k^2 \bar{E}_k^* - (\sum_{k=1}^{K} x_k \bar{E}_k^*)^2/O_+}. \qquad (3.12)$$

In situations in which the categories are merely ordered, and there is no specific quantitative exposure, it suffices to set $x_k = k$. Formal justification for both (3.11) and (3.12) stems from the fact that they are efficient score tests under various sets of assumptions, including the log linear models for Poisson variables discussed in the next chapter (Tarone & Gart, 1980).

Example 3.5

Returning to the Montana data, the standard rates shown in Table 3.2 were used in conjunction with the data in Appendix V to produce expected numbers of deaths and SMR_ks for each exposure category using equations (3.2) and (3.3). With the exception of the highest dose category for the post-1924 cohort, the SMR_ks are in reasonable agreement with the corresponding CMF_ks (Table 3.3). However, the CMF for this category is not comparable to the others since there are no data for the earliest calendar period for two age groups. To alleviate this difficulty, we could, of course, restrict all CMFs to those age × calendar period strata for which full data are available. Relative risks obtained by dividing each SMR_k by the SMR for 0–0.9 years exposed indicate that workers hired before 1925 who had 15 or more years of moderate to heavy arsenic exposure have mortality rates from respiratory cancer that are approximately three times higher than the rates among workers who remained in areas of the plant where only light exposures occurred.

The penultimate rows in both parts of Table 3.3 show the adjusted expected values $\bar{E}_k^*$ for the four exposure categories. These were obtained in accordance with equation (3.4), multiplying the expected numbers shown in the sixth row of each part of the table by the overall SMR. In the $0 - 0.9$ years exposure group for pre-1925 employees, for example, we have $21.47 \times (115/31.62) = 78.10$ cases expected after adjustment. The global test (3.11) yields

$$\chi_3^2 = \frac{(51 - 78.10)^2}{78.10} + \frac{(17 - 10.71)^2}{10.71} + \frac{(13 - 10.02)^2}{10.02} + \frac{(34 - 16.17)^2}{16.17} = 33.7$$

as shown at the bottom of the first part of Table 3.3. Likewise, the trend statistic (3.12) is

$$\chi_1^2 = \frac{\{1 \times (51 - 78.10) + 2 \times (17 - 10.71) + 3 \times (13 - 10.02) + 4 \times (34 - 16.17)\}^2}{(1 \times 78.10 + 4 \times 10.71 + 9 \times 10.02 + 16 \times 16.17) - (78.10 + 2 \times 10.71 + 3 \times 10.02 + 4 \times 16.17)^2/115} = 30.5$$

Note the use of the coded levels $x_k = k$ in this example.

(d) Trend test for exposure effect versus trend test for dose-response

The object of a dose-response analysis is to demonstrate a continuously increasing response to increasing dose or, in the present context, a continuously increasing (relative) risk with increasing exposure. While the trend statistic (3.12) is designed to detect such alternatives to the null hypothesis (no effect of exposure), it may sometimes give a significant result even if the relative risks are not continuously increasing. This could happen, for example, if the risk were increased for any amount of exposure relative to no exposure but the risks among the different exposure levels remained constant. The causal inference linking exposure and disease is less secure in such cases, because of the greater possibility that a dose-response function that jumps up initially and then remains flat could be produced by bias or confounding. For example, the weak relationship between coffee drinking and bladder cancer observed in several case-control studies was interpreted as noncausal on just such a basis (§3.2 of Volume 1). One may wish to restrict the trend statistic to a comparison of positive dose or duration levels and exclude the baseline nonexposed category when testing specifically for a dose-response effect.

Example 3.6

Returning to Table 3.3, we noted significant 'trends' in relative risk with increasing duration of heavy/medium arsenic exposure for both the pre-1925 and post-1925 sub-cohorts ($\chi_1^2 = 30.5$ and 8.74, respectively). However, the relative risk estimates in fact showed little variation among the three highest categories of exposure. Restricting the trend analyses to the categories 1.0–4.9 years duration, 5.0–14.9 years, and 15+ years, this being accomplished by adjusting the expected values to agree with the total observed for the three categories, and applying the usual statistic (3.12), we find $\chi_1^2 = 1.67$ ($p = 0.19$) for the pre-1925 cohort and $\chi_1^2 = 0.60$ ($p = 0.44$) for the post-1925 cohort. This confirms what is already apparent from an examination of the relative risks, namely, that there is no evidence for an increasing dose-response trend with exposure duration above one year.

If the object of the analysis is primarily to test for a possible carcinogenic effect, however, the baseline or lowest dose level should definitely be included in calculation of the trend. An issue that then arises is whether the intercept of the regression line of SMR on dose, the slope of which is implicitly being tested in a trend analysis, necessarily passes through unity or instead through some other value that represents the true position of the cohort vis-à-vis the standard population. If the true SMR at zero dose were somehow known a priori to be equal to one, although this is unlikely in practice, this would permit a more powerful analysis and yield a more significant result on average (Gilbert, 1983).

The trend statistic (3.12) implicitly assumes that the intercept is being estimated from the data. One argument in favour of estimating the intercept is that the cohort may have higher death rates than expected even in the low dose range, due to the effects of other risk factors. Or the initial SMR may be less than 1 due to a 'healthy worker' selection effect. A trend analysis that assumed it was equal to 1 would yield a trend test statistic that was too large in the first case and too small in the second. With the Montana study, for example, the SMR_ks for respiratory cancer in the lowest dose groups are 237.5% and 134.9% for the pre- and post-1925 cohorts, respectively (Table 3.3). It is unclear whether the excess is due to generally higher levels of smoking in the study population or to the effects of arsenic exposures that even 'low dose' persons may receive. Thomas, D.C. and McNeill (1982) note that other reasons for the regression line not to pass through unity at zero dose, besides the possible noncomparability of the standard population, are that the assumed dose-response function is wrong or that random errors in dose measurement have led to a slope estimate that is too shallow. In the face of such uncertainty, it does not seem prudent to make a strong assumption about the intercept.

(e) Selection of the dose metameter

In order to carry out the test for trend we must assign quantitative values to each exposure category. Underlying the test is the implicit assumption that some transformation of the disease rate is a linear function of a dose variable x. It is the slope of this relation that is being tested (Tarone & Gart, 1980). Thought should be given to the most appropriate values, since the choice sometimes can have a substantial influence on the significance of the result. Often one will want to choose the dose scale so that there is an approximately linear relationship between disease rates and exposures, at least at low doses. Multistage models of carcinogenesis (Chapter 6) suggest a low-order polynomial relationship of the form $\lambda(d) = \beta_0 + \beta_1 d + \beta_2 d^2 + \ldots$, where all coefficients are positive. These imply that there is an approximately linear relationship between relative risk and exposure at low (measured) doses. Other assignments of x values to exposure categories may be tried also, although problems of interpretation will arise if a large number of separate tests are carried out on the same data.

Example 3.7

Table 3.7 shows numbers of deaths from haematological malignancies among workers at the Portsmouth (US) Naval Shipyard, according to the cumulative radiation exposure received by the time of death (Najarian, 1983). Also shown are person-years denominators by dose category. In order to test for a trend in the Poisson rates with increasing dose, we use Armitage's (1955) statistic, which has the same form as (3.12) except that the expected deaths $\bar{E}_k$ are obtained by allocating the total deaths in proportion to the person-years in each category. Both observed and expected deaths are shown in Table 3.7.

Note that the intervals used for grouping the data into exposure categories are approximately logarithmic. After the initial control category, each group of radiation doses is approximately ten times larger than the preceding one. Thus, the usual assignment of coded values $x_k = k$ to the $K = 7$ exposure categories effectively means that a log dose metameter is being used. An alternative would be to use a linear dose metameter, assigning to each exposure category the average of the doses included within it. Someone who believed that the true dose-response curve was discontinuous and that there was a threshold at 1 rad might

Table 3.7 Observed and expected deaths from haematological malignancies among Portsmouth (USA) Naval Shipyard workers, by cumulative radiation dose[a]

Lifetime dose (rems)	No. of observed deaths	No. of person-years	No. of expected deaths[b]	Dose metameters		
				Linear	Log	Threshold
0.000	2	24 232	3.36	0.0	1	0
0.001–0.030	2	14 810	2.06	0.015	2	0
0.030–0.100	0	15 960	2.22	0.065	3	0
0.100–0.500	4	24 138	3.35	0.30	4	0
0.500–1.00	1	10 418	1.45	0.75	5	0
1.00–5.00	7	21 769	3.02	3.0	6	1
5.00+	1	11 128	1.54	6.0	7	1
Total	17	122 455	17.00			
Test for trend (χ_1^2):				1.19	2.25	3.53
p value (one-sided):				0.14	0.07	0.03

[a] From Najarian (1983)
[b] Assuming constant rate in all dose groups

assign $x_k = 0$ for $k = 1, 2, 3, 4, 5$, and $x_k = 1$ for $k = 6$ and 7. We would have to be suspicious of this choice for the threshold, however, since setting it at 1 rad for these particular data obviously maximizes the difference in relative risks one will observe between the 'exposed' ($x_k = 1$) and 'unexposed' ($x_k = 0$).

The three dose metameters lead to rather different trend statistics in this example. The logarithmic scale yields $\chi^2 = 2.25$ ($p = 0.07$; one-sided), whereas the value on the arithmetic scale is somewhat lower at $\chi^2 = 1.19$ ($p = 0.14$). The most significant result is obtained from the threshold model comparing doses over and under 1 rad ($\chi^2 = 3.53$, $p = 0.03$). Setting the threshold at 0.5 rads reduces χ^2 from 3.53 to 2.32, indicating the sensitivity to a basically arbitrary threshold. Since the results obtained with the continuous scales do not attain statistical significance, one would conclude little more than that the situation perhaps warranted further investigation. No excess of deaths due to cancer nor specifically to cancer of the blood or blood-forming tissues was found in the analysis of these data performed by Rinsky et al. (1981). It seems likely that the positive results reported from the earlier proportional mortality study (Najarian & Colton, 1978) were biased by the incomplete ascertainment of deaths that had occurred among workers at the facility (Committee on the Biological Effects of Ionizing Radiation, 1980). See also the discussion in §1.6.

(f) Alternative tests for trend

The statistic (3.12) that we have suggested for a trend test relies heavily on the assumed Poisson variability of the observed numbers of deaths. In some situations in which there are a large number of different comparison groups, it may be more prudent to carry out a standard regression analysis of the SMR_ks or their logarithms on the quantitative dose levels. Especially when the SMR_ks are calculated for different intervals of calendar time, the observed variation in numbers of deaths between adjacent time intervals may be greater than would be expected from Poisson sampling variation. It is then more appropriate to evaluate the linear time trend against the observed background of year-to-year variation rather than against the smaller theoretical variance. The issue is complicated by the fact that the estimate of residual variation from the regression analysis may be heavily dependent on the particular regression model chosen, or may be unstable because the number of different dose categories does not provide a sufficient number of 'degrees of freedom' for error estimation. Furthermore, there is some controversy regarding the extent to which one should account for the underlying Poisson variability by giving greater weight in the regression analysis to SMR_ks based on large numbers of deaths.

The ideal solution is probably intermediate between an unweighted analysis, in which most of the observed variability is attributed to extraneous factors rather than sampling, and an analysis based entirely on Poisson sampling theory (Pocock et al., 1981; Breslow, 1984a). A practical alternative is to carry out both Poisson and unweighted regressions and compare results.

Example 3.8

Table 3.8 presents data from the study of Rocky Mountain uranium miners quoted by Thomas, D.C. and McNeill (1982). There is a reasonably linear relationship between the logarithm of the SMR and the logarithm of the average cumulative radiation exposure, measured in working level months (WLM) (Fig. 3.2). As noted in equation (2.9), the (Poisson) variance of the log SMR is estimated approximately by the reciprocal of the number of deaths, which suggests we use the number of deaths to weight the individual observations. A weighted linear regression analysis of log SMR on log WLM yields a residual (weighted) sum of squares of 6.68 on six degrees of freedom. We conclude that the extra-Poisson variability in this case is minor or nonexistent, since, otherwise, the residual mean square would be substantially larger than one. The corresponding F statistic for the significance of the linear trend is 57.4 on one and six degrees of freedom. An unweighted analysis yields $F_{1,6} = 59.8$. Both results confirm the highly significant $\chi_1^2 = 95$ that is found from the usual trend test (3.12).

If one considers instead a linear regression of the SMR_k on dose x_k, weighting each observation by $(E_k^*)^2/O_k$, where E_k^* is the expected and O_k the observed number of deaths, the residual mean square is $11.09/6 = 1.85$. In view of the preceding results, the excess above unity is probably due more to the lack of fit of the linear model than to non-Poisson variation. The F statistics are 41.9 for the weighted analysis and 261.4 for the unweighted. The discrepancy between the weighted and unweighted test statistics on the arithmetic scale results from the data point for the highest dose category being far removed from the others and having a much greater influence on the unweighted analysis than the weighted one. This instability reminds us of the dangers of the uncritical use of least-squares regression techniques, especially with small samples, and suggests that they are best reserved for situations in which there is a large number of dose categories. Alternatively, modern techniques of robust regression (Huber, 1983) may be used.

Table 3.8   Lung cancer risk in US uranium miners[a]

Cumulative WLM[b]		Person-years	Lung cancers		SMR (%)
Range	Midpoint		Observed	Expected	
0–119	60	5 183	3	3.96	76
120–239	180	3 308	7	2.24	312
240–359	300	2 891	9	2.24	402
360–599	480	4 171	19	3.33	571
600–839	720	3 294	9	2.62	344
840–1 799	1 320	6 591	40	5.38	743
1 800–3 719	2 760	5 690	49	4.56	1 075
>3 719	7 000 (est)	1 068	23	0.91	2 727
All	1 180 (mean)	32 196	159	25.24	

[a] From Committee on the Biological Effects of Ionizing Radiation (1980) as quoted by Thomas, D.C. and McNeill (1982)
[b] WLM, working-level-month measure of cumulative exposure

Fig. 3.2   Log–log plots of SMRs for US uranium miners from Table 3.8

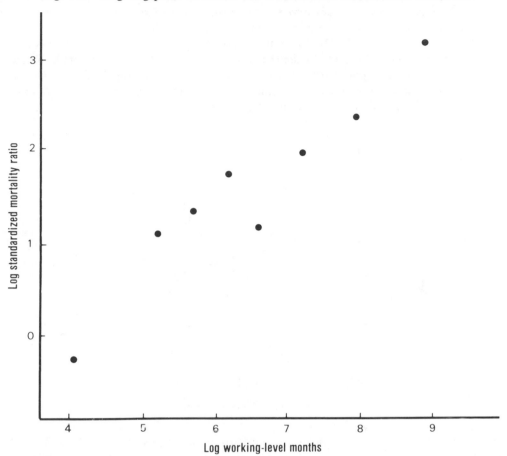

(g) Some examples from the literature

Doll and Peto (1976) reported results of the 20-year follow-up of British doctors to study cigarette smoking and mortality. Most of their analyses compared cause-specific mortality rates among exposure categories determined by smoking history, using methods of internal standardization that are described below. However, the authors also wanted to see whether the fact that doctors gave up smoking more rapidly than members of the general population was reflected in an improvement in their relative survival. Thus, mortality rates for all of England and Wales were used as a standard for computation of SMR_ks for each calendar year for two causes of death (Fig. 3.3). The evident decline in the relative rates of lung cancer was confirmed by a least-squares linear regression analysis of the $20\,SMR_k$s on calendar year.

Another example illustrates more specifically the use of the Poisson trend statistic. Table 3.9 presents leukaemia mortality rates during various intervals following first

Fig. 3.3   Trend in number of deaths certified in British male doctors as percentage of
number expected from experience of all men in England and Wales of the
same ages. Results are given from the second to the twentieth years of study
for lung cancer (●) (459 deaths observed *versus* 931.9 expected) and all
other cancers (○) (1238 deaths observed *versus* 1630.7 expected). Regression lines on time were calculated from data for the fourth to the twentieth
years of study (regression coefficients: −1.4 for lung cancer and 0.0 for all
other cancers). From Doll and Peto (1976)

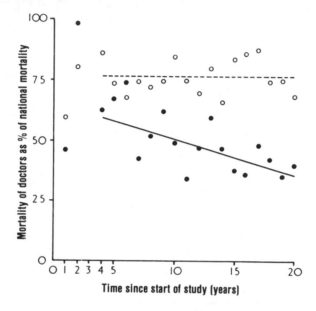

treatment for a cohort of ankylosing spondylitis patients (Smith & Doll, 1982). The
expected numbers shown were also obtained from mortality rates for England and
Wales specific for sex, age and calendar year. In this example, the statistic (3.12) gives
a value of $\chi_1^2 = 10.40$ and provides clear evidence for a decline in the observed:
expected ratios with increasing time since exposure.

Finally, Table 3.10 presents data from a cohort study of US and Canadian insulation

Table 3.9 Observed and expected leukemia deaths among
ankylosing spondylitis patients, by time since initial treatment[a]

	Time since treatment (years)							Total
	0–2	3–5	6–8	9–11	12–14	15–17	18+	
Observed	6	10	6	3	1	4	1	31
Expected	1.00	0.89	0.87	0.90	0.96	0.90	0.95	6.47
SMR	6.00	11.24	6.90	3.33	1.04	4.44	1.05	4.79

[a] From Smith and Doll (1982)

Table 3.10 Lung cancer deaths and person-years among asbestos and insulation workers according to duration of time since initial exposure[a]

Duration (years)	Number of men	Person-years	No. of observed deaths	No. of expected deaths	SMR (%)
0–9	8 190	26 393	0	0.7	—
10–14	9 063	29 003	7	2.7	255
15–19	9 948	34 066	29	8.5	340
20–24	8 887	31 268	59	17.0	348
25–29	6 596	20 657	105	21.0	500
30–34	3 547	11 598	112	18.4	608
35–39	2 020	5 403	65	11.5	568
40–44	1 108	3 160	40	8.1	493
45+	1 448	5 305	69	17.8	389

[a] From Selikoff et al. (1980)

workers (Selikoff et al., 1980). Ratios of observed to expected lung cancer deaths reached a peak between 30–35 years from the initial exposure to asbestos. This does not mean, of course, that the absolute rates of lung cancer decline after 35 years, although this is a common misconception. The death rates continue to increase as the exposed workers grow older, but at a slightly lower rate in comparison to the general population than was true during earlier years. Because the SMRs first rise and then fall, one could well expect the trend statistic not to yield a significant result in this example. Various possible explanations have been suggested for the decline. One is that the combined exposure to asbestos and cigarettes was so lethal that heavy smokers were eliminated from the study cohort at an even faster rate than they were eliminated from the general population. Another possibility is that the termination of exposure following retirement, which would start to occur 35 years or so after initial employment, led to an attenuation of subsequent relative risk but at a much slower pace than that noted for ex-smokers (Table 3.5). Thirdly, it should be noted that there is a strong confounding effect in this cohort between period of initial exposure, when different types of asbestos fibres may have been used or the exposure intensity different, and the time since first exposure. Finally, the SMR_ks reflect any difference in smoking patterns between asbestos workers and the general population, and these also may have been changing over time.

3.5 Comparison of internally standardized mortality ratios

The methods of analysis discussed so far rely on standard rates that are external to the study cohort in order to make comparisons between exposure groups. Questions about the appropriateness of the particular standard selected and the comparability of the resulting SMR_ks suggest that a more satisfactory approach would be to use the observed data, without consideration of any outside rates, when making internal comparisons.

From a theroretical viewpoint, the method of internal standardization is probably best regarded as a rough and ready approximation to the more complicated but more appropriate methods of grouped data analysis that are presented in the next section. If there are only two exposure categories, it tends to yield mildly conservative tests and estimates in typical practice (Bernstein *et al.*, 1981; see also Fig. 4.3). The conservatism could be substantial if age and calendar time or other stratification variables strongly confound the exposure-disease relationship. Nevertheless, the method of internal standardization enjoys a considerable following due to its relative simplicity and strong intuitive appeal.

If there are more than two exposure categories, internal standardization does not eliminate the problem that was discussed at length in §2.3 concerning the comparability of SMRs. Although the external standard is replaced by an internal standard consisting of the combination of all exposure groups, in particular examples this pooled group may be dominated by one or two large exposure groups. When comparing the ratios of SMR_ks for two other exposure groups, therefore, it is possible for the same type of bias to occur.

The calculations required for internal standardization are surprisingly easy. Referring to the data layout in Table 3.4, the stratum-specific death rates calculated without regard to exposure category are $\lambda_j = D_j/N_j$. It follows that the expected number of deaths in the kth exposure class, assuming that exposure had no effect on the rates, is

$$E_k = \sum_{j=1}^{J} n_{jk}\lambda_j = \sum_{j=1}^{J} n_{jk}D_j/N_j. \qquad (3.13)$$

These internally derived fitted values share with the adjusted expected numbers (3.4) the property that their sum is equal to the total number of observed deaths. They are used in place of the $\bar{E}_k^*$ in equations (3.7), (3.8), (3.11) and (3.12) in order to make approximate estimates of the relative risks for each exposure category and approximate tests of their heterogeneity and trend. As already noted, these tests and estimates tend to be somewhat conservative, more so if there is a high degree of association between the stratum variables and the exposures. However, this feature is not well illustrated by the data on the Montana workers, since, as often happens in practice, the degree of confounding is rather slight.

Example 3.9

By pooling the respiratory cancer deaths and person-years shown in Appendix V over period of hire and duration of exposure, one obtains the pooled death rates shown in Table 2.8 by ten-year intervals of age and calendar period. Table 3.11 presents the expected numbers of deaths calculated for each exposure category by multiplying the pooled rates by the appropriate number of person-years and summing in accordance with equation (3.13). Separate analyses were carried out according to period of employment. Note the similarity between the internally fitted values and the adjusted expected values shown in Table 3.3. The latter are slightly more extreme and therefore indicate a slightly steeper dose-response relationship. For example, the estimated relative risk for the highest exposure category among those employed prior to 1925 is 3.22 for external standardization *versus* 3.09 for internal standardization.

Inserting the observed and expected values from Table 3.11 in equations (3.11) and (3.12), following exactly the same method of calculation as in Example 3.5, the values of the tests for heterogeneity and trend are $\chi_3^2 = 31.7$ and $\chi_1^2 = 28.3$, respectively, for the pre-1925 subgroup. These are less than the values found with external standardization, but they are still highly significant ($p < 0.0001$). A similar result holds for the post-1925 subgroup.

Table 3.11 Dose-response analysis of respiratory cancer deaths among Montana smelter workers, based on internal standardization

	Cumulative years of moderate/heavy arsenic exposure				
	0–0.9	1.0–4.9	5.0–14.9	15+	Total
Workers employed before 1925					
No. of observed deaths	51	17	13	34	115
No. of expected deaths (adjusted for age and calendar year)	77.58	10.51	10.18	16.73	115.00
Relative risk (using ratios of Observed/Expected)	1.0	2.46	1.94	3.09	
Relative risk (Mantel-Haenszel)	1.0	2.49	2.00	3.14	

Approximate test for homogeneity, $\chi_3^2 = 31.7$; test for trend, $\chi_1^2 = 28.3$
  (using observed and expected numbers only with equations (3.11) and (3.12))
Complete test for homogeneity, $\chi_3^2 = 31.9$; test for trend, $\chi_1^2 = 28.5$
  (using full variances with equations (3.24) and (3.25))

Workers employed in 1925 or after					
No. of observed deaths	100	38	15	8	161
No. of expected deaths (adjusted for age and calendar year)	122.12	22.20	11.04	5.64	161.00
Relative risk (using ratios of Observed/Expected)	1.0	2.09	1.66	1.73	
Relative risk (Mantel-Haenszel)	1.0	2.13	1.64	1.73	

Approximate test for homogeneity, $\chi_3^2 = 17.7$; test for trend, $\chi_1^2 - 10.1$
  (using observed and expected numbers only with equations (3.11) and (3.12))
Complete test for homogeneity, $\chi_3^2 = 17.8$; test for trend, $\chi_1^2 = 10.2$
  (using full variances with equations (3.24) and (3.25))

Table 3.12 Number of men developing nasal sinus cancer by age at first employment and number expected after standardization for year of employment and calendar year of observation[a]

Age at first employment (years)	No. of men developing nasal sinus cancer		Observed as proportion of expected
	Observed	Expected[b]	
Under 20	2	5.36	0.37
20–24	9	11.30	0.80
25–29	13	12.26	1.06
30–34	8	6.34	1.26
35+	8	4.73	1.69
All ages	40	39.99	

χ^2 for trend = 5.2; degrees of freedom (df) = 1; $p = 0.03$

[a] From Doll *et al.* (1970)
[b] If age at first employment had no effect on susceptibility to cancer induction

An example from the literature

A classic example of the use of internal standardization to examine the effect of various time factors on mortality rates is the report of the study of nickel refinery workers in South Wales by Doll *et al.* (1970). The study design is discussed in detail in Appendix ID. Cancer deaths and person-years denominators were classified simultaneously by year of employment (a fixed variable), by age at employment (fixed), and by calendar year of occurrence (time-varying). The effect of each factor was then examined according to the methods described above, using simultaneous stratification on the other two factors. The results shown in Table 3.12 indicate that age at first employment had an influence on the relative incidence of nasal sinus cancer even after the effect of years since exposure (as determined by year of employment and calendar year of observation) had been accounted for. However, calendar year had little effect following adjustment for the other two variables (Table 3.13). The authors concluded: 'The results suggest that, so far as nasal cancer is concerned, susceptibility to induction increases with age and that the risk remains approximately constant for between 15 and 42 years after the carcinogen has been removed from the environment.' The last statement is a reference to the fact that no nasal sinus cancer death was observed among men first employed after 1925, when the manufacturing process was changed. We can agree with these conclusions, provided we bear in mind that they refer to relative risks of cancer mortality rather than absolute ones. Additional analyses of these data which incorporate more recent follow-up are used in Chapters 4, 5 and 6 to illustrate some principles of model fitting.

Table 3.13 Number of men developing nasal sinus cancer by calendar period of observation and number expected after standardization for year and age at first employment[a]

Calendar period of observation	No. of men developing nasal sinus cancer		Observed as proportion of expected
	Observed	Expected[b]	
1939–1941	7	3.63	1.93
1942–1946	8	7.28	1.10
1947–1951	9	9.66	0.93
1952–1956	5	9.34	0.54
1957–1961	6	6.28	0.96
1962–1966	5	3.82	1.31
All years	40	40.01	

χ^2 for trend $= 0.95$; degrees of freedom (df) $= 1$; $0.3 < p < 0.5$

[a] From Doll *et al.* (1970)
[b] If year of observation had no effect on risk of developing cancer

3.6 Preferred methods of analysis of grouped data

We repeatedly emphasized in Volume 1 that the goal of a case-control study conducted in a given population was to obtain the same estimates of relative risk as would have been found in a cohort study of that population, had one been performed. Furthermore, methods of analysis of case-control studies were virtually identical to those of cohort studies *vis-à-vis* estimation and testing of hypotheses about relative risk. Thus, it should come as no surprise that the preferred methods of cohort analysis, which we now describe, are nearly identical to those presented in the earlier volume.

The correspondence between case-control and cohort data is easily seen by comparing the data layout of Table 3.4 with that shown in equation (4.40) of Volume 1. There, we considered the joint distribution of cases (a_{ki}) and controls (c_{ki}) in K exposure groups and I strata; here we deal with deaths and person-years cross-classified into K exposure groups and J strata. Making the substitution of j for i, denoting the cases (deaths) by d_{jk} rather than a_{ki} and considering a fixed number n_{jk} of person-years rather than a random number c_{ki} of controls in each cell, the formal identity of the two situations is complete. All of the test and estimates derived in Volume 1 for a dose-response analysis of case-control data have analogues for use with cohort data. Moreover, the calculations required for cohort data are in most respects even simpler than those for case-control data.

Consider the methods of estimating the relative risk associated with the kth exposure level. For both cohort and case-control studies, these parameters represent the rate ratios for the kth level relative to the first level – ratios that are assumed to remain constant across the various strata. For case-control studies, the odds ratios $(a_{ki}c_{1i})/(a_{1i}c_{ki})$ are good estimates of the corresponding stratum-specific relative risks, and, hence, the analysis may be carried out in terms of summary estimates and tests for heterogeneity and trend in the odds ratios (§2.8, Volume 1). Precisely the same is true of cohort studies, except that the 'odds ratios' $(d_{jk}n_{j1})/(d_{j1}n_{jk})$, rather than being mere approximations to the desired rate ratios, are in fact best estimates of those ratios for the indicated stratum and exposure level.

Some differences between the test statistics used for case-control and cohort studies arise from the different sampling schemes that generate the basic data. In cohort analyses, we regard the observed deaths d_{jk} as having Poisson distributions with means $\psi_k\lambda_{j1}n_{jk}$, where λ_{j1} denotes the baseline death rate in stratum j, and ψ_k is the relative risk associated with exposure at level k. (A more complete statement of this model, its rationale, and its consequences is presented in the next chapter.) If follows that the conditional distribution of the deaths $(d_{j1}, \ldots, d_{jK})$ in each stratum is multinomial with denominator D_j and cell occupancy probabilities $\pi_{jk} = \psi_k n_{jk}/\sum_l \psi_l n_{jl}$. For the case-control study, the conditional distribution of the cases $(a_{1i}, \ldots, a_{Ki})$, given the marginal totals in the $2 \times K$ table (equation 4.40 in Volume 1), was multidimensional hypergeometric with noncentrality parameter depending on the relative risk ψ_k. Differences between the variances of the multinomial and hypergeometric distributions lead to slight differences in the corresponding test statistics. The cohort statistics are simpler because one does not need to consider the marginal totals $d_{jk} + n_{jk}$ at all. By substituting n_{jk} for both c_{ki} and m_i, N_j for both n_{0i} and N_i and d_{jk} for a_{ki}, many of the statistics developed in §4.5 of Volume 1 are converted into precisely the form needed for cohort analyses. Furthermore, just as the tests presented there were derived as efficient score tests based on linear logistic models for binomially distributed case-control data, the versions of those same tests presented here are derived as efficient score tests for analogous hypotheses based on log-linear models for Poisson distributed cohort data.

(a) Two dose levels: exposed versus unexposed

Let us start by considering once again the simple problem of comparing death rates for exposed *versus* unexposed without any stratification. We regard O_1 and O_2 as

Poisson variables with means λN_1 and $\psi\lambda N_2$, respectively, where λ represents the background rate, ψ the relative risk, and N_1 and N_2 are the corresponding person-years. Conditional on the total $O_+ = O_1 + O_2$, O_2 is binomially distributed with parameters O_+ and $\pi = \psi N_2/(N_1 + \psi N_2)$. The situation is formally identical to that already considered in §3.4; E_1^* and E_2^* have simply been replaced by N_1 and N_2. Hence, one may apply the same procedures for exact and approximate inferences about π using the binomial distribution and its normal approximation. These are the analogues for cohort analysis of the exact and approximate methods for case-control data developed in §§4.2 and 4.3 of Volume 1.

Example 3.10

Suppose that $O_1 = 5$ lung cancer deaths are observed among a cohort of unexposed persons with $N_1 = 7300$ person-years of observation, whereas $O_2 = 14$ such deaths occur among the exposed with $N_2 = 5500$ person-years of observation. These are precisely the numbers of deaths considered in Example 3.4, and the person-years $N_1 : N_2$ and expected numbers $E_1^* : E_2^*$ are likewise in equal proportion. Consequently, the calculations made earlier apply here as well: $\hat{\psi} = 3.72$ with exact 95% limits of $(1.26, 13.2)$ and approximate ones of $(1.25, 11.8)$.

In more realistic situations, the deaths and person-years are stratified into a series of J 2×2 tables $(j = 1, \ldots, J)$ representing different age strata, as shown in Table 3.4. Conditional on fixed values for the total D_j of deaths in the jth stratum, the number of these that occur at the second exposure level is binomially distributed with parameters D_j and $\pi_j = \psi n_{j2}/(n_{j1} + \psi n_{j2})$. Exact inferences about ψ could, in principle, be made from the convolution of these J binomial distributions in the same fashion that exact inferences about the odds ratio in case-control studies are made from the convolution of the corresponding hypergeometric distributions (Gart, 1971). However, the usual normal approximations are entirely satisfactory for most practical purposes.

(b) Summary test of significance

A test of the null hypothesis $\psi = 1$ is obtained by referring the standardized deviate

$$\chi = \frac{|O_2 - E(O_2)| - 1/2}{\{\mathrm{Var}\,(O_2)\}^{1/2}} = \frac{|O_2 - \sum_{j=1}^{J} n_{j2}D_j/N_j| - 1/2}{\{\sum_{j=1}^{J} D_j n_{j1} n_{j2}/N_j^2\}^{1/2}} \tag{3.14}$$

to tables of the normal distribution. When squared, this is the analogue of the summary statistic used to test for a relative risk of unity in case-control studies (equation 4.23 in Volume 1). Note the use of the continuity correction to improve the normal approximation.

(c) The maximum likelihood estimate

In large samples the most accurate estimator of ψ is the maximum likelihood estimate, obtained by setting the observed number of deaths O_2 equal to its expected value

$$O_2 = E(O_2; \psi) = \sum_{j=1}^{J} D_j \psi n_{j2}/(n_{j1} + \psi n_{j2}). \tag{3.15}$$

Since solution of (3.15) requires iterative calculations, its use is generally restricted to computer analyses and in particular those which involve the fitting of log-linear models. Note that the problems with maximum likelihood estimation of the common odds ratio in a large series of small 2×2 tables (Breslow, 1981) do not apply to the present situation. Under the Poisson model, conditional and unconditional maximum likelihood estimators are identical (Haberman, 1974).

(d) The Mantel–Haenszel estimate and its standard error

The Mantel–Haenszel estimate for cohort data is a simple and robust alternative to maximum likelihood. It is written

$$\hat{\psi}_{MH} = \frac{\sum_{j=1}^{J} R_j}{\sum_{j=1}^{J} S_j} = \frac{\sum_{j=1}^{J} d_{j2} n_{j1}/N_j}{\sum_{j=1}^{J} d_{j1} n_{j2}/N_j}, \tag{3.16}$$

where R_j and S_j are defined by the numerator and denominator terms on the right-hand side of the equation. Clayton (1982) has shown that this estimate arises at the first stage of iteration of one of the computational methods used to find the maximum likelihood estimate. Numerical examples presented below indicate a very good agreement between the two.

A robust variance formula for the Mantel–Haenszel estimate was lacking at the time Volume 1 was written, but the situation has since been remedied both for cohort (Breslow, 1984b) and case-control studies (Robins et al., 1986b). Because of the skewness of the distribution of $\hat{\psi}_{MH}$ it is more appropriately applied on the log scale. Using the fact that $\hat{\psi}_{MH} - \psi = \sum_j (R_j - \psi S_j)/\sum_j S_j$, we have the asymptotic

$$\text{Var} (\hat{\psi}_{MH}) = \frac{\sum_{j=1}^{J} \text{Var} (R_j - \psi S_j)}{\{\sum_{j=1}^{J} E(S_j)\}^2},$$

and thus that the estimated variance of $\hat{\beta}_{MH} = \log(\hat{\psi}_{MH})$ of the log relative risk parameter $\beta = \log(\psi)$ is

$$\text{Var} (\hat{\beta}_{MH}) = \hat{\psi}_{MH}^{-2} \text{Var} (\hat{\psi}_{MH}) = \frac{\sum_{j=1}^{J} n_{j1} n_{j2} D_j / N_j^2}{\hat{\psi}_{MH} \left\{ \sum_{j=1}^{J} \dfrac{n_{j1} n_{j2} D_j}{N_j(n_{j1} + \hat{\psi}_{MH} n_{j2})} \right\}^2}. \tag{3.17}$$

Equations (3.16) and (3.17) are symmetric in the sense that interchanging the role of exposed and unexposed subcohorts has the effect of transforming $\hat{\psi}_{MH}$ into $1/\hat{\psi}_{MH}$ and $\hat{\beta}_{MH}$ into $-\hat{\beta}_{MH}$, but leaves the estimate of $\text{Var} (\hat{\beta}_{MH}) = \text{Var} (-\hat{\beta}_{MH})$ unchanged. Equation (3.17) applies only to Poisson distributed data as collected in a cohort study. The recommended Mantel–Haenszel variance estimate for case-control studies (Robins et al., 1986b) is more complicated.

One important use of any variance estimate is to set approximate confidence intervals on the estimated parameter. Using the interval $\hat{\beta}_{MH} \pm Z_{\alpha/2} \{\text{Var} (\hat{\beta}_{MH})\}^{1/2}$ for β, we have

$$\psi_L = \hat{\psi}_{MH} \exp \{-Z_{\alpha/2}(\text{Var} \, \hat{\beta}_{MH})^{1/2}\}$$

and

$$\psi_U = \hat{\psi}_{MH} \exp \{+Z_{\alpha/2}(\text{Var} \, \hat{\beta}_{MH})^{1/2}\}, \tag{3.18}$$

where $\text{Var}\,\hat{\beta}_{\text{MH}}$ is given by (3.17). Alternatively, we could solve iteratively the equations

$$O_2 - 1/2 - \sum_{j=1}^{J} \frac{\psi_L D_j n_{j2}}{(n_{j1} + \psi_L n_{j2})} = +Z_{\alpha/2}\left[\sum_{j=1}^{J} \frac{\psi_L D_j n_{j1} n_{j2}}{(n_{j1} + \psi_L n_{j2})^2}\right]^{1/2}$$

and   (3.19)

$$O_2 + 1/2 - \sum_{j=1}^{J} \frac{\psi_U D_j n_{j2}}{(n_{j1} + \psi_U n_{j2})} = -Z_{\alpha/2}\left[\sum_{j=1}^{J} \frac{\psi_U D_j n_{j1} n_{j2}}{(n_{j1} + \psi_U n_{j2})^2}\right]^{1/2},$$

which are based on the notion that $\{O_2 - E(O_2; \psi)\}/\{\text{Var}\,(O_2; \psi)\}^{1/2}$ has an approximate unit normal distribution. These equations are the analogues of equation (4.27) in Volume 1.

Example 3.11

In order to estimate the relative risk associated with 15 or more years moderate or heavy exposure to arsenic among men first employed prior to 1925 in the Montana study, we abstracted 13 2×2 tables from Appendix V giving deaths and person-years for exposure levels 1 and 4. These are shown in Table 3.14. While for most ages, rates are higher in the heavily exposed group, the effect is concentrated particularly in the earlier calendar periods among men aged 50–69. Overall, there are 34 deaths in the higher exposure category, whereas 15.36 would be expected under the null hypothesis that the death rates for the two exposure levels were equal within each of the 13 strata. Since the null variance is 12.42, the summary test statistic (3.14) is $\chi = (34 - 15.36)/\sqrt{12.42} = 5.29$ ($p < 0.0001$). The estimate $\hat{\beta}_{\text{MH}} = \log(\hat{\psi}_{\text{MH}})$ is $1.144 = \log(3.138)$ and has a standard error calculated according to (3.17) of $\sqrt{\text{Var}\,(\hat{\beta}_{\text{MH}})} = 0.2239$. These values are quite close to those of the maximum likelihood estimate (MLE) $\hat{\beta}_{\text{ML}} = 1.126$ and its standard error $\text{SE}(\hat{\beta}_{\text{ML}}) = 0.2238$ that were obtained as a by-product of fitting the corresponding model. Approximate confidence limits based on (3.18) are (2.02, 4.87), while those obtained by solving equations (3.19) are (1.94, 4.65). Mantel–Haenszel estimates of relative risk for each of the other exposure categories are shown in Table 3.11.

(e) Testing for heterogeneity of relative risk (effect modification)

A fundamental assumption underlying the use of the Mantel–Haenszel or other estimators of relative risk is that the ratio of disease rates between the two exposure categories is constant over the various age groups, calendar years, or other groupings used for stratification of the sample. If there are substantial discrepancies or trends in the disease rate ratios, use of a summary relative risk measure is generally not advisable. Instead, one wants to describe how the effects of exposure as measured by relative risk are modified by age or year. Simple test statistics are available to evaluate this assumption by comparing the observed numbers of deaths among the exposed and unexposed in each stratum with expected numbers calculated using the summary estimate of relative risk. These are closely related to the statistics developed to test for differences between the odds ratios in a series of 2×2 tables formed from case-control data (equations 4.30 and 4.31 in Volume 1).

Setting $\hat{\pi}_j = \hat{\psi} n_{j2}/(n_{j1} + \hat{\psi} n_{j2})$, we denote by $\hat{d}_{j2} = D_j \hat{\pi}_j$, the expected or fitted number of deaths among the exposed and by $\hat{d}_{j1} = D_j(1 - \hat{\pi}_j)$, the number among the unexposed. The maximum likelihood estimator should be used in these calculations, in which case the total number of exposed deaths and the total fitted numbers will agree (equation (3.15)). However, the MH estimator is often sufficiently close to the MLE

Table 3.14 Series of 2 × 2 tables used in example 3.11. Low exposure (−) means less than 1 year of heavy or moderate arsenic exposure; high exposure (+) means 15+ years

Age (years)		Calendar period							
		1938–1949		1950–1959		1960–1969		1970–1977	
	Exposure	−	+	−	+				
40–49	$d/\hat{d}$	2/1.50	0/0.50	0/0.00	0/0.00				
	n	3075.27	337.29	936.75	121.00				
	$\hat{\psi}$	0.00		—					
	Exposure	−	+	−	+	−	+		
50–59	$d/\hat{d}$	2/3.58	4/2.42	3/4.02	3/1.98	3/2.52	1/1.48		
	n	2849.76	626.72	2195.59	349.53	747.77	142.33		
	$\hat{\psi}$	9.0		6.3		1.8			
	Exposure	−	+	−	+	−	+	−	+
60–69	$d/\hat{d}$	2/5.52	9/5.48	7/7.73	7/6.27	10/8.65	3/4.35	1/1.17	1/0.83
	n	2085.43	672.09	1675.91	441.10	1501.73	244.82	440.21	100.64
	$\hat{\psi}$	14.0		3.8		1.8		4.4	
	Exposure	−	+	−	+	−	+	−	+
70–79	$d/\hat{d}$	3/1.98	1/2.02	6/4.32	2/3.68	6/4.40	1/2.60	6/5.62	2/2.38
	n	833.61	277.25	973.32	268.27	1027.12	197.20	674.44	92.75
	$\hat{\psi}$	1.0		1.2		0.9		2.4	

d = observed deaths; $\hat{d}$ = fitted deaths under ML estimate of common rate ratio; n = person-years denominator; $\hat{\psi}$ = rate ratio in each table

that fitted values based on it yield nearly identical results. Moreover, if $O_2 = \sum_j d_{j2}$ and $\sum_j \hat{d}_{j2}$ based on MH differ, say by more than 1%, a 'one-step' correction of $\hat{\beta}_{MH}$ towards the MLE is available as

$$\hat{\beta}_C = \hat{\beta}_{MH} + \frac{\sum_{j=1}^{J} d_{j2} - \sum_{j=1}^{J} \hat{d}_{j2}}{\sum_{j=1}^{J} \hat{d}_{j1}\hat{d}_{j2}/D_j} . \qquad (3.20)$$

Fitted values $\hat{d}_{j1}$ and $\hat{d}_{j2}$ determined from the corrected MH estimator $\hat{\psi}_C = \exp(\hat{\beta}_C)$ should be adequate for use in what follows if the MLE itself is not available.

To test for a general difference among the rate ratios in the J strata, we compare the observed and fitted values using the standard chi-square statistic

$$\chi^2_{J-1} = \sum_{j=1}^{J} \left\{ \frac{(d_{j1} - \hat{d}_{j1})^2}{\hat{d}_{j1}} + \frac{(d_{j2} - \hat{d}_{j2})^2}{\hat{d}_{j2}} \right\}, \tag{3.21}$$

which has $J - 1$ degrees of freedom. A test for a trend in the stratum-specific ratios with quantitative variables z_j, representing, for example, the age level in stratum j, is accomplished using the statistic

$$\frac{\{\sum_j z_j (d_{j2} - \hat{d}_{j2})\}^2}{\sum_j z_j^2 \hat{d}_{j1} \hat{d}_{j2}/D_j - (\sum_j z_j \hat{d}_{j1} \hat{d}_{j2}/D_j)^2/(\sum_j \hat{d}_{j1} \hat{d}_{j2}/D_j)}. \tag{3.22}$$

This is referred to tables of chi-square on one degree of freedom. If the z_j are equally spaced, the numerator may be reduced in absolute value before squaring by half the distance between adjacent z values in order to correct for the discontinuity of the actual distribution.

Example 3.11 (cont)

Table 3.14 also presents fitted values of $\hat{d}_{j1}$ and $\hat{d}_{j2}$ for the respiratory cancer deaths determined by inserting the MLE $\hat{\psi}_{ML} = \exp(1.126) = 3.083$ in the expressions $\hat{d}_{j1} = D_j n_{1j}/(n_{1j} + \hat{\psi}_{ML} n_{2j})$ and $\hat{d}_{j2} = D_j \hat{\psi}_{ML} n_{2j}/(n_{1j} + \hat{\psi}_{ML} n_{2j})$, respectively. The summary chi-square statistic (3.21) comparing observed and fitted values yields $\chi^2_{12} = 12.9$ ($p = 0.37$), with the largest contribution

$$\frac{(9 - 5.48)^2}{5.48} = 2.25$$

coming from the 60–69-year age group in calendar period 1938–1949. Thus, in spite of the wide range of rate ratios for individual strata observed in this example, the variation is well within the limits expected under the hypothesis that the true ratio is constant across strata.

Example 3.12

Table 3.15 presents data on coronary deaths from the British doctors study (Doll & Hill, 1966) that have been used by Rothman and Boice (1979) and Breslow (1984b) to illustrate methods of cohort analysis. From (3.16) we find a summary relative risk estimate of $\hat{\psi}_{MH} = 1.4247$. The fitted frequencies determined from it

Table 3.15 Deaths from coronary disease among British male doctors[a]

Age group (years)	No. of person-years		No. of observed deaths		No. of expected deaths[b]		Rate ratio	Rate difference per 100 000 person-years
	Non-smokers	Smokers	Non-smokers	Smokers	Non-smokers	Smokers		
j	n_{j1}	n_{j2}	d_{j1}	d_{j2}	$\hat{d}_{j1}$	$\hat{d}_{j2}$		
35–44	18 790	52 407	2	32	6.83	27.17	5.73	50.4
45–54	10 673	43 248	12	104	17.12	98.88	2.14	128.0
55–64	5 710	28 612	28	206	28.74	205.26	1.47	229.6
65–74	2 585	12 663	28	186	26.81	187.19	1.36	385.7
75–84	1 462	5 317	31	102	21.51	111.49	0.90	−202.0
Totals	39 220	142 247	101	630	101.00	630.00	1.72	185.4

[a] Data from Doll and Hill (1966) as quoted by Rothman and Boice (1979)
[b] Estimated by maximum likelihood under the hypothesis of a common rate ratio

total $\sum_j \hat{d}_{2j} = 629.9487$, which agrees very closely with the observed total $\sum_j d_{j2} = 630$. Thus, we know that the MH and MLE estimates are already almost equal, and a correction to the MH estimate would not normally be needed in such circumstances. Nevertheless, in order to illustrate the use of equation (3.20), we further calculate (using fitted values based on $\hat{\psi}_{MH}$) $\sum_j \hat{d}_{1j}\hat{d}_{j2}/D_j = 88.7729$ and thus find

$$\hat{\beta}_C = 0.35395 + \frac{630 - 629.9487}{88.7729} = 0.35454,$$

which agrees with $\hat{\beta}_{ML}$ to the number of decimal places shown.

The sixth and seventh columns of Table 3.15 show the final fitted values $\hat{d}_{j1}$ and $\hat{d}_{j2}$ based on $\hat{\psi}_{ML} = \exp(0.3545) = 1.426$. Inserting these in equations (3.21) and (3.22), and using $z_j = j$ to examine the trend with age, we obtain heterogeneity and (corrected) trend statistics of $\chi_4^2 = 11.1$ and $\chi_1^2 = 10.0$ on four and one degrees of freedom, respectively. Thus, most of the heterogeneity in relative risk is explained by the linear decrease with age. Rothman and Boice (1979) note that these data are more consistent with an additive effect model than with a multiplicative one. In §4.4 we show that an even better fit is obtained using a square-root function to relate age and smoking effects.

In this example, the standard error of $\hat{\beta}_{MH}$ estimated from the square root of (3.17) is 0.1073, almost identical with $SE(\hat{\beta}_{ML}) = 0.1074$. This illustrates once again the generally high efficiency of the MH estimator. However, in other applications the discrepancy may be found to be greater.

(f) Extensions to $K > 2$ exposure classes

In §3.4, we described the use of externally standardized mortality ratios to evaluate the relative risk of disease associated with each of K exposure categories, for example, the $K = 4$ levels of duration of heavy/moderate exposure to arsenic in both cohorts of the Montana study. A similar approach is taken with the methods of this section. First, Mantel–Haenszel estimates are computed for each of the $k = 2, \ldots, K$ exposure categories relative to baseline. These may be tested for significance individually using the summary chi-square (3.14). The stability of the relative risk estimates from one stratum to another is evaluated using the methods just presented.

In order to test the global null hypothesis that death rates for none of the K exposure classes differ, we require a multivariate extension of (3.14). As in §4.5 of Volume 1, this follows from consideration of the joint distribution, under the null hypothesis, of the deaths $\mathbf{d}_j = (d_{j1}, \ldots, d_{jK})$ in each stratum. Using the Poisson sampling model, the null distribution of $\mathbf{d}_j$ conditional on the total number of deaths D_j in stratum j is easily shown to be multinomial, with a covariance matrix the (k, ℓ) element of which $(1 \leq k, \ell \leq K)$ is

$$\|V_j\|_{k\ell} = \begin{cases} n_{jk}(N_j - n_{jk})D_j/N_j^2, & \text{if } k = \ell \\ -n_{jk}n_{j\ell}D_j/N_j^2, & \text{if } k \neq \ell. \end{cases} \tag{3.23}$$

Under the null hypothesis, the summary vector $\mathbf{O} = (O_1, \ldots, O_K)$ has expectation $\mathbf{E} = (E_1, \ldots, E_K)$ (see equation 3.13) and covariance matrix $\mathbf{V} = \sum_j V_j$. The global test for equality of death rates compares $\mathbf{O}$ and $\mathbf{E}$ using the criterion

$$\chi_{K-1}^2 = (\mathbf{O} - \mathbf{E})^\mathsf{T} \mathbf{V}^- (\mathbf{O} - \mathbf{E}), \tag{3.24}$$

where $\mathbf{V}^-$ denotes a generalized inverse of $\mathbf{V}$ (Rao, 1965) and T denotes a matrix transpose. In practice, this is calculated by restricting $\mathbf{O}$ and $\mathbf{E}$ to the first $K - 1$ components and replacing $\mathbf{V}$ by the corresponding $(K - 1) \times (K - 1)$ dimensional covariance matrix. For the special case $K = 2$, the test is obtained either as

$(O_1 - E_1)^2/V_1$ or $(O_2 - E_2)^2/V_2$ where $V_1 = \text{Var}(O_1)$ and $V_2 = \text{Var}(O_2)$. It thus reduces to the square of the two-group statistic (3.14), without correction for continuity.

The K group statistic based on indirect standardization, namely (3.11) with the internal fitted values E_k replacing the adjusted external expected, does not require calculation of the variances. It may be recognized as the analogue of the conservative test (equation 4.42 in Volume 1) proposed for case-control data. It always yields smaller values than (3.24), and the degree of conservatism depends on the extent to which the stratum variables confound the disease-exposure relationship (Armitage, 1966; Peto, R. & Pike, 1973).

The test for a trend in relative risk with increasing exposure is obtained from the regression of the observed − expected differences on the dose levels x, namely $\sum_k x_k(O_k - E_k)$. This has a variance of $(\mathbf{x}^T \mathbf{V} \mathbf{x})$. The test statistic is written

$$\chi_1^2 = \frac{\{\sum_{k=1}^K x_k(O_k - E_k)\}^2}{\sum_{k=1}^K x_k^2 E_k - \sum_{j=1}^J (\sum_{k=1}^K x_k e_{jk})^2/D_j}, \tag{3.25}$$

where $e_{jk} = n_{jk} D_j/N_j$ denotes the expected value in the component $2 \times K$ table. This is the analogue of equation (4.43) in Volume 1 for cohort data. Once again, the corresponding statistic based on internal standardization (equation (3.12) using E_k) provides a conservative approximation.

Example 3.13

The last lines in each part of Table 3.11 show the values of the heterogeneity and trend statistics (3.24) and (3.25) obtained with the data in Appendix V. These are slightly greater than the approximating statistics (3.11) and (3.12) calculated from the observed and expected values only, without consideration of the variances. While this is not atypical of what one observes in practice, more serious discrepancies must be anticipated when there is strong confounding.

(g) Conservatism of indirect standardization

The impression one might get from our analysis of the Montana smelter workers data, namely, that indirect standardization always yields results close to those obtained with the Mantel–Haenszel methodology, is of course mistaken. The degree of conservatism depends on the degree of statistical confounding between the stratum variables and the exposures. In situations in which the confounding is marked, the conservatism may be also, as the following hypothetical data make clear.

Consider two strata in which the relative risk of exposure is 2, but the pooled risk is considerably less:

	Stratum I		Stratum II		Combined sample	
	Unexposed	Exposed	Unexposed	Exposed	Unexposed	Exposed
Cases	25	5	5	25	30	30
Person-years	10 000	1 000	4 000	10 000	14 000	11 000

	Stratum I	Stratum II	Combined sample
Relative risk ($\hat{\psi}$)	2.0	2.0	1.27
$E_2 = E(O_2)$	27.273	8.571	35.844
$E_1 = E(O_1)$	2.727	21.429	24.156
$V_2 = \text{Var}(O_2)$	2.479	6.122	8.602

The chi-square test for $\psi = 1$ based on internal standardization calculated without continuity correction is

$$\chi^2 = \frac{(30 - 24.156)^2}{24.156} + \frac{(30 - 35.844)^2}{35.844} = 2.37, \quad (p = 0.13),$$

whereas the chi-square test that uses the actual variances from each component table is

$$\chi_1^2 = \frac{(30 - 24.156)^2}{8.602} = 3.97, \quad (p = 0.047).$$

Due to the moderately strong confounding, the approximate statistic is substantially smaller and yields a nonsignificant result. Similarly, the relative risk estimate based only on observed and expected values, namely $(O_2 E_1)/(O_1 E_2) = (30 \times 35.844)/(30 \times 24.156) = 1.48$, is less than that of the estimate $\hat{\psi}_{MH} = 2.0$.

3.7 Proportional mortality and dose-response analyses

Occasionally one is called upon to conduct a dose-response analysis using only the deaths observed in a defined cohort, without consideration of the corresponding person-years denominators. These may be the only data available. Or, complete exposure histories may have been reconstructed first for dead subjects, for example, and one wants to make an initial evaluation of the probable magnitude of the relative risks before proceeding with the collection of data on those persons who are still alive. The available information consists only of numbers of deaths classified by age at death and other stratification factors, by level of exposure, and by cause of death. Once again, we denote by d_{jk} the number of deaths in stratum j and exposure group k for the cause of interest, by t_{jk} the total deaths from all causes in that stratum and exposure category, and by $D_j = \sum_k d_{jk}$ and $T_j = \sum_k t_{jk}$ the subtotals cumulated over categories. We may also have available a quantitative variable x giving the dose level x_k in exposure class k.

The object of the analysis is to determine whether the proportion of deaths due to the cause of interest increases systematically with increasing levels of exposure, while adjusting for age and other potentially confounding factors by stratification into J strata. The major weakness of the approach is the fact that some of the other causes of death may also be affected by the exposure, thus obscuring the association of interest and hindering precise quantitative estimation of its magnitude. If one is reasonably confident that the other causes of death included in the analysis are not related to the exposure, at least not after accounting for the stratification factors, then the data are best viewed as arising from a type of case-control study in which the deaths from other causes are assumed to represent an unbiased sample (vis-à-vis the exposures) of the population at risk within each stratum. This means that the most appropriate analysis of proportional mortality data is to treat them as arising from a case-control study in which the controls died from other causes (Miettinen & Wang, 1981).

In practice, it is useful to exclude from the control sample deaths from those causes that are already known to be related to the exposures. This enhances confidence in the critical assumption that underlies the methodology, namely that the 'controls' are representative of the population at risk. If one is uncertain about its validity – and this is usually the case – the inferences drawn must necessarily be more tentative than those from an actual case-control study of incident cases in which random sampling methods have been used to select controls from the population in an unbiased fashion.

Although case-control methodology is preferred for the analysis of proportional mortality data, it has been common practice in the past to apply techniques of indirect standardization analogous to those presented in §3.4 and 3.5. One first computes expected numbers of deaths e_{jk} from the cause of interest in the (j, k) stratum/exposure cell under the hypothesis that exposure has had no effect on the death rates. In symbols,

$$e_{jk} = t_{jk} D_j / T_j. \tag{3.26}$$

These values are cumulated to give $E_k = \sum_j e_{jk}$ as the total number expected at level k after adjustment. It would be tempting to insert such E_k into equations (3.8), (3.11) and (3.12) in order to estimate and make tests on the relative risk. If the disease is common, however, such ad-hoc methods may lead to results that are at considerable variance from those obtained using the proper case-control methods. The main difficulty is the fact that the disease of interest is making a contribution to the totals t_{jk} and T_j used to calculate the expected numbers, so that these are closer to the observed numbers than they are for the analogous cohort data. Even under the proportionality assumption that justified dose-response analysis of SMR_k, the equivalent proportional mortality analysis may not be valid.

Example 3.14

The sixth column of Appendix V shows the total numbers of deaths among the Montana workers classified by age, calendar period, date of employment and exposure duration. These were used in a case-control dose-response analysis according to the methods presented in Chapter 4 of Volume 1. There were 18 age × calendar period strata and four exposure levels for the pre-1925 cohort, and 16 strata and four exposure levels for the post-1925 cohort. Table 3.16 presents the results. The Mantel–Haenszel estimates of relative risk are in reasonable agreement with those found from the entire set of cohort data (Table 3.11), except for the highest exposure duration category in the early cohort (2.62 versus 3.14). Here, the proportional mortality analysis yields a substantially lower estimate of relative risk, suggesting that causes of death other than respiratory cancer may be affected by lengthy exposures to arsenic. The Mantel–Haenszel estimates are in good agreement with those obtained by (unconditional) maximum likelihood according to the methods presented in Chapter 6 of Volume 1, namely, the fitting of linear logistic models to the binomial proportions of cause-specific deaths divided by total deaths. The statistics (4.41) and (4.43) in Volume 1 for testing for heterogeneity and trend in the relative risks are substantially less than the corresponding statistics shown in the sixth row of Table 3.11 for the full cohort data. This is not surprising in view of the reduced value for the relative risk estimate for the highest exposure category.

Also shown in Table 3.16 for each subcohort are the expected numbers of respiratory deaths obtained by multiplying the total deaths in each age-stratum-exposure cell by the proportion of respiratory deaths in that stratum as shown in equation (3.26), and then summing across strata. When these are inserted in equation (3.8) to estimate the 'relative risk' for each exposure level, the results are considerably more conservative than were the results based on indirect standardization using the complete set of cohort data (Table 3.11). For example, the estimate of relative risk from proportional mortality data for the 15+ years exposure duration category in the pre-1925 cohort is $\hat{\psi} = 2.38$ based on observed/expected values versus $\psi = 2.62$ for Mantel–Haenszel. The corresponding figures from cohort data were 3.09 versus 3.14. Similarly, whereas the test statistics (3.11) and (3.12) yielded only slightly conservative results when used with internally standardized expected numbers based on the person-years denominators, when used with the proportional expected values from equation (3.26) that depend only on the proportional mortality data, the results are

Table 3.16 Dose–response analysis of respiratory cancer deaths among Montana smelter workers, based on proportional mortality

	Cumulative years of moderate/heavy arsenic exposure				
	0–0.9	1.0–4.9	5.0–14.9	15+	Total
Workers employed prior to 1925					
Observed deaths	51	17	13	34	115
Total deaths (All causes)	636	100	93	195	1024
Expected deaths (Internal adjustment for age and calendar year)	72.47	11.84	10.41	20.29	115.00
Relative risk (using ratios of Observed/Expected)	1.0	2.04	1.77	2.38	
Relative risk (Mantel-Haenszel)	1.0	2.30	2.12	2.62	
Relative risk (Maximum likelihood)	1.0	2.32	1.98	2.82	

Approximate test for homogeneity, $\chi_3^2 = 18.5$; test for trend, $\chi_1^2 = 16.6$ (using observed and expected values in equations (3.11) and (3.12))
Case-control test for homogeneity, $\chi_3^2 = 21.6$; test for trend, $\chi_1^2 = 19.4$ (equations 4.41 and 4.43 from Volume 1)

	0–0.9	1.0–4.9	5.0–14.9	15+	Total
Workers employed 1925 or later					
Observed deaths	100	38	15	8	161
Total deaths (All causes)	1389	274	143	68	1874
Expected deaths (Internal adjustment for age and calendar year)	118.47	24.47	11.83	6.25	161.00
Relative risk (using ratios of Observed/Expected)	1.0	1.84	1.50	1.52	
Relative risk (Mantel-Haenszel)	1.0	2.06	1.54	1.58	
Relative risk (Maximum likelihood)	1.0	2.02	1.57	1.61	

Approximate test for homogeneity, $\chi_3^2 = 11.7$; test for trend, $\chi_1^2 = 6.3$ (using observed and expected values in equations (3.11) and (3.12))
Case-control test for homogeneity, $\chi_3^2 = 13.2$; test for trend, $\chi_1^2 = 7.0$ (equations 4.41 and 4.43 from Volume 1)

noticeably different from those obtained with proper case-control techniques. This illustrates the basic point that indirect standardization techniques should not be used in the context of proportional mortality unless one is dealing with a very rare disease. Whereas they may or may not yield conservative results with cohort data depending on the degree of statistical confounding, they are bound to produce conservative results with proportional mortality (case-control) data.

Nothing has yet been said about the possibility of incorporating information from the external standard population into the dose-response analysis of proportional mortality data. The reason is that the elementary methods presented in §3.4 for cohort studies have no suitable analogue when death records are the only data available, nor do the indirect standardization techniques of §3.5, as shown in the preceding example. Suppose we were to calculate expected numbers of deaths for each exposure category using the formula $E_k^* = \sum_j t_{kj} p_j^*$, where p_j^* denotes the standard proportion of deaths in stratum j due to the cause of interest. Even under the assumption of proportionality, in which the stratum-specific mortality rates for both cause-specific and general deaths in each exposure category are constant multiples of the stratum-specific standard rates, inserting these expected numbers into equations (3.8), (3.11) and (3.12) may yield badly biased estimates and tests if more than a few percent of total deaths are due to the cause of interest. Although it is possible to use the external standard proportions by incorporating them into an appropriate model, none of the standard estimates or tests based on the model have simple closed form expressions. Therefore, we defer further discussion of this approach to proportional mortality analysis until the next chapter.

4. FITTING MODELS TO GROUPED DATA

CHAPTER 4

FITTING MODELS TO GROUPED DATA

A major goal of the statistical procedures considered in the preceding two chapters was to condense the information in a large set of incidence or mortality rates into a few summary measures so as to estimate the effects that a risk factor has on the rates. A secondary goal was to evaluate the statistical significance of the effect estimates at different levels of exposure in order to rule out the possibility that the observed differences in rates were due simply to the play of chance. Some attention was devoted also to determining whether the effect measures used (relative risks) were reasonable summary measures in the sense of remaining relatively constant from one age stratum to the next, or whether, instead, it was necessary to describe how the effect was modified by age or other variables used for stratification.

Role of statistical modelling

Estimation of risk factor effects and tests of hypotheses about them are also the goals of statistical modelling. The statistician constructs a probability model that explicitly recognizes the role of chance mechanisms in producing some of the variation in the rates. Observed rates are regarded as just one of many possible realizations of an underlying random process. Parameters in the model describe the systematic effects of the exposures of interest, and estimates of those parameters, obtained during the process of fitting the model to the data, serve as summary statistics analogous to the SMR or Mantel–Haenszel estimates of relative risk. Evaluation of dose-response trends is conducted in terms of tests for the significance of regression coefficients for variables representing quantitative levels of exposure. Additional parameters may be incorporated in order to model variations of the exposure effects with age, calendar year or other stratum variables.

Statistical modelling has several advantages over standardization and related techniques. It facilitates consideration of the simultaneous effects of several different exposure variables on risk. Applied to the study of nasal sinus and lung cancers in Welsh nickel workers, for example, the effects of period of employment, age at employment and years since employment may be estimated in a single model equation (see §4.3) rather than in separate stratified analyses (Tables 3.12 and 3.13). If quantitative variables are available that specify the timing and degree of exposure, then a more economical description of the data often may be given in terms of dose-time-response relationships rather than by making separate estimates of risk for each exposure category. Such quantitative expression of the results facilitates the interpolation of risk estimates for intermediate levels of exposure. It is essential for extrapolation beyond the range of the available data, although this is usually a hazardous undertaking. Examination of the goodness-of-fit of the model to the observed rates alerts the investigator to situations in which the simple model description is inadequate or in which important features of the data are being overlooked. Estimates of relative risk obtained by model fitting generally have greater numerical stability than those computed from standardized rates.

There are, of course, some apparent drawbacks to model fitting that need to be considered along with the advantages. Perhaps the greatest problem lies in the parametric specification of the model. While explicit theories about the nature of the disease process are sometimes available to suggest models with a particular mathematical form (see Chapter 6), more often the models used in statistical data analysis are selected on the basis of their flexibility and because the associated fitting procedures are well understood and convenient. Alternative models may have quite different epidemiological interpretations. Examining the relative goodness-of-fit of two distinct model structures enables one to judge whether the evidence favours one interpretation over another, or whether they are both more or less equally in agreement with the observed facts. Unfortunately, epidemiological data are rarely extensive enough to be used to discriminate clearly between closely related models, and some uncertainty and arbitrariness in the process of model selection is to be anticipated. Nevertheless the very act of thinking about the possible biological mechanisms that could have produced the observations under study can be beneficial. Consideration of possible model structures is not strictly necessary when applying the elementary techniques, but even these implicitly assume some regularity in the basic data and, as we have seen, may yield misleading answers if it is absent.

Scope of Chapter 4

This chapter develops methods for the analysis of grouped cohort data that are based on maximum likelihood estimation in Poisson models for the underlying disease rates. Additive and multiplicative models are introduced in §4.1 as a means of summarizing the basic structure in a two-dimensional table of rates. It is again shown that the ratio of two CMFs appropriately summarizes age-specific rate ratios under the multiplicative model, but that the ratio of two SMRs does not unless additional assumptions are met. The basic process of model fitting is illustrated by an analysis of Icelandic breast cancer rates classified by age and birth cohort.

Section 4.2 contains more technical material that justifies the use of the Poisson model as the basis for maximum likelihood analysis of grouped cohort data. It may be omitted on a first reading.

Methods of fitting multiplicative models to grouped cohort data consisting of a multidimensional cross-classification of cases (or deaths) and person-years denominators are developed in §4.3. The computer program GLIM is shown to offer particularly convenient features for fitting Poisson regression models. Quantities available from the GLIM fits are easily converted into 'deletion diagnostics' that aid in assessing the stability of the fitted model under perturbations of the basic data. These techniques are by no means limited to the analysis of relative risk: §4.4 shows that GLIM may be used also to fit a class of generalized linear models that range from additive to multiplicative. Methods for selecting the model equation that best describes the structure in the data are illustrated by application to a rather simple problem involving coronary deaths among smoking and nonsmoking British doctors.

The Montana smelter workers data from Appendix V are reanalysed in §§4.5, 4.6 and 4.7 in order to demonstrate the close connection between multiplicative models and the elementary techniques of standardization and Mantel–Haenszel estimation introduced in §§3.4, 3.6 and 3.7. Section 4.5 considers internal estimation of background rates from study data, whereas §4.6 develops analogous models that incorporate external standard rates. Proportional mortality analyses based on fitting of logistic regression models to case-'control' data, both with and without reference to external standard proportions, are developed in §4.7.

More comprehensive analyses of the Montana data, using original records not published here, appear in §§4.8 and 5.5. Some additional models that do not fall strictly under the rubric of the generalized linear model are considered in the last two sections of the chapter. Foremost among these is the additive relative risk model whereby different exposures act multiplicatively on the background rates, but combine additively in determining the relative risk. This is illustrated in §4.9 by application to data on lung cancer deaths among British doctors. GLIM macros are presented for fitting a general class of relative risk models which includes both the additive and multiplicative as special cases. In §4.10, grouped data from the Welsh nickel refiners study are used to illustrate the fitting of a model in which the excess risk of lung cancer (over background based on national rates) is expressed as a mutliplicative combination of exposure effects. These results are contrasted with those of a more conventional multivariate analysis of the SMR under the multiplicative model.

Some familiarity with the principles of likelihood inference and linear models is assumed. Readers without such background are referred to §§6.1 and 6.2 of Volume 1, and the references contained therein, for an appropriate introduction.

4.1 Additive and multiplicative models for rates

Most of the essential concepts involved in statistical modelling can be introduced by considering the simple example of a two-dimensional table of rates. The data layout (Table 3.4) consists of a table with J rows ($j = 1, \ldots, J$) and K columns ($k = 1, \ldots, K$). Within the cell formed by the intersection of the jth row and kth column, one records the number of incident cases or deaths d_{jk} and the person-years denominators n_{jk}. For concreteness, we may think of j as indexing J age intervals and k as representing one of K exposure categories.

The observed rate in the (j, k)th cell may be written $\hat{\lambda}_{jk} = d_{jk}/n_{jk}$. This is considered as an estimate of a true rate λ_{jk} that could be known exactly only if an infinite amount of observation time were available. In order to account for sampling variability, the d_{jk} are regarded as independent Poisson variables with means and variances $E(d_{jk}) = \mathrm{Var}\,(d_{jk}) = \lambda_{jk}n_{jk}$. The denominators n_{jk} are assumed to be fixed. The rationale for this Poisson assumption is discussed in §§4.2 and 5.2.

The goal of the statistical analysis is to uncover the basic structure in the underlying rates λ_{jk}, and, in particular, to try to disentangle the separate effects of age and exposure. This is accomplished by introducing one set of parameters or summary indices which describe the age effects and another set for the exposures. However, such a simple description makes sense only if the age-specific rates display a degree of consistency such that, within defined limits of statistical variation, the relative position of each exposure group remains constant over the J age levels (see Chapter 2, Volume 1). If one exposure group has higher death rates among young persons, but lower rates among the elderly, use of a single summary rate (or the analogous parameter in a statistical model) to represent the exposure effect will obscure the fact that the effect depends on age.

(a) The model equations

Various possible structures for the rates satisfy the requirement of consistency. In particular, it holds if the effect of exposure at level k is to add a constant amount β_k to the age-specific rates λ_{j1} for individuals in the baseline or nonexposed category ($k = 1$). The model equation is

$$\lambda_{jk} = \alpha_j + \beta_k, \tag{4.1}$$

where $\alpha_j = \lambda_{j1}$ and β_k ($\beta_1 = 0$) are parameters to be estimated from the data.

If additivity does not hold on the original scale of measurement, it may hold for some transformation of the rates. The log transform

$$\log \lambda_{jk} = \alpha_j + \beta_k \tag{4.2}$$

yields the multiplicative model

$$\lambda_{jk} = \theta_j \psi_k,$$

where now $\alpha_j = \log \theta_j = \log \lambda_{j1}$ and $\beta_k = \log \psi_k$. In this case, ψ_k represents the relative risk (rate ratio) of disease for exposure at level k relative to a baseline at level 1 ($\psi_1 = 1$).

The excess (additive) and relative (multiplicative) risk models are the two most commonly used to describe the relationship between the effects of exposure and the effects of age and other 'nuisance' factors that may account for background or spontaneous cases. Both have been used to describe different aspects of radiation carcinogenesis in human populations (Committee on the Biological Effects of Ionizing Radiation, 1980). The upper two panels of Figure 4.1 contrast the age-incidence curves that result from the two models when a given dose of radiation produces a constant effect that persists for life after a latent period. Due to the sharp rise in background incidence with age, relative risk estimates derived from current data generally predict a greater lifetime radiation risk than do estimates of additive effect. The two lower panels of Figure 4.1 illustrate the effect of age at irradiation on risk for a multiplicative model in which the radiation effect itself is concentrated in the period from l_1 to l_2 years after exposure. However, this complication of a limitation of the period of effect is not considered further in this section.

Fig. 4.1   Radiation-induced cancer effect superimposed on spontaneous cancer incidence by age. Illustrations of various possibilities; X_e, age at exposure; l,
minimal latent period. From Committee on the Biological Effects of Ionizing
Radiation (1980)

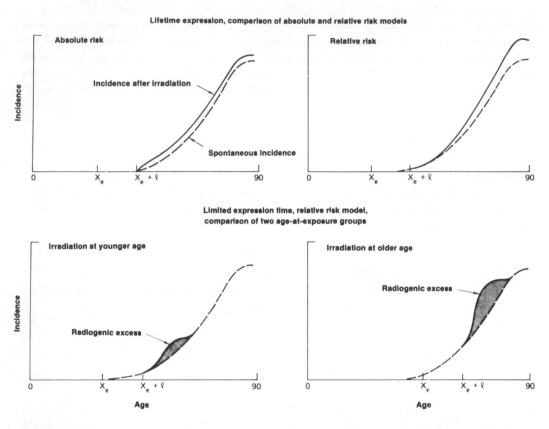

Considerable attention has been given in recent years to the problems of dis-
criminating between additive and multiplicative models using epidemiological data
(Gardner & Munford, 1980; Thomas, D.C., 1981; Walker & Rothman, 1982; Breslow
& Storer, 1985). One possible approach is presented in §4.5. Unless the data are quite
extensive and the effect of exposure pronounced, however, random sampling errors
may make such discriminations difficult. Furthermore, errors of misclassification of the
exposure variable may operate to distort the true relationship (Tzonou *et al.*, 1986). In
view of such uncertainties, the choice of model is legitimately based as much on
a-priori considerations as it is on goodness-of-fit tests, unless of course these show one
or the other model to be markedly superior. As with the report of the Committee on
the Biological Effects of Ionizing Radiation, some authors follow the prudent course of
examining and presenting their data using several alternative model assumptions.

(b) Biological basis for model selection

Sections 2.4–2.7 of Volume 1 gave both empirical and logical reasons for the usually greater convenience in cancer epidemiology of measuring the effects of exposures in terms of the relative risk parameters of the multiplicative model rather than the excess risk parameters of the additive model. Incidence and death rates for cancers of epithelial tissue are known to rise rapidly with age, the age-incidence curves approximating a power function with exponent between four and five (Doll, 1971). When plotted on log paper for different exposure or population groups, the age-incidence curves are therefore roughly linear with a common slope but varying intercept (Fig. 2.2). This implies a multiplicative relationship.

If the two dimensions of the table correspond to two different exposure factors, however, then various models for the disease process suggest that their individual effects on the age-specific rates or on the lifetime risks may combine additively, multiplicatively or in some other fashion. Models based on the multistage theory of carcinogenesis lead to approximately additive structures if the two risk factors affect the same stage of the process and to multiplicative structures if two distinct stages are affected (Lee, 1975; Siemiatycki & Thomas, 1981; Hamilton, 1982). A detailed discussion of quantitative theories of carcinogenesis and how they may be used to suggest appropriate dose-time-response relationships involving one or more agents is given in Chapter 6. Under Rothman's (1976) component-sufficient cause paradigm of disease causation, which is perhaps of greater relevance to other areas of epidemiology, 'independent' factors or those which contribute to different disease pathways have effects that combine in a nearly additive fashion, whereas the effects of 'complementary' factors or those that contribute different parts to the same pathway combine in a manner that is close to multiplicative (Koopman, 1982).

(c) Standardization and multiplicative models

The CMF and the SMR (see Chapter 2) were originally developed from a general, intuitive perspective, in the absence of any formal assumption about the structure that might be present in the underlying age-specific disease rates. Nevertheless, considerable insight into the properties of such statistical measures is gained by investigating their performance under well-defined and plausible models for the basic data. Here, we compare the performance of the CMF and SMR in the multiplicative environment and develop an interesting relationship between the iterative fitting of multiplicative models and the calculation of the indirectly standardized SMR. Similar investigations have been undertaken by Freeman and Holford (1980), Anderson *et al.* (1980) and Hoem (1987).

Suppose, for simplicity, that there are only two exposures categories ($k = 1$ or 2) and denote by $w_j = n_{j0}/N_0$ and $\lambda_j^* = d_{j0}/n_{j0}$ the standard weights and rates that enter into the calculation of the summary measures. According to (4.2) the ratio of age-specific rates for the two categories is equal to ψ_2/ψ_1, or just ψ_2 if $\psi_1 = 1$ as is generally assumed, regardless of the age interval. Thus, the ratio of the two corresponding summary measures should tend towards ψ_2 in large samples if the measures are to reflect accurately the basic regularity in the rates. An easy calculation shows this is indeed true for direct standardization:

$$\frac{\mathrm{CMF}_2}{\mathrm{CMF}_1} \to \frac{\sum_{j=1}^{J} w_j \lambda_{j2}}{\sum_{j=1}^{J} w_j \lambda_{j1}} = \frac{\psi_2 \sum_{j=1}^{J} w_j \theta_j}{\psi_1 \sum_{j=1}^{J} w_j \theta_j} = \psi_2.$$

For the ratio of two SMRs, however, we have

$$\frac{\mathrm{SMR}_2}{\mathrm{SMR}_1} \to \frac{\sum_{j=1}^{J} n_{j2} \lambda_{j2} / \sum_{j=1}^{J} \lambda_j^* n_{j2}}{\sum_{j=1}^{J} n_{j1} \lambda_{j1} / \sum_{j=1}^{J} \lambda_j^* n_{j1}} = \psi_2 \times \frac{\sum_{j=1}^{J} n_{j2} \theta_j / \sum_{j=1}^{J} \lambda_j^* n_{j2}}{\sum_{j=1}^{J} n_{j1} \theta_j / \sum_{j=1}^{J} \lambda_j^* n_{j1}}. \qquad (4.3)$$

The second term in this expression generally does not equal 1 unless we also have $\theta_j = \text{const} \times \lambda_j^*$ or else $n_{j2} = \text{const} \times n_{j1}$; that is, unless the age-specific rates for exposure categories 1 and 2 are both proportional to the external standard rates, in addition to being proportional to each other, or else the two age distributions are identical. The bias in the ratio of SMRs can be severe if these conditions are grossly violated, as Table 2.13 makes clear.

The condition of proportionality with the external standard automatically holds for the multiplicative model if one takes for the 'standard' either one of the two sets of age-specific rates that are being compared. If the first exposure group ($k = 1$) is taken as standard for computation of the CMF, and the second group ($k = 2$) as standard for the SMR, then the ratios of CMFs and SMRs are identical (Anderson *et al.*, 1980, Section 7A.4). Using the pool of the two comparison groups as an internal standard, however, generally does not satisfy the proportionality condition, and the ratio of SMRs computed on this basis does not estimate the ratio of age-specific rates. Nevertheless, use of the pooled population seems to avoid some of the more severe biases that can arise with a completely external standard population. Moreover, the SMR calculated with the pooled groups as standard arises naturally at the first cycle of iteration in one of the numerical procedures for fitting the multiplicative model. These features are illustrated in a cohort analysis of Icelandic breast cancer incidence rates.

(d) Effects of birth cohort on breast cancer incidence in Iceland

Table 4.1 shows the numbers of female breast cancer cases diagnosed in Iceland during 1910–1971 according to five-year interval and decade of birth (Bjarnason *et al.*, 1974). These data can be considered as arising from a large-scale retrospective cohort study that was made possible by the existence of good records and the fact that all diagnoses in a nearly closed population were made by a small number of pathologists. Also shown are the person-years denominators as estimated from census data and the expected number of cases after fitting of the multiplicative model (4.2). Note that the cells in the lower left- and upper right-hand corners of the table are empty, a consequence of the limited period of case ascertainment. This means that the age distributions of the different birth cohorts are extremely different, and, since the cohort effects are strong also, the age-specific rates for the pooled population will not be proportional to the rates for any particular cohort. Thus, we should not expect that SMRs computed using the pooled population as standard will provide very accurate estimates of the relative risk parameters.

Table 4.1 Observed (O) and expected (E) numbers of female breast cancer cases in Iceland during 1910–1971 by age and year of birth, with approximate person–years (P–Y) at risk[a]

Age group (years)		Year of birth										
		1840–1849	1850–1859	1860–1869	1870–1879	1880–1889	1890–1899	1900–1909	1910–1919	1920–1929	1930–1939	1940–1949
20–24	O						2	—	1	1	1	2
	E						0.42	0.52	0.74	0.85	1.30	3.16
	P–Y						41 380	43 650	49 810	58 105	57 105	76 380
25–29	O						—	2	1	1	5	5
	E						1.10	1.37	1.96	2.27	3.47	3.83
	P–Y						39 615	42 204	48 315	57 685	55 965	33 955
30–34	O					1	1	3	7	12	10	
	E					2.38	3.37	4.22	6.12	7.06	10.84	
	P–Y					29 150	38 430	40 810	47 490	55 720	55 145	
35–39	O					6	11	9	14	20	14	
	E					6.01	8.61	10.84	15.88	18.30	14.36	
	P–Y					27 950	37 375	39 935	46 895	54 980	27 810	
40–44	O				7	14	22	25	29	37		
	E				10.13	12.28	17.72	22.56	33.11	38.21		
	P–Y				25 055	27 040	36 400	39 355	46 280	54 350		
45–49	O				21	11	29	33	57	24		
	E				15.21	18.68	27.03	34.75	51.05	28.29		
	P–Y				24 040	26 290	35 480	38 725	45 595	25 710		
50–54	O			15	8	22	27	38	52			
	E			9.71	15.88	19.25	27.96	36.09	53.41			
	P–Y			22 890	23 095	25 410	34 420	37 725	44 740			
55–59	O			10	15	2	26	47	31			
	E			10.61	17.22	21.43	31.45	40.58	29.70			
	P–Y			21 415	21 870	24 240	33 175	36 345	21 320			
60–64	O		8	11	17	23	31	38				
	E		5.68	10.44	17.01	21.47	32.06	41.34				
	P–Y		17 450	19 765	20 255	22 760	31 965	34 705				
65–69	O		8	10	24	30	53	26				
	E		7.71	14.44	23.67	30.32	46.16	28.71				
	P–Y		15 350	17 720	18 280	20 850	29 600	15 635				
70–74	O	5	3	10	18	22	30					
	E	2.92	5.14	9.74	16.21	21.23	32.77					
	P–Y	9 965	12 850	15 015	15 725	18 345	26 400					
75–79	O	1	7	11	26	32	17					
	E	3.62	6.64	12.80	21.83	28.75	20.37					
	P–Y	8 175	11 020	13 095	14 050	16 480	10 885					
80–84	O	5	8	17	32	31						
	E	4.46	8.85	16.28	31.19	32.23						
	P–Y	7 425	10 810	12 260	14 780	13 600						

[a] From Breslow and Day (1975)

Methods of fitting the multiplicative model by maximum likelihood using the computer program GLIM (Baker & Nelder, 1978) are described below in a more general context. This program uses a modification of the Newton–Raphson algorithm to solve the nonlinear likelihood equations; standard errors of the parameter estimates arise as a by-product of these calculations. For the particular model (4.2), however, there is an alternative fitting algorithm, use of which provides greater insight into the relationship between model fitting and the technique of indirect standardization (Breslow & Day, 1975). The equations that determine the maximum likelihood solution may be written

$$\theta_j = \frac{D_j}{\sum_{k=1}^{K} \psi_k n_{jk}} \quad (j = 1, \ldots, J)$$

and   (4.4)

$$\psi_k = \frac{O_k}{\sum_{j=1}^{J} \theta_j n_{jk}} \quad (k = 1, \ldots, K),$$

where $D_j = \sum_k d_{jk}$ are the total deaths at age j and $O_k = \sum_j d_{jk}$ the total deaths at exposure level k (Table 3.4). Inserting initial values $\psi_k^{(0)} = 1$ in the first equation leads to $\theta_j^{(1)} = D_j/N_j$, the marginal death rate in the jth age group, as the initial estimate of θ_j. Here, $N_j = \sum_k n_{jk}$ denotes the total person-years in the jth group. Substituting $\theta_j^{(1)}$ in the second equation gives an initial estimate for ψ_k of $\psi_k^{(1)} = O_k/\sum_j (n_{jk}D_j/N_j)$. Thus, the first-cycle estimate of ψ_k is simply the SMR for the kth exposure group, computed using the age-specific rates for the pooled exposure groups as the standard. Refinements to the initial estimate are obtained by sutstituting $\psi_k^{(1)}$ in the first equation to obtain $\psi_k^{(2)}$, and continuing until convergence when both sets of equations are satisfied simultaneously. If $\hat{\psi}_k$ and $\hat{\theta}_j$ denote the maximum likelihood estimates found at convergence, $\hat{\psi}_k$ may be interpreted as an SMR using the estimated rates $\hat{\theta}_j$ as standard.

Model (4.2) is over-parametrized in the sense that if a particular set of $J + K$ numbers θ_j and ψ_k satisfy the model equation, then so do the sets $\alpha\theta_j$ and $(1/\alpha)\psi_k$ for any positive α. Statisticians refer to such a situation, in which there are more free parameters than can be estimated from the data, as the problem of nonidentifiability. The usual means of solving the problem is to impose constraints on the parameters that are consistent wih a desired interpretation. For the usual choice $\psi_1 = 1$, the remaining ψ_k may be interpreted as relative risks using the first exposure category ($k = 1$) as baseline. The θ_j then correspond to age-specific rates in that baseline category. Of course, the $\hat{\theta}_j$ are actually determined using the data for all the exposure groups, a fact that is especially apparent in this example since for the baseline 1840–1849 cohort data are available for only three age groups.

Another possible resolution of the nonidentifiability problem (Mantel & Stark, 1968) is to choose the normalizing constant α in such a way that when the $\hat{\theta}_j$, interpreted as adjusted age-specific rates, are applied to the pooled population at risk in each age interval, the expected number of deaths is equal to the observed number. Thus,

$$\sum_{j=1}^{J} \hat{\theta}_j N_j = D_+,$$ (4.5)

Table 4.2 Results of fitting the multiplicative model to the data in Table 4.1 (10 iterations)[a]

(a) *Adjusted SMR by cohort*
Year of birth

1840–	1850–	1860–	1870–	1880–	1890–	1900–	1910–	1920–	1930–	1940–
0.252	0.345	0.558	0.886	0.995	1.067	1.257	1.568	1.541	2.392	4.350

(b) *Adjusted age-specific incidence rates per 100 000 person–years*
Age (years)

20–	25–	30–	35–	40–	45–	50–	55–	60–	65–	70–	75–	80–
1.0	2.6	8.2	21.6	45.7	71.4	76.1	88.8	94.8	146.1	116.3	175.3	238.1

[a] From Breslow and Day (1975)

where $D_+ = \sum D_j$ denotes total deaths. This ensures that the $\hat{\theta}_j$ will be roughly comparable in magnitude to the pooled rates $\hat{\lambda}_j = D_j/N_j$ determined from the marginal totals.

Table 4.2 presents the parameter estimates $\hat{\theta}_j$ and $\hat{\psi}_k$ that arise from fitting model (4.2) under the constraint (4.5). Goodness-of-fit is evaluated by comparing the observed d_{jk} and fitted $\hat{d}_{jk} = \hat{\theta}_j \hat{\psi}_k n_{jk}$ numbers of cases in each cell, both of which are shown in Table 4.1. A summary of the goodness-of-fit is provided by the chi-square statistic

$$\chi^2 = \sum_{j=1}^{J} \sum_{k=1}^{K} (d_{jk} - \hat{d}_{jk})^2/\hat{d}_{jk}, \tag{4.6}$$

Fig. 4.2 Crude ($\times$) and fitted ($\bullet$) age-specific incidence rates for female breast cancer in Iceland, 1911–1972. From Breslow and Day (1975)

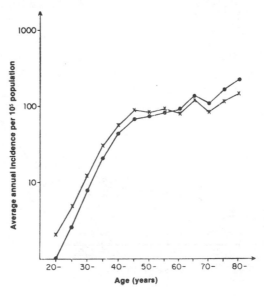

in which the degrees of freedom equal the number of cells with non-zero denominators $(n_{jk} > 0)$, minus the number of independently estimated parameters. For our example, (4.6) yields $\chi^2 = 49.0$ with $77 - 23 = 54$ degrees of freedom ($p = 0.67$). It is important that the contributions to chi-square $(d_{jk} - \hat{d}_{jk})^2/\hat{d}_{jk}$ exceed the 95% critical value of 3.84 for a squared normal deviate for only one cell: in the youngest age group in the 1890–1899 cohort there were two cases observed *versus* only 0.42 expected. Thus, the fit appears remarkably good.

The estimates $\hat{\theta}_j$ are plotted on a semilogarithmic scale in Figure 4.2 together with the marginal rates $\hat{\lambda}_j = D_j/N_j$. It is clear that pooling several heterogeneous birth cohorts has overemphasized the change in slope of the age-incidence curve that occurs around the time of the menopause. This is because the marginal rates at older ages are based on earlier birth cohorts which had lower incidence, whereas the marginal rates at younger ages are based on recent cohorts with high incidence. The fitted values $\hat{\theta}_j$ give an impression of the shape of the age relationship for breast cancer that is more comparable to those seen in other populations (Moolgavkar *et al.*, 1980).

A similar disparity between the SMR_ks determined using the marginal rates as standard and the fitted parameters $\hat{\psi}_k$ representing birth cohorts effects is shown in Figure 4.3 (Hoem, 1987). Here, the expected numbers of cases for recent birth cohorts are too high since only marginal rates for young women are used in their calculation, whereas the expected numbers for the earliest cohorts use only the rates at the oldest

Fig. 4.3 Comparison of indirect standardization and multiplicative model fitting in cohort analysis of female breast cancer in Iceland; ○, standardized mortality ratio; ●, multiplicative parameter. From Hoem (1987)

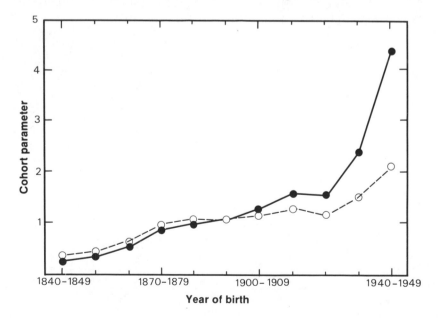

ages. The estimated effect for the 1940–1949 cohort should probably be ignored as it is based on only seven cases occurring at young ages.

4.2 The Poisson assumption[1]

The Poisson model is used throughout this monograph for purposes of making statistical inferences about rates. Specifically, the number of deaths d occurring in a particular age-time-exposure cell is assumed to take on the values $x = 0, 1, 2, \ldots$ with probabilities

$$\text{pr}\,(d = x) = \exp\,(-\lambda n)(\lambda n)^x / x!, \qquad (4.7)$$

where λ denotes the unknown rate and n is the person-years denominator. Furthermore, the numbers of deaths occurring in different cells are regarded as statistically independent, even if the same individuals contribute person-years observation time to more than one of them. In this section, we explore the assumptions required for (4.7) to provide a reasonably accurate description of the statistical fluctuations in a collection of rates. Pocock *et al.* (1981) and Breslow (1984a) have developed some alternative models and techniques that may be used in cases in which the observed variation in rates is greater than that predicted by Poisson theory.

(a) Exponential survival times

Suppose, for simplicity, that there is a single study interval or cell to which I individuals $(i = 1, 2, \ldots, I)$ contribute person-years observation times t_i. Set $\delta_i = 1$ if the ith person dies from (or is diagnosed with) the disease of interest in that cell after observation for t_i years; otherwise, $\delta_i = 0$. We further suppose (although this may be unrealistic in certain applications) that there is a fixed maximum time T_i for which the ith individual will be observed if death does not occur. Most frequently, T_i represents the limitation on the period of observation imposed by the person's entry in the middle of the study or his withdrawal from observation at its end (see Fig. 2.1). Thus, $t_i = T_i$ if $\delta_i = 0$, in which case we say that the observation t_i is censored on the right by T_i.

Inferences are to be made about the death rate λ, defined as the instantaneous probability $\lambda\,dt$ that someone dies in the infinitesimal interval $(t, t + dt)$ of time, given that he was alive and under observation at its start. We assume that the rate λ remains constant for the entire period that each individual is under observation. While obviously only an approximation to the true situation, in practice this means that the cell should be constructed to represent a reasonably short interval of age and/or calendar time and that the corresponding exposure category should be fairly homogeneous. Thus, for example, thinking of duration of employment as a measure of exposure, a particular cell might refer to deaths and person-years that occurred between the ages of 55 and 59 during the years 1960–1964 for persons who had been employed for at least 25 and no more than 30 years. We also make the entirely

---

[1] This section treats a specialized and rather technical topic. Since it presumes greater familiarity with probability theory and statistical inference than the other sections, it may be omitted at first reading.

plausible assumption that the death of one individual has no effect on the outcome for another, or in other words that the two outcomes are statistically independent. Under these conditions the exact distribution of the data (t_i, δ_i) for $i = 1, \ldots, I$ is that of a series of censored exponential survival times.

The exponential distribution has a long history of use in the fields of biometrics, reliability and industrial life testing (Little, 1952; Epstein, 1954; Zelen & Dannemiller, 1961). The ith individual contributes a factor $\lambda e^{-\lambda t_i}$ to the likelihood if he is observed to die during the study interval $(t_i < T_i, \delta_i = 1)$ and a factor $e^{-\lambda t_i}$ (or $e^{-\lambda T_i}$) if he survives until withdrawal $(t_i = T_i, \delta_i = 0)$. Thus, the log-likelihood function is written

$$L(\lambda) = \sum_{i=1}^{I} (\delta_i \log \lambda - t_i \lambda) = d \log (\lambda) - n\lambda, \qquad (4.8)$$

where $d = \sum_i \delta_i$ denotes the total number of events observed and $n = \sum_i t_i$ the total person-years observation time in the specified cell. The elementary estimate $\hat{\lambda} = d/n$ introduced in Chapter 2 is thus seen to be maximum likelihood; it satisfies the likelihood equation $\partial L/\partial \lambda = d/\lambda - n = 0$.

The exact probability distribution of $\hat{\lambda}$ is extremely complicated due to the presence of the censoring times T_i (Kalbfleisch & Prentice, 1980). Mendelhall and Lehman (1960) and Bartholomew (1963) have investigated the first few moments of the distribution, or rather that of the estimated mean survival time $1/\hat{\lambda}$, under the restriction that the censoring times are constant $(T_i = T$ for all $i)$. Approximations to the first two moments are available when the T_i vary. However, these results are all sufficiently complex as to discourage their application to routine problems. One tends to rely instead on large sample normal approximations to the distribution that are based on the log-likelihood (4.8).

(b) The Poisson model

One reason for the complexity of the exact distribution of d/n is the fact that the observation time is terminated at $t_i < T_i$ for individuals who die. Much simpler distributional properties would obtain if each such subject were immediately replaced by an 'identical' one at the time of death, a type of experimental design that is possible in industrial life testing. For then, considering the ith individual and all subsequent replacements as a single experimental unit, the times of death or failure for that unit constitute observations on a single Poisson process on the interval $0 \leqslant t \leqslant T_i$. The δ_i, which could then take on the values $0, 1, 2, \ldots$ rather than just 0 or 1, would have exact Poisson distributions with means λT_i. Since the sum of independent Poisson variables is also Poisson, it follows that the sampling distribution of $d = \sum_i \delta_i$ would be given precisely by (4.7) with $n = \sum_i T_i$, a fixed quantity.

Noting the problems caused by the random observation times t_i, Bartholomew (1963) proposed simply to ignore them in order to obtain an alternative estimate of λ with a more tractable sampling distribution. The only random variables are then the δ_i, which have independent Bernoulli (0/1) distributions with probabilities $p_i = \text{pr}\,(\delta_i = 1) = 1 - \exp\,(-\lambda T_i)$. If all $T_i = T$, $d = \sum_i \delta_i$ follows the binomial law exactly. If the T_i vary, but either they or λ are sufficiently small that $\text{pr}\,(d = 1)$ is moderate, then an extension of the usual Poisson approximation to the binomial distribution (Armitage, 1971) shows that d is approximately Poisson with mean $\lambda \sum_i T_i$.

Both lines of reasoning suggest that the Poisson approximation to the exact sampling distribution of d/n, i.e., treating d as Poisson with fixed mean λn as in (4.7), will be adequate, provided that λ is sufficiently small and that only a fraction of the cohort members are expected to become incident cases or deaths during the period in question. Then, the withdrawal of such cases from observation will have a negligible effect on the total observation time and $\sum_i t_i$ will approximate $\sum_i T_i$. From another point of view, the number of 'units' that experience more than one event in the fictitious experiment described above will be negligible. Thus, when the number of deaths or cases d is small in comparison with the total cohort size, a condition which holds for many of the cohort studies of particular cancers that we have in mind, the Poisson model should provide a reasonable approximation to the exact distribution of the rate. Under these same conditions, moreover, the numbers of deaths occurring in different cells may be regarded as statistically independent. Due to their rarity, deaths occurring in one interval will have negligible effects on the probability that a specified number of deaths occurs in the next interval, even though they remove the individuals in question from risk. Hoem (1987) provides a formal statement and proof of this property that is based on unpublished work of Assmussen.

(c) Asymptotic normality

If the cases are numerous enough to make up a considerable fraction of the total cohort, the arguments just used to justify the Poisson approximation do not apply. One would probably tend not to use exact Poisson probabilities when the events are numerous anyway, but would instead rely on the approach to normality of estimators and tests based on the Poisson model. This point of view provides some reassurance regarding our reliance on approximate methods of inference based on the likelihood function. Since the log-likelihoods for the Poisson and exponential distributions, both being given by equation (4.8), are identical, it makes no difference which sampling framework we adopt for purposes of making likelihood inferences. The usual large-sample distributions of the maximum likelihood estimates and associated statistics are the same, whether we regard the number of deaths as random and the observation times as fixed, the times as random and the number of deaths as fixed, or both times and number of deaths as random.

This conclusion holds also for problems with multiple cells and rates. Suppose there are J cells with associated death rates λ_j, and let δ_{ij} denote whether ($\delta_{ij} = 1$) or not ($\delta_{ij} = 0$) the ith individual dies in the jth cell, while t_{ij} denotes his contribution to the observation time n_j in that cell. According to the general theory of survival distributions (Kalbfleisch & Prentice, 1980; see also §5.2), the log-likelihood of the data may be written

$$L(\lambda) = L(\lambda_1, \ldots, \lambda_J) = \sum_{i=1}^{I} \sum_{j=1}^{J} \delta_{ij} \log \lambda_j - t_{ij}\lambda_j = \sum_{j=1}^{J} d_j \log \lambda_j - n_j\lambda_j. \tag{4.9}$$

This likelihood also arises when the d_j are independent Poisson variables with means

$n_j\lambda_j$ or when the t_{ij} form a censored sample of independent exponential survival times with death rate parameters λ_j (Holford, 1980). However, because of the dependencies between deaths that occur in different intervals and the fact that the n_j are random variables, neither of these exact sampling models is strictly correct. While they are adequate for large-sample likelihood inferences, such as made in this section, other properties based on the Poisson model (such as the standard errors given by equations (2.6) and (2.7)) may require also that the deaths be only a small fraction of the total persons in each cell in order that these be reasonably accurate (Hoem, 1987).

In the sequel, log-likelihood functions similar to (4.9) will be considered as functions of a relatively small number of unknown parameters that describe the structure in the rates. The shape of the log-likelihood function can change drastically depending upon the model selected or even upon the choice of parameters used to describe a given model. As an example, suppose that ten deaths are observed in a single cell with 1000 person-years of observation. Figure 4.4 contrasts the shape of the log-likelihood (4.9) of these data considered as a function of: (i) the death rate λ itself; (ii) the expected

Fig. 4.4   Exact (——) and approximate (- - - -) log-likelihoods for various parametrizations of the death rate, λ, when $d = 10$ and $n = 1000$

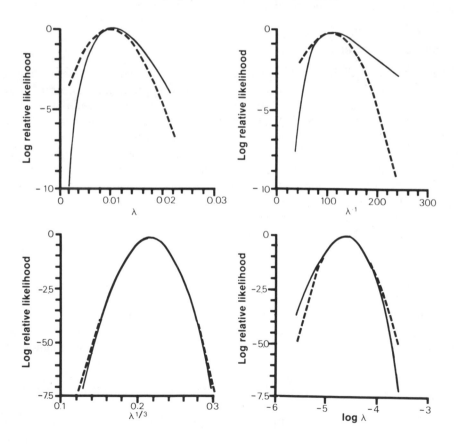

lifetime $1/\lambda$; (iii) the cube-root transform $\lambda^{1/3}$, and (iv) the log death rate $\log \lambda$. Also shown are quadratic approximations to each likelihood that would apply if the data were normally distributed with a mean value equal to the unknown parameter and a fixed variance given by the observed information[1] function evaluated at the maximum likelihood estimate. Comparison of the four figures shows that the cube-root and log parametrizations yield the most 'normal' looking likelihoods, whereas those for λ and especially $1/\lambda$ are rather skewed. The cube-root transform, which also occurred in Byar's approximation to Poisson error probabilities (equations (2.11) and (2.13)), has the property that it exactly eliminates the cubic term in a series expansion of L about the maximum likelihood estimate (Sprott, 1973). Empirical work by Schou and Vaeth (1980) has confirmed that the sampling distributions of $\log \hat{\lambda}$ and $\hat{\lambda}^{1/3}$ are more nearly normal in finite samples than those of $\hat{\lambda}$ or its inverse.

The implication of these results for the statistician is that statistical inferences that rely on asymptotic normal theory are better carried out using procedures that are invariant under transformations of the basic parameters. The maximum likelihood estimate itself satisfies this requirement, as do likelihood ratio tests, score tests computed with expected information, and confidence intervals obtained by inverting such invariant tests. However, procedures based on a comparison of the point estimate with its standard error as obtained from the normal (quadratic) approximation to the log-likelihood are not generally reliable and should be used only if the normal approximation is known to be good (Vaeth, 1985). This condition is met for parameters in the standard multiplicative models considered below, as it was for the logistic models discussed in Volume 1. It is not met for other models, as we shall see.

4.3 Fitting the multiplicative model

Most of the features of the multiplicative model for rates are already present in the two-dimensional table considered in §4.1. We continue to think of the basic data as being stratified in two dimensions. The first dimension corresponds to nuisance factors such as age and calendar time, the effects of which on the baseline rates are conceded in advance and are generally of secondary interest in the study at hand. The second dimension corresponds to the exposure variables, the effects of which we wish to model explicitly. The total number of cells into which the data are grouped is thus the product of J strata and K exposure categories. The basic data consist of the counts of deaths d_{jk} and the person-years denominators n_{jk} in each cell, together with p-dimensional row vectors $\mathbf{x}_{jk} = (x_{jk}^{(1)}, \ldots, x_{jk}^{(p)})$ of regression variables. These latter may represent either qualitative or quantitative effects of the exposures on the stratum-specific rates, interactions among the exposures and interactions between exposure variables and stratification (nuisance) variables.

---

[1] Recall from §6.4 of Volume 1 or elsewhere that the information is defined as minus the second derivative of L. Since we consider some models in this volume for which the information depends on the data, a distinction is made between the observed information and its expectation. The latter is also known as Fisher information.

(a) *The model equation*

A general form of the multiplicative model is

$$\log \lambda_{jk} = \alpha_j + \mathbf{x}_{jk}\boldsymbol{\beta}, \tag{4.10}$$

where the λ_{jk} are the unknown true disease rates, the α_j are nuisance parameters specifying the effects of age and other stratification variables, and $\boldsymbol{\beta} = (\beta_1, \ldots, \beta_p)^T$ is a p-dimensional column vector of regression coefficients that describe the effects of primary interest. An important feature of this and other models introduced below is that the disease rates depend on the exposures only through the quantity $\alpha_j + \mathbf{x}_{jk}\boldsymbol{\beta}$, which is known as the linear predictor. If the regression variables $\mathbf{x}_{jk}$ depend only on the exposure category k and not on j, (4.10) specifies a purely multiplicative relationship such that the ratio of disease rates $\lambda_{jk}/\lambda_{jk'}$ for two exposure levels k and k', namely $\exp\{(\mathbf{x}_k - \mathbf{x}_{k'})\boldsymbol{\beta}\}$, is constant over the strata. Evaluation of the goodness-of-fit of such models informs us as to whether a summary of the data in terms of relative risk is reasonably plausible. If the ratios $\lambda_{jk}/\lambda_{jk'}$ change with j, additional variables x_{jk} which depend on both j and k and describe interactions between stratum and exposure effects may be needed to provide a comprehensive summary of the data.

The simple multiplicative model (4.2) for the two-dimensional table of rates is expressed by taking the x variables to be dummy or indicator variables with a value of 1 for a particular exposure category and 0 elsewhere. A total of $K - 1$ such indicator variables is needed to express the relative risks associated with the different exposure categories, the first level ($k = 1$) typically being used as a reference or baseline category. The advantage of the more general model (4.10) is that it allows us to quantify the relative risks according to measured dose levels, impose some structure on the joint effects of two or more exposures, and relax the strict multiplicative hypothesis through the introduction of interaction terms. These features are developed below in a series of examples. However, we first discuss implementation of the methodology using the Royal Statistical Society's GLIM program for fitting generalized linear models (Baker & Nelder, 1978).

(b) *Fitting the model with GLIM*

Input to GLIM or other standard programs will consist of up to JK data records containing the counts d_{jk} of disease cases or deaths, the person-years denominators n_{jk}, the values $x_{jk}^{(1)}, \ldots, x_{jk}^{(p)}$ of the regression variables to be included in the model, and sufficient additional data to identify each stratum (j) and exposure category (k). Records for (j, k) cells with no person-years of observation ($n_{jk} = 0$) are usually omitted.

If some or all of the exposures are to be analysed as qualitative or discrete variables, it is not necessary to construct the 0/1 indicators explicitly for each exposure category or stratum, since GLIM makes provision in its FACTOR command for designating certain input variables as qualitative. Their values $(1, 2 \ldots)$ are then presumed to designate the factor level. By default, the first level is taken as baseline, binary indicator variables being constructed by the program for each higher level.

According to §4.2 the numbers of deaths d_{jk} from a specific cause may be regarded as independent Poisson variables with mean values $E(d_{jk}) = n_{jk}\lambda_{jk}$. In view of (4.10) we have

$$\log E(d_{jk}) = \log (n_{jk}) + \alpha_j + \mathbf{x}_{jk}\boldsymbol{\beta}. \tag{4.11}$$

Since the log transform of the mean is a linear function of the unknown parameters $\boldsymbol{\alpha}$ and $\boldsymbol{\beta}$, the model conforms to the usual log-linear model for Poisson variables and as such is easily fitted using standard features of GLIM. Note that the constants $\log (n_{jk})$ offset the model equation (4.11) from the origin in the sense that the log mean equals $\log (n_{jk})$ when the α and β parameters are zero. This means that a variable containing the log person-years denominators is declared an OFFSET when invoking the program. In order to fit a separate α_j for each stratum level, it is easiest to create a stratum variable taking values $j = 1, \ldots, J$ and declare it as a FACTOR. When the strata are formed by combinations of two or more variables, these may each be declared FACTORs and included in the model with all their interactions. The exposures are treated as either variables or factors, depending upon whether quantitative or qualitative (categorical) effects are to be specified.

An alternative GLIM approach is to define the dependent or y variable as the observed rate $\hat{\lambda}_{jk} = d_{jk}/n_{jk}$ and to declare the person-years denominator n_{jk} as a prior WEIGHT. Then, no OFFSET is needed. This approach also applies with the additive (identity) and power 'link' functions considered in §4.4, whereas the approach that declares $\log (n_{jk})$ to be an OFFSET does not. See Frome and Checkoway (1985).

(c) Summary measures of fit

Summary measures of fit give an overall evaluation of the agreement between observed and fitted values. Two are in common use. One is the χ^2 statistic already defined in (4.6) as the sum of the squared residuals. The other is the log-likelihood ratio statistic that compares the observed and fitted values *via*

$$G^2 = 2\left\{\sum_{j=1}^{J} \sum_{k=1}^{K} d_{jk} \log (d_{jk}/\hat{d}_{jk}) + (\hat{d}_{jk} - d_{jk})\right\}. \tag{4.12}$$

G^2 is known as the deviance in GLIM. G^2 and χ^2 are referred to tables of the chi-square distribution in order to ascertain the overall goodness-of-fit. They tend to give similar values in most applications. Both may overstate the degree of departure from the fitted model when many cells contain small counts (Fienberg, 1980) and when they are interpreted as chi-square statistics; a correction factor for G^2 is available (Williams, 1976).

The degrees of freedom associated with these statistics equal the number of cells with nonzero person-years of observation minus the number of linearly independent parameters in the model, namely $J + p$ in the above formulation. When the value of G^2 or χ^2 exceeds its degrees of freedom by an amount significantly greater than expected under chi-square sampling, we conclude that the fit is inadequate. Either there are systematic effects that have not been accounted for by the model, or else the random variation in disease rates among neighbouring cells is greater than that specified by the Poisson assumption. Agreement between the deviance and its degrees of freedom does not guarantee that the fit is good, however, particularly when the degrees of freedom are large. Systematic patterns or trends in the residuals that may be indicative of departures from model assumptions, and large residual values for individual cells, often are not reflected adequately in the summary measure. Also, a good fit for a model based on a cross-classification that ignores relevant covariables does not imply that such variables are unimportant or should not be considered.

(d) Adding variables to the model equation

The most common remedy for the lack of fit of a given model equation, or for examining whether systematic departures from model assumptions are being obscured by the global goodness-of-fit statistic, is to add regression variables. Indeed, the process of model building generally involves fitting a hierarchy of model equations that represent increasing degrees of complexity in the relationship between the relative risk and the exposure variables, or increasingly complex interaction (modifying) effects of the stratification variables with the exposure variables. Comparison of the goodness-of-fit measures for two different models, one of which is contained within the other, provides a formal test of the statistical significance of the additional variables. Thus, if G_1^2 and G_2^2 are the deviances for models 1 and 2, where model 2 contains q more independent parameters than model 1, the difference $G_1^2 - G_2^2$ is treated as a chi-square statistic with q degrees of freedom for testing the significance of the additional variables. Two other commonly used tests, one based on the estimated regression coefficients and the other on the efficient score (first derivative of the log-likelihood), are briefly described in §6.4 of Volume 1.

(e) Further evaluation of goodness-of-fit: analysis of residuals

The extent to which the model summarizes the data can be evaluated globally by an overall goodness-of-fit test, but often a more informative approach is to examine how well the number of deaths in each cell is predicted. This is accomplished by comparing the observed numbers of deaths d_{jk} in each cell with the fitted number $\hat{d}_{jk} = n_{jk} \exp(\hat{\alpha}_j + \mathbf{x}_{jk}\hat{\beta})$, where $\hat{\alpha}_j$ and $\hat{\beta}$ denote the maximum likelihood estimates. In order to get some idea of whether the deviations between observed and fitted values are greater than would be expected from sampling (Poisson) variability, we calculate the standardized residuals $r_{jk} = (d_{jk} - \hat{d}_{jk})/\sqrt{\hat{d}_{jk}}$. Since they have the form of the difference between an observation and its estimated mean, divided by the estimated standard deviation under the Poisson model, the r_{jk} may be regarded roughly as equivalent normal deviates when assessing the fit for any particular cell. A refinement, taking account of the number of fitted parameters, is to consider as equivalent normal deviates the adjusted residuals

$$\tilde{r}_{jk} = \frac{r_{jk}}{(1 - h_{jk})^{1/2}} = \frac{d_{jk} - \hat{d}_{jk}}{\{\hat{d}_{jk}(1 - h_{jk})\}^{1/2}}, \qquad (4.13)$$

where the h_{jk} denote the diagonal element of the 'hat' or projection matrix that arises in the theory of linear regression (Hoaglin & Welsh, 1978). These are available in

GLIM as the product of the 'iterative weights', which equal $\hat{d}_{jk}$ for the multiplicative Poisson model, times the variances of the linear predictors. In other words, for the multiplicative model,

$$h_{jk} = \hat{d}_{jk} \operatorname{Var}(\hat{\alpha}_j + \mathbf{x}_{jk}\hat{\boldsymbol{\beta}}). \tag{4.14}$$

The sum of the h_{jk} equals the number of parameters estimated, namely $J + p$.

Modern texts on regression anslysis (e.g., Cook & Weisberg, 1982) devote considerable attention to graphical methods of residual analysis. Certain patterns in the residuals are indicative of specific types of departures from model assumptions. For example, a tendency for the absolute values $|r_{jk}|$ to increase with $\hat{d}_{jk}$ would indicate that the equality of mean and variance specified by the Poisson model was inadequate and that the variability increased faster than as a linear function of the mean. Correlations between the residuals and regression variables not yet included in the model equation would indicate that the model was incomplete, whereas correlations with certain functions of the fitted values may indicate that the log-linear specification (4.11) is inadequate and that the death rates λ_{jk} are better modelled by some other function of the linear predictors (Pregibon, 1980). We present some examples of graphical residual analyses in the sequel, but systematic discussion of their rationale and use is beyond the scope of this monograph.

(f) Gauging the influence of individual data points

Another aspect of model checking, apart from examination of residuals, is to determine the influence that individual data points have on the estimated regression coefficients $\hat{\alpha}_j$ and $\hat{\boldsymbol{\beta}}$. The investigator needs to be aware whenever elimination of one of the (j, k) cells from the analysis would lead to a particularly marked change in the fitted model. Sometimes, such influential cells are also 'outliers', in the sense that the multivariable observation $(d_{jk}, n_{jk}, \mathbf{x}_{jk})$ is far removed from the rest of the data. It is important to check that such data have been correctly recorded and are not in error. The same is true for data points that give rise to large residuals. 'Robust' regression methods have been developed specifically to reduce the influence of such outlying observations (Huber, 1983); however, the rationale for their use is not entirely clear when the data in question are known to be valid. A concerted effort to understand why the particular observation does not conform to the rest of the data may be more important than finding the model that best fits when that point is removed.

Influential data points are often reasonably well fitted by the model and not amenable to detection by an examination of their residuals. More sensitive measures of influence can be developed using a combination of the residuals and the diagonal elements h_{jk} of the 'hat' matrix (equation 4.14). A rough rule of thumb for general applications is to regard an individual observation as having a particularly heavy influence on the overall fit if the corresponding h_{jk} exceeds twice the average value (Hoaglin & Welsh, 1978). This rule is not applicable in the present context, however, since cells with large person-years and expected numbers of cases will necessarily have a large impact on the fit. Rather, we use the h_{jk} diagnostics in a descriptive and comparative manner to identify those cells that have the greatest overall influence on the fit and to demonstrate that the relative influence of different cells on the regression coefficients can depend on the transformation linking the rates λ_{jk} to the linear predictor.

Measures of the influence of individual cells on particular regression coefficients involve these same basic quantities (Pregibon, 1979, 1981). In particular, an approximation to the change in the estimated regression coefficients $(\hat{\alpha}, \hat{\beta})$ that is occasioned by deletion of the (j, k) cell from the statistical analysis is given by

$$\Delta(\hat{\alpha}, \hat{\beta})_{-jk} \simeq -\Sigma \, \mathbf{x}_{jk}^*(d_{jk} - \hat{d}_{jk})/(1 - \hat{h}_{jk}), \qquad (4.15)$$

where Σ denotes the asymptotic covariance matrix of the estimates $(\hat{\alpha}, \hat{\beta})$ and $\mathbf{x}_{jk}^* = (0, \ldots 1, \ldots, 0, \mathbf{x}_{jk})$ denotes an augmented vector of regression variables preceded by J stratum indicators of which the jth equals one.

Example 4.1

Appendix VI contains grouped data from a recent update (Peto, J. *et al.*, 1984) of the Welsh nickel refinery workers study that is described in detail in Appendix ID. Previously published data from this study (Doll *et al.*, 1970) were used in §3.5 to illustrate techniques of internal standardization. The latest follow-up through 1981 uncovered 137 lung cancer deaths among men aged 40–85 years and 56 deaths from cancer of the nasal sinus.

Nasal sinus cancer deaths and person-years of observation are classified in Appendix VI by three risk factors: (i) age at first employment (AFE) in four levels (1 = <20; 2 = 20–27.4; 3 = 27.5–34.9; and 4 = 35+ years); (ii) calendar year of first employment (YFE) in four levels (1 = <1910; 2 = 1910–1914; 3 = 1915–1919; and 4 = 1920–1924); and (iii) time since first employment (TFE) in five levels (1 = 0–19; 2 = 20–29; 3 = 30–39; 4 = 40–49; and 5 = 50+ years). Since less than one case of nasal sinus cancer would have been expected from national rates, it was deemed unnecessary to account for the background rates. Instead, the object was to study the evolution of nasal sinus cancer risk as a function of time since first exposure, and to determine whether this was influenced by the age and year in which that exposure began.

Table 4.3 displays the GLIM commands needed to read the 72 data records, fit the log-linear model with main effects for factors AFE, YFE and TFE, and print the results shown in Tables 4.5 and 4.6. Models involving a number of other combinations of these same factors were investigated also. Their deviances, displayed in Table 4.4, demonstrate that the three factors have strong, independent effects on rates of nasal sinus cancer. The log-likelihood ratio statistics of 95.6 − 58.2 = 37.4 for AFE, 83.5 − 58.2 = 25.3 for YFE and 70.8 − 58.2 = 12.6 for TFE, with 3, 3 and 4 degrees of freedom, are all highly significant. The parameter estimates in Table 4.5 indicate that nasal sinus cancer risk increases steadily with both age at and time since first exposure, and that it peaks for men who were first employed in the 1910–1914 period. Since the global tests for two-factor interactions are of at most borderline significance, the largest being 16.4 (9 degrees of freedom, $p = 0.06$) for YFE × TFE, we conclude that the simple multiplicative model provides a reasonable description of the data. Further support for this conclusion is obtained by comparing observed and fitted numbers of cases classified by AFE × TFE collapsing over YFE (Table 4.6), and similarly for the other two-factor combinations. The greatest discrepancy is observed for the YFE × TFE cross-classification (not shown), where four cases are observed in the cell with YFE = <1910 and TFE = 20–29 years, whereas only 1.30 are expected under the model ($\chi_1^2 = 5.6$). We are inclined to interpret this aberrant value as a chance occurrence.

The marginal totals of expected numbers of deaths in Table 4.6 agree exactly with the observed numbers, which confirms this as a defining characteristic of the maximum likelihood fitting of the log-linear model (Fienberg, 1980). Inclusion of the main effects of AFE, YFE and TFE in the model ensures that the fitted values for each of these factors, when summed over the levels of the other two, will agree with the subtotals of observed values. (Inclusion of the AFE × TFE interactions in the model in addition to the main effects would result in subtotals of fitted values for the AFE × TFE two-dimensional marginal table that agree with the corresponding observed subtotals.) Table 4.6 also illustrates a fundamental property of the 'hat' matrix elements, h, namely, that their grand total equals the number of independent parameters in the model. In this example, there is one parameter associated with the constant term or grand mean (see Table 4.5), three

Table 4.3 GLIM commands used to analyse the data in Appendix VI

$UNITS 72 ! 72 DATA RECORDS IN FILE IN APPENDIX VI; EQUATE TO FORTRAN UNIT 1
$DATA AFE YFE TFE CASE PY! NAMES OF 5 VARIABLES TO BE READ FROM FILE
$DINPUT 1 80 ! READ DATA FROM FORTRAN UNIT 1
$FACTOR 72 AFE 4 YFE 4 TFE 5 ! DECLARE FACTORS WITH 4 AND 5 LEVELS EACH
$CAL LPY = %LOG(PY) ! CALCULATE LOG PERSON–YEARS
$OFFSET LPY ! DECLARE LOG PERSON–YEARS AS OFFSET TO MODEL EQUATION
$ERR P ! POISSON MODEL WITH DEFAULT (LOG-LINEAR) LINK
$YVAR CASE ! NO. OF NASAL CANCERS (CASE) AS DEPENDENT VARIABLE
$FIT AFE + YFE + TFE ! FIT LOG-LINEAR MODEL WITH MAIN EFFECTS FOR EACH FACTOR
$ACC 5 ! CHANGE NO. OF DECIMALS IN PRINTOUT
$REC 10 $FIT . ! REFIT SAME MODEL FOR GREATER ACCURACY
$DIS M E$! DISPLAY MODEL AND PARAMETER ESTIMATES. SEE TABLE 4.5
$EXT %VL %PE ! EXTRACT VARIANCE OF LINEAR PREDICTOR AND PARAMETER ESTIMATES
$VAR 11 PR ! DECLARE REL RISK RR AS VARIABLE OF DIMENSION 11
$CAL RR = %EXP(%PE) $LOOK RR $! CALCULATE AND PRINT REL RISKS FOR TABLE 4.5
$CAL H = %WT*%VL ! CALCULATE DIAGONAL ELEMENTS OF 'HAT' MATRIX H
$CAL I = 5*(AFE-1) + TFE ! SET UP INDEX FOR CELLS IN AFE BY TFE MARGINAL TABLE
$VAR 20 CAST EXPT PYT HT ! SET UP VARIABLES OF DIMENSION 20
$CAL CAST = 0 : EXPT = 0 : PYT = 0 : HT = 0 ! INITIALIZE ARRAYS
$CAL CAST(I) = CAST (I) + CASE : EXPT(I) = EXPT(I) + %FV : PYT(I) + PYT(I) + PY$
$CAL HT(I) = HT(I) + H ! CULULATE SUBTOTALS OF CASES, FITTED VALUES ETC. OVER YFE
$LOOK CAST EXPT PTY HT ! PRINTOUT FOR TABLE 4.6
$STOP

Table 4.4 Goodness-of-fit statistics (deviances) for a number of multiplicative models fitted to the data on Welsh nickel refinery workers in Appendix VI

Factors in model[a]	Degrees of freedom	Deviance
—	71	135.7
AFE	68	109.1
YFE	68	100.6
TFE	67	120.6
AFE + YFE	65	70.8
AFE + TFE	64	83.5
YFE + TFE	64	95.6
AFE + YFE + TFE	61	58.2
AFE*YFE[b] + TFE	52	49.2
AFE*TFE + YFE	50	48.5
YFE*TFE + AFE	50	41.8

[a] AFE, age at first employment; YFE, year of first employment; TFE, time since first employment

[b] AFE*YFE indicates, in standard GLIM notation, that both main effects and first-order interactions involving the indicated factors are included in the model equation.

Table 4.5 Regression coefficients, standard errors and associated relative risks for the multiplicative model fitted to data on nasal sinus cancers in Welsh nickel refinery workers (Appendix VI)

Factor[a]	Level	Regression coefficient ± standard error	Relative risk[b]
AFE	<20	—	1.0
	20.0–27.4	1.67 ± 0.75	5.3
	27.5–34.9	2.48 ± 0.76	12.0
	35+	3.43 ± 0.78	30.8
YFE	<1910	—	1.0
	1910–14	0.62 ± 0.37	1.9
	1915–19	0.05 ± 0.47	1.1
	1920–24	−1.13 ± 0.45	0.3
TFE	<20	—	1.0
	20–29	1.60 ± 1.05	4.9
	30–39	1.75 ± 1.06	5.8
	40–49	2.35 ± 1.07	10.5
	50+	2.82 ± 1.12	16.7
Constant term		−9.27 ± 1.32	Estimated baseline[c] rate of nasal sinus cancer deaths: 9.42 per 100 000 person–years

Deviance: $G^2 = 58.2$ on 61 degrees of freedom

[a] AFE, age at first employment; YFE, year of first employment; TFE, time since first employment
[b] Exponentiated regression coefficients
[c] For AFE < 20, YFE < 1910 and TFE < 20

each with AFE and YFE and four with TFE, for a total of 11. Note that the larger values of h_+ are generally associated with the cells with the largest number of observed deaths.

4.4   Choosing between additive and multiplicative models

If a good fit is obtainable with the multiplicative model only by introducing complicated interaction terms involving baseline and exposure factors, re-examination of the basic multiplicative relationship is usually in order. It may be that the effects of exposure are better and more easily expressed on another scale. Formal evaluation of the relative merits of the multiplicative and additive models for any particular set of regression variables is made possible by embedding them in a wider class of models that contain both as special cases. One useful class of models for this purpose is the power family

$$\lambda_{jk}^{\rho} = \alpha_j + \mathbf{x}_{jk}\boldsymbol{\beta} \tag{4.16}$$

that relates the disease rates to the linear predictors $\alpha_j + \mathbf{x}_{jk}\boldsymbol{\beta}$ by means of the power transform with exponent ρ (Aranda–Ordaz, 1983). The additive model corresponds to the case $\rho = 1$, whereas, since $(\lambda^{\rho} - 1)/\rho$ tends to $\log \lambda$ in the limit as ρ tends towards zero, the multiplicative model corresponds to $\rho = 0$.

Power models may be fitted easily using GLIM. The dependent or y observations, assumed to have a Poisson error structure, are the rates $\hat{\lambda}_{jk} = d_{jk}/n_{jk}$ rather than

Table 4.6 Results of fitting the multiplicative model to the data on Welsh nickel refinery workers in Appendix VI: observed (O) and expected (E) numbers of nasal sinus cancer deaths, person–years (P–Y) and summed regression diagnostics h by age at first employment and time since first employment

Age at first employment (years)		Years since first employment					
		0–19	20–29	30–39	40–49	50+	Total
<20	O	0	1	0	1	0	2
	E^a	0.02	0.34	0.43	0.58	0.63	2.00
	P–Y	353.0	806.6	832.4	652.1	445.0	3089.1
	$h_+{}^b$	0.03	0.22	0.26	0.36	0.41	1.28
20.0–27.4	O	0	3	6	7	4	20
	E	0.21	4.40	5.61	5.97	3.80	20.00
	P–Y	1107.9	2044.2	2094.9	1281.8	536.1	7064.9
	h_+	0.23	0.69	0.85	0.94	0.91	3.62
27.5–34.4	O	0	8	5	5	2	20
	E	0.31	6.30	6.62	5.19	1.57	20.00
	P–Y	732.7	1303.8	1098.6	481.4	95.3	3711.8
	h_+	0.34	0.89	0.94	0.86	0.43	3.46
35+	O	1	7	6	0	—	14
	E	0.46	7.96	4.33	1.25	—	14.00
	P–Y	392.4	622.9	303.4	46.1	—	1364.8
	h_+	0.49	1.10	0.78	0.28	—	2.65
Total	O	1	19	17	13	6	56
	E	1.00	19.00	17.00	13.00	6.00	56.00
	P–Y	2586.0	4777.5	4329.3	2461.4	1076.4	15 230.6
	h_+	1.09	2.90	2.83	2.44	1.75	11.00

[a] Expected values adjusted also for year of first employment
[b] Regression diagnostics h summed over levels of year of first employment. These values should *not* be substituted in the expression for adjusted residuals (equation 4.13).

the numbers of deaths; the person-years denominators are treated as prior weights, using the WEIGHT command. The model (4.16) is available as an alternative GLIM 'link' for Poisson observations.

Diagonal elements of the 'hat' matrix are obtained at convergence as

$$h_{jk} = n_{jk} w_{jk} \operatorname{Var}(\hat{\eta}_{jk}),$$

where w_{jk} is the GLIM iterated weight for the power model and $\hat{\eta}_{jk} = \hat{\alpha}_{jk} + \mathbf{x}_{jk}\hat{\boldsymbol{\beta}}$ is the linear predictor. The approximate change in the regression coefficients upon deletion of the (j, k)th cell of data is given by

$$\Delta(\hat{\alpha}, \hat{\boldsymbol{\beta}})_{-jk} = -\boldsymbol{\Sigma} \, \mathbf{x}_{jk}^* \, n_{jk} w_{jk}(y_{jk} - \hat{\eta}_{jk})/(1 - h_{jk}), \qquad (4.17)$$

where $\mathbf{x}_{jk}^*$ is the vector of augmented regression variables, y_{jk} denotes the GLIM 'working variable', and $\boldsymbol{\Sigma}$ is again the covariance matrix of the estimated parameters.

Example 4.2

The data on coronary deaths among British male doctors shown in Table 3.15 offer a simple example for examining some of these issues regarding goodness-of-fit and model selection. The rate ratios for smokers *versus* nonsmokers decrease with advancing age, while the rate differences generally increase. This suggests

Fig. 4.5   Goodness-of-fit statistics (G^2) for a variety of power models fitted to the data
in Table 3.15

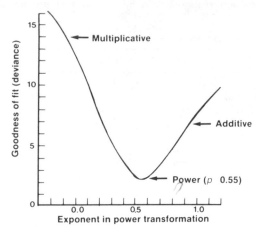

that neither the multiplicative nor the additive model is completely appropriate for expressing the effect of
smoking in a single number, and that some intermediate power model might work better. Accordingly,
several models of the form (4.16) were fitted with a single binary exposure variable coded 0 for nonsmokers
and 1 for smokers. Figure 4.5 shows that the minimum value of the deviance G^2, nominally a
chi-square-distributed statistic with $10 - 6 = 4$ degrees of freedom, occurs in the vicinity of $\rho = 0.55$,
intermediate between the additive and multiplicative models. Neither of these extremes provides a
satisfactory fit, since one finds $G^2 = 12.1$ for the multiplicative and $G^2 = 7.4$ for the additive structure,
compared with $G^2 = 2.1$ for the best power transform.

Table 4.7 presents estimates and standard errors for the five α_j parameters and the single smoking
coefficient β under each of the three models. When suitably transformed, the α's represent the fitted death
rates among nonsmokers per 1000 person-years of observation. Under the additive model, for example, the
fitted rate for men aged 55–64 years is 6.2 deaths per 1000 population per year. For the power model the rate
per 1000 person-years is $(2.180)^{(1/0.55)} = 4.1$, and for the multiplicative model it is $\exp(1.616) = 5.0$. Smoking
is estimated to increase (add to) the death rate by 0.59 deaths per 1000 person-years under the additive
model, while under the multiplicative model smoking multiplies the death rate by $\exp(0.355) = 1.43$ at all
ages. The smoking effect is not so conveniently expressed on the power scale, but since ρ and β are each
about equal to 0.5 it may be roughly described as increasing the square root of the death rate per 1000
person-years by one-half. Note that t statistics of the form $t = \hat{\beta}/SE(\hat{\beta})$ yield roughly comparable values for
all three models with these data. The likelihood ratio (deviance) tests for smoking $(\beta = 0)$ are obtained by
subtracting the goodness-of-fit deviances in Table 4.7 from the deviance for the model with age effects only,
which equals 23.99 regardless of the value of ρ. Best agreement between the t test and deviance test of
smoking effect is found for the multiplicative model.

Table 4.7 also shows the fitted numbers of deaths $\hat{d}_{jk}$ for smokers and nonsmokers under the three models.
These were combined with the diagnostic values h_{jk} to calculate adjusted residuals $\bar{r}_{jk}$ (equation 4.13). The
'hat' matrix elements h_{jk}, approximate changes in the smoking coefficient from equation 4.15 or 4.17 and
adjusted residuals $\bar{r}_{jk}$ are all displayed in Table 4.8.

Examination of the entries in the first two parts of Table 4.8 shows that the data for the youngest age
group, which contains a small number of deaths observed in a rather large population, have the greatest
influence on the estimated rate difference in the additive model. More of the information about the rate ratio
under the multiplicative model comes from older age groups where there are larger numbers of deaths. The
power model occupies an intermediate position vis-à-vis the diagnostics h_{jk}, and deletion of single cells has
little effect on the smoking parameter. The residual patterns are in the anticipated direction, the death rates

Table 4.7 Parameter estimates and fitted values for three statistical models for the data on coronary deaths among British male doctors in Table 3.15

Age range (years)	Parameter	Statistical model[a]		
		Additive ($\rho = 1$)	Power ($\rho = 0.55$)	Multiplicative ($\rho = 0$)
		Parameter estimates $\pm$ SE[b]		
35–44	α_1	0.084 ± 0.066	0.276 ± 0.092	-1.012 ± 0.192
45–54	α_2	1.641 ± 0.218	1.115 ± 0.110	0.472 ± 0.130
55–64	α_3	6.304 ± 0.456	2.456 ± 0.132	1.616 ± 0.115
65–74	α_4	13.524 ± 0.964	3.859 ± 0.180	2.338 ± 0.116
75–84	α_5	19.170 ± 1.704	4.763 ± 0.257	2.688 ± 0.125
Smoking	β	0.591 ± 0.125	0.493 ± 0.098	0.355 ± 0.107
$t^2 = (\hat{\beta}/\text{SE}(\hat{\beta}))^2$		19.3	25.3	11.0

		Fitted values[c]					
		Non-smokers	Smokers	Non-smokers	Smokers	Non-smokers	Smokers
35–44		1.59	35.37	1.81	32.53	6.83	27.17
45–54		17.51	96.50	13.00	102.56	17.12	98.88
55–64		35.99	197.25	29.26	204.49	28.74	205.26
65–74		34.96	178.73	30.12	183.61	26.81	187.19
75–84		28.03	105.07	24.97	108.65	21.51	111.49

	Additive	Power	Multiplicative
Goodness-of-fit (deviance) χ_4^2	7.43	2.14	12.13
Deviance test for smoking effect χ_1^2	16.56	21.85	11.86

[a] Exponent (ρ) of power function relating death rates and linear predictor
[b] Person–years denominators expressed in units of 1000
[c] See Table 3.15 for observed values

for smokers being seriously underestimated by the multiplicative model in the youngest age group and seriously overestimated in the oldest group. By contrast, in spite of the heavy influence of this age group on the estimated regression coefficients, the death rate among 35–44-year-old smokers is seriously overestimated by the additive model. With the power model, the residuals are all quite small, indicative of the good fit, and none of them shows statistically significant deviations when referred to tables of the standard normal distribution.

An alternative method of examining the goodness-of-fit is *via* the introduction of regression variables representing the interaction of smoking and age. For this purpose we defined a single quantitative interaction term in coded age and exposure levels, namely $x_{jk} = (j - 3)(k - 1.5)$ for $j = 1, 2, \ldots, 5$ and $k = 1, 2$. The constants 3 and 1.5 were subtracted before multiplying in order that the interaction variable be not too highly correlated with the main effects for age and smoking (see §6.10, Volume 1). Table 4.9 shows the estimated regression coefficient $\hat{\gamma}$ of the interaction variable, its standard error, and the goodness-of-fit statistic G^2 for each of the three basic models. The deviances at the bottom of Table 4.7 show that introduction of the interaction term results in a marked improvement in fit for both additive and multiplicative models. Note that the estimated interaction term is positive in the additive model, indicating that the rate difference increases with age, and negative in the multiplicative model, indicating that the rate ratios decline. These

Table 4.8 Regression diagnostics and adjusted residuals for three statistical models fitted to the data on coronary deaths among British male doctors (Table 3.15)

Age range (years) (j)	Statistical model					
	Additive ($\rho = 1$)		Power ($\rho = 0.55$)		Multiplicative ($\rho = 0$)	
	Non-smokers ($k = 1$)	Smokers ($k = 2$)	Non-smokers ($k = 1$)	Smokers ($k = 2$)	Non-smokers ($k = 1$)	Smokers ($k = 2$)
Diagonal elements of hat matrix (h_{jk})						
35–44	0.98	0.93	0.67	0.86	0.25	0.81
45–54	0.31	0.77	0.42	0.85	0.29	0.88
55–64	0.19	0.82	0.28	0.85	0.38	0.91
65–74	0.18	0.83	0.22	0.84	0.36	0.91
75–84	0.22	0.78	0.24	0.79	0.34	0.87
Approximate change in β coefficient for smoking after deletion of each observation						
35–44	0.855	0.855	0.026	0.026	−0.060	−0.060
45–54	−0.058	−0.058	−0.021	−0.021	−0.072	−0.072
55–64	−0.020	−0.020	−0.010	−0.010	−0.012	−0.012
65–74	−0.008	−0.008	−0.010	−0.010	0.018	0.018
75–84	0.002	0.002	0.023	0.023	0.138	0.138
Adjusted residuals ($\bar{r}_{jk}$)						
35–44	2.17	−2.17	0.25	−0.25	−2.14	2.14
45–54	−1.58	1.58	−0.36	0.36	−1.47	1.47
55–64	−1.47	1.47	−0.27	0.27	−0.17	0.17
65–74	−1.30	1.30	−0.44	0.44	0.29	−0.29
75–84	0.64	−0.64	1.38	−1.38	2.51	−2.51

Table 4.9 Fitting of a quantitative interaction variable in age × smoking to the data on coronary deaths among British male doctors (Table 3.15): regression coefficients ± standard errors for three statistical models

	Statistical model		
	Additive ($\rho = 1$)	Power ($\rho = 0.55$)	Multiplicative ($\rho = 0$)
Coefficient γ	0.732 ± 0.301	-0.024 ± 0.095	-0.309 ± 0.097
Goodness-of-fit G^2 on 3 degrees of freedom	2.16	2.08	1.55

features are of course already evident from the original data (Table 3.15). The fit to the power model was improved scarcely at all by the interaction terms. Thus, for these simple data, inclusion of interaction variables to measure lack of fit gives the same result as when lack of fit is evaluated *via* the power model.

4.5 Grouped data analyses of the Montana cohort with the multiplicative model

We now turn to a re-examination of the data on Montana smelter workers analysed in Chapter 3, in order to illustrate how the results of model fitting compare with the techniques of standardization. Appendix V contains the data records from the Montana smelter workers study that were analysed earlier using standardization and related techniques (Tables 3.3, 3.11 and 3.16). There are $J = 16$ strata formed by the combination of four ten-year age groups and four calendar periods of variable length. The $K = 8$ 'exposure' categories are defined by the combination of two periods of first employment or date of hire (1 = pre-1925, 2 = post-1925) and four categories of duration of employment in work areas with high or medium exposure to arsenic (1 = <1 years, 2 = 1–4 years, 3 = 5–14 years, 4 = 15+ years). The coded levels for these four factors (AGE, YEAR, PERiod and EXPosure duration) appear as the first four columns (variables) in the data set. For 14 of the $4 \times 4 \times 2 \times 4 = 128$ combinations of these factors, no person-years of observation, and hence no deaths, occurred and no data record is included. These include the combinations with AGE = 1 (40–49 years), YEAR = 3 or 4 (1960–1977), and PER = 1 (pre-1925) and those with AGE = 2, YEAR = 4 and PER = 1. Individuals in these categories, being under 50 years of age in 1960, would have been aged 14 or less in 1925 and unlikely to have started work earlier. Likewise, there is no observation at AGE = 4 (60–79 years), YEAR = 1 (1938–1949), PER = 2 (post-1925) and EXP = 4 (15+ years).

(a) Estimation of relative risk

Our first goal is to reproduce as closely as possible the results obtained in the last chapter. Recall that relative risks of respiratory cancer for each duration of arsenic exposure were obtained separately for the pre-and post-1925 cohorts by three methods: (i) external standardization (Table 3.3); (ii) internal standardization (Table 3.11); and (iii) the Mantel–Haenszel procedure (Table 3.11). Maximum likelihood estimates of these same relative risks, using a multiplicative model with three binary exposure variables to represent the effect of each exposure category *versus* baseline (0–0.9 years heavy/medium arsenic exposure) and a varying number of stratum parameters α_j to represent the effects of age and calendar year, are shown in Table 4.10. Differences in the degrees of freedom for the goodness-of-fit statistics used with each subcohort are due to the fact that information on person-years was available for different combinations of age-year-exposure. For the pre-1925 cohort there were 13 age × year strata, and each of these had a data record for the full complement of four exposure categories. Thus, the total number of data records is $4 \times 13 = 52$ and the degrees of freedom are $52 - 13 - 3 = 36$. For the post-1925 cohort, two of the $4 \times 16 = 64$ possible exposure-age-year combinations were missing, and since there were $16 + 3 = 19$ parameters estimated, the degrees of freedom numbered $62 - 19 = 43$.

(b) Testing for heterogeneity and trend in the relative risk with exposure duration

The relative risk estimates and likelihood ratio (deviance) tests for heterogeneity and trend obtained *via* maximum likelihood fitting (Table 4.10) agree reasonably well with those based on Mantel–Haenszel methodology (Table 3.11). The Mantel–Haenszel style test statistics (3.24) and (3.25) are in fact efficient score tests based on the multiplicative model (4.2), as were the analogous statistics developed in Volume 1 for case-control data (Day & Byar, 1979). When interpreting the individual relative risk estimates by comparing each exposure group with baseline, it is important to

Table 4.10 Fitting of multiplicative models to grouped data from the Montana smelter workers study: internal estimation of baseline rates

Variable fitted	Relative risk (exponentiated regression coefficient) and standardized regression coefficient (in parentheses)			
	Employed prior to 1925	Employed 1925 or after	Combined cohort	
			Four levels of exposure	Two levels of exposure
Exposure duration (years)				
Under 1	1.0	1.0	1.0	1.0
1–4	2.43 (3.20)	2.10 (3.88)	2.21 (5.04)	
5–14	1.96 (2.15)	1.67 (1.84)	1.77 (2.77)	2.19 (6.45)
15+	3.12 (5.10)	1.75 (1.52)	2.58 (5.25)	
Pre-1925 employment	—	—	1.62 (3.23)	1.66 (3.46)
Deviance (G^2)	32.9	56.0	96.8	99.2
Degrees of freedom	36	43	94	96
Tests of significance of exposure based on G^2				
Global	$\chi_3^2 = 28.3$	$\chi_3^2 = 15.8$	$\chi_3^2 = 42.4$	$\chi_1^2 = 39.7$
Trend	$\chi_1^2 = 24.7$	$\chi_1^2 = 8.9$	$\chi_1^2 = 32.7$	

remember that they utilize information from all the exposure categories, and not just the two in question. For example, the estimated risk ratio of $\hat{\psi}_2 = 2.43$ comparing rates in the 1–4-year exposure duration category to those in the under-1-year category uses some information from the comparisons of the 1–4 *versus* 5–9 and under 1 *versus* 5–9 categories, and so on. Were we to estimate the relative risks for pairwise comparisons of exposure categories using only the data for each pair, whether by Mantel–Haenszel or maximum likelihood, the resulting estimates would fail to be consistent with each other. The product of estimated relative risks for under 1 *versus* 1–4 and 1–4 *versus* 5–9 years would not necessarily equal the relative risk for under 1 *versus* 5–9. The same phenomenon was noted also for case-control studies (§§4.5 and 5.5, Volume 1). Consistency is achieved only by building it into the fitted model.

(c) Evaluating the goodness-of-fit of the multiplicative model

An evaluation of the goodness-of-fit of the multiplicative model was made by examination of residuals and the addition of interaction terms to the model equation. While the goodness-of-fit statistic for the pre-1925 cohort is slightly less than its degrees of freedom, indicating that the model fits reasonably well overall, that for the post-1925 cohort is larger ($G^2 = 56.0$, degrees of freedom $= 43$, $p = 0.09$). The corresponding chi-square statistic is $\chi_{43}^2 = 54.9$. However, examination of the observed and fitted numbers of deaths for the 62 age-year-exposure cells for this cohort reveals no particular pattern to the lack of fit. The greatest contribution to chi-square is from the 15+ year exposure category for ages 50–59 and years 1950–1959 where two respiratory cancer deaths were observed *versus* 0.24 expected from the multiplicative model. Elimination of this one cell would markedly improve the fit. The example also serves as

Table 4.11 Evaluating the goodness-of-fit of the multiplicative model of Table 4.10; deviance test statistics for interaction effects

Interaction effect	Degrees of freedom	Employed prior to 1925	Employed 1925 or after	Combined cohort
Year × exposure				
Qualitative	9	8.2	18.0	15.3
Quantitative (linear × linear)	1	2.7	2.5	6.5
Age × exposure				
Qualitative	9	9.1	14.0	13.2
Quantitative (linear × linear)	1	3.3	3.7	3.5

a reminder that the usual asymptotic approximations for χ^2 and G^2 statistics may not apply when the data are sparse and expected values for some cells are small (McCullagh, 1986).

In order to look more systematically for possible trends in the relative risks with age and year, we examined a number of additional models with both qualitative and quantitative interaction terms. The results, summarized in Table 4.11, do not suggest that the relative risks estimated for different exposure durations change systematically with either age or year in the pre-1925 cohort. However, even in the absence of a definite trend, there is considerable variation in the exposure effects from one calendar period to another for the post-1925 cohort. Some caution needs to be exercised, therefore, in interpreting the relative risks shown in Table 4.10 for the latter cohort.

Table 4.12 lists the deviances for several models that we fitted to the full set of cohort data in the process of obtaining the results shown in the right-hand columns of

Table 4.12 Goodness-of-fit (deviance) statistics for a series of models fitted to the data on Montana smelter workers: internal estimation of baseline rates

Model number	Terms included in the model[a]	Degrees of freedom	Deviance
1	—	98	155.4
2	PER	97	138.9
3	EXP	95	107.0
4	PER + EXP	94	96.8
5	PER + EXP0 + PER . EXP	91	94.6
6	PER + EXP1	96	99.2
7	PER + EXP1 + PER . EXP1	95	97.5
8	PER + EXP1 + AGE . EXP1	93	90.0
9	PER + EXP1 + YEAR . EXP1	93	95.2

[a] In addition to 16 terms for stratum (age and year) effects. The variables are coded as follows: PER, period of employment (pre- *versus* post-1925); EXP, four-level factor for duration of exposure; EXP1, binary indicator of one or more years of heavy/medium arsenic exposure

Table 4.10. (Models 4 and 6 in Table 4.12 correspond to columns 3 and 4 of Table 4.10.) The first four lines of Table 4.12 show that both period of first employment and exposure to heavy-medium arsenic had marked and relatively independent effects on risk. The addition of period × exposure interaction terms (model 5) does not significantly improve the fit. Relative risks for the three exposure duration levels are estimated by model 5 to be 2.43, 1.99 and 3.22 for those first employed before 1925 and 2.03, 1.63 and 1.62 for those employed afterwards, which results compare well to those obtained when the two subcohorts are analysed separately (columns 1 and 2 of Table 4.10).

An important advantage of model fitting is the flexibility it offers for looking at the same data in a number of different ways. Examination of the relative risk estimates in Table 4.10 suggests that they do not change much either with increasing duration of exposure or with period of first employment. In order to study the issue further, we constructed a new binary exposure variable EXP1 to indicate whether or not a full year of heavy/medium arsenic exposure had yet been experienced, and fitted several additional models to the complete set of cohort data. The most interesting aspect of Table 4.12 is the comparison of models 5 and 6. Constraining the relative risk estimates for arsenic exposure to be constant regardless of period or duration of exposure leads to nearly as good a summary of the data as allowing them to vary ($99.2 - 94.6 = 4.6$, 5 degrees of freedom, $p = 0.47$). The estimated effect of exposure for a year or more to heavy/medium levels of arsenic is to increase the subsequent respiratory cancer death rate by a factor of 2.2. There is little evidence that this estimate of arsenic effect changes with additional exposure or according to the date of hire. The improved fit from model 8 suggests, however, that it may depend on age ($99.2 - 90.0 = 9.2$, 3 degrees of freedom, $p = 0.03$), the estimated relative risks being 1.68, 3.07, 2.50 and 1.10 for the four age groups. Using EXP1 rather than EXP gives less evidence for an interaction with calendar year; the separately estimated relative risks for the four decades are 2.57, 3.23, 1.92 and 1.76.

In order to determine whether one or two data records might have had an undue influence on the fit, we computed the 'hat' matrix elements and approximate changes in regression coefficients for model 6 of Table 4.12. (This model is also shown in the last column of Table 4.10.) GLIM was used to carry out the calculations of h and $\Delta \hat{\beta}$ using equations 4.14 and 4.15. As expected, the records with the largest effects on the overall fit were generally those with the largest person-years of observation: record 17 with seven lung cancer cases and over 12 000 person-years gave $h = 0.617$; record 21 with one case and 7151 person-years gave $h = 0.634$; and record 49 with 89 cases and 8495 person-years gave $h = 0.590$. The total value of h summed over all 114 records is 18, the number of parameters being estimated.

Other data records had the largest influence on the estimated effect of arsenic exposure as evaluated by the change in the coefficient of EXP1. The maximum change occurred with record 56 (9 cases observed *versus* 4.00 expected), the deletion of which would reduce the relative risk associated with heavy/moderate arsenic exposure by a factor of approximately $\exp(-0.086)$, i.e., from 2.19 to 2.01. None of these results suggests any serious instability in the fitted model.

4.6 Incorporating external standard rates into the multiplicative model

Up to now we have considered that the stratum-specific parameters α_j in the model equation (4.10), which represent the log death rates for unexposed $(x_{jk} = 0)$ individuals in that stratum, were unknown 'nuisance' parameters to be estimated internally from the study data. The spirit of this approach is similar to that discussed in §§3.5 and 3.6. It avoids the problems caused by the noncomparability of external standard rates, namely, that relative risk estimates for different exposure groups will fail to summarize adequately the stratum-specific rate ratios.

While this ability of multivariate modelling to accommodate the internal estimation of baseline rates is desirable, incorportion of external standard rates into the analysis may be advantageous in some circumstances. Suppose the baseline rates are specified up to a scale factor θ, say $\lambda_j = \theta\lambda_j^*$ where the λ_j^* are known from vital statistics or other sources. The model equation analogous to (4.10) is

$$\log \lambda_{jk} = \alpha_j^* + \mu + \mathbf{x}_{jk}\boldsymbol{\beta}, \qquad (4.18)$$

where $\mu = \log(\theta)$ is a parameter (the grand mean) which represents the log SMR for the unexposed $(x_{jk} = 0)$, and $\alpha_j^* = \log \lambda_j^*$. If follows that the mean values $E(d_{jk})$ for the number of deaths in the (j, k) cell satisfy

$$\log E(d_{jk}) = \log(n_{jk}\lambda_j^*) + \mu + \mathbf{x}_{jk}\boldsymbol{\beta},$$

so that now the log expected standard deaths are declared as the OFFSET in a GLIM analysis, rather than the log person-years (compare equation 4.11).

One advantage of (4.18) is that it provides in the parameter μ an overall measure of how the baseline cohort rates compare with those for the general population. Also, since the number of parameters to be estimated from the data is reduced considerably in comparison to (4.11), there could theoretically be an improvement in the efficiency of estimation of the β parameters of most interest. However, this improvement is not likely to be great for many practical problems (see Example 4.7). Perhaps more important is the fact that when the x variables depend only on exposure (k) and not on stratum (j), the likelihood for the model (4.18) is a function of the totals $O_k = \sum_j d_{jk}$ and $E_k^* = \sum_j n_{jk}\lambda_j^*$ of observed and expected deaths in each of the K exposure categories. (In fact, if a separate parameter β_k is attached to each exposure category, the $\text{SMR}_k = O_k/E_k^*$ are maximum likelihood estimates.) This permits a much more economical presentation of the basic data needed for the regression analysis than is true for the models considered in the preceding section. For tests of goodness-of-fit, however, the full set of data records for all $J \times K$ cells are needed.

Since the β parameters describe how the log SMR varies as a function of the exposures, (4.18) extends the method of indirect standardization into the domain of multivariate regression analysis. If $\boldsymbol{\beta}$ indexes K different exposure classes, the efficient score statistic of the hypothesis $\boldsymbol{\beta} = \mathbf{0}$ developed from this model corresponds to the statistic (3.11) previously proposed for testing heterogeneity of risk. Likewise, for a single quantitative regression variable the score test of $\boldsymbol{\beta} = \mathbf{0}$ is identical with the trend test (3.12). Finally, the maximum likelihood estimate of μ in the model where $\boldsymbol{\beta} = \mathbf{0}$ is precisely $\hat{\mu} = \log(O_+/E_+^*) = \log(\text{SMR})$, where O_+ and E_+^* denote totals of observed and expected values. These results provide the essential link between the elementary methods of cohort analysis considered in Chapter 3 and those based on the multiplicative model.

The drawbacks of indirect standardization noted earlier of course apply also to an uncritical application of the regression model. However, the process of model fitting encourages the investigator to evaluate the assumptions of proportionality that are essential in order that the estimated β parameters have the intended interpretation. The usual goodness-of-fit machinery may be applied to validate these assumptions. Additional terms may be incorporated in the model to account for confounding of the SMR/exposure relationship by age, year or other stratification factors. The estimates of the exposure effects as expressed in $\hat{\beta}$ will then start to approximate those obtained with the model (4.10), wherein the baseline rates are estimated internally. See §4.8 for an example.

Example 4.3

To illustrate the process of multivariate modelling using external standard rates, we return to the problem of estimating relative risks of respiratory cancer associated with duration of heavy/medium arsenic exposure in the Montana cohort. The basic data needed to fit the models consist of just eight records containing observed (O_k) and expected (E_k^*) numbers of deaths by period of employment and exposure duration (Table 3.3).

Table 4.13 summarizes the results of fitting the same models as in Table 4.10, but where the baseline rates are obtained from Table 3.2 rather than estimated internally. There is good agreement between the two analyses as far as the arsenic effects are concerned, but the pre- *versus* post-1925 period effect is overestimated when the comparison is made using the external standard rates. Goodness-of-fit using external

Table 4.13   Fitting of multiplicative models to grouped data from the Montana smelter workers study: external baseline rates

Regression variable	Relative risk (exponentiated regression coefficient) and standardized regression coefficient (in parentheses)			
	Employed prior to 1925	Employed 1925 or after	Combined cohort	
			Four levels of exposure	Two levels of exposure
Constant (SMR)	2.38 (6.18)	1.35 (2.99)	1.28 (2.65)	1.26 (2.55)
Duration heavy/medium arsenic exposure (years)				
Under 1	1.0	1.0	1.0	1.0
1–4	2.43 (3.17)	2.05 (3.78)	2.16 (4.89)	
5–14	1.99 (2.21)	1.63 (1.76)	1.76 (2.73)	2.16 (6.36)
15+	3.22 (5.28)	1.62 (1.31)	2.58 (5.28)	
Pre-1925 employment	—	—	2.03 (5.59)	2.09 (5.99)
Deviance (G^2)	39.0	70.4	112.3	114.7
Degrees of freedom	48	58	109	111
Tests of significance of exposure based on G^2				
Global	$\chi_3^2 = 29.6$	$\chi_3^2 = 14.4$	$\chi_3^2 = 41.0$	$\chi_1^2 = 38.6$
Trend	$\chi_1^2 = 26.1$	$\chi_1^2 = 7.6$	$\chi_1^2 = 32.4$	

standard rates appears no worse than when the rates are estimated. Note that we have considered the fit of the model to the original data from Appendix VI rather than to the summary data in Table 3.3 in order to be able to evaluate goodness-of-fit.

The relative risk estimates shown separately for the two employment periods in Table 4.13 are identical to those given in Table 3.3, and the coefficients $\exp(\hat{\mu}) = 2.38$ for the pre-1925 cohort or $\exp(\hat{\mu}) = 1.35$ for the post-1925 cohort also agree with the SMRs of 238% and 135% found earlier for the baseline exposure duration category (under 1 year). This is a numerical confirmation of the fact that the maximum likelihood estimates of parameters in these simple qualitative models are log (SMR)s, or differences between log (SMR)s.

4.7 Proportional mortality analyses

Regression analyses similar to those already considered for grouped cohort data with person-years denominators can also be carried out using information only for persons who have died. As mentioned in §3.7, the data are best considered as arising from a case-control study in which the persons who die from the cause of interest are regarded as the 'cases', while those who die of other causes (or some subset thereof) are the 'controls'. They are classified into precisely the same J strata and K exposure classes as are the cases and person-years in the corresponding cohort analysis. The observations in stratum j and exposure class k consist of the number d_{jk} of deaths or cases, the total t_{jk} of cases and controls (all deaths) and the associated covariables $\mathbf{x}_{jk}$.

(a) Derivation of the logistic regression model

As usual we denote the death rate from the cause of interest in the (j, k) cell by λ_{jk}. We denote the death rate from the other causes by v_{jk} so that the total death rate is given by $\lambda_{jk} + v_{jk}$. Let us suppose that each of these satisfies the multiplicative model (4.10), say

$$\log \lambda_{jk} = \alpha_j + \mathbf{x}_{jk}\boldsymbol{\beta}$$

$$\log v_{jk} = \gamma_j + \mathbf{x}_{jk}\boldsymbol{\delta}. \tag{4.19}$$

It follows that the conditional probability p_{jk} that a death in the (j, k) cell is from the cause of interest, given that one occurred at all, is given by

$$p_{jk} = \frac{\lambda_{jk}}{\lambda_{jk} + v_{jk}} = \frac{\exp\{(\alpha_j - \gamma_j) + \mathbf{x}_{jk}(\boldsymbol{\beta} - \boldsymbol{\delta})\}}{\exp\{(\alpha_j - \gamma_j) + \mathbf{x}_{jk}(\boldsymbol{\beta} - \boldsymbol{\delta})\} + 1}.$$

In other words, the probability that a death is from the specific cause satisfies the linear logistic model

$$\text{logit } p_{jk} = \log \frac{p_{jk}}{1 - p_{jk}} = (\alpha_j - \gamma_j) + \mathbf{x}_{jk}(\boldsymbol{\beta} - \boldsymbol{\delta}). \tag{4.20}$$

Furthermore, if the exposures have no effect on the rate of death from the other causes ($\boldsymbol{\delta} = \mathbf{0}$), the regression parameters of the covariables $\mathbf{x}_{jk}$ estimated from this linear logistic relationship correspond precisely to the log relative risks of principal interest. This provides a formal confirmation of the well-known fact that proportional mortality analyses are valid only if the controls are selected from among deaths due to causes

Table 4.14 Fitting of multiplicative models to grouped data from the Montana smelter workers study: proportional mortality analysis with internal control

Variable fitted	Relative risk (exponentiated regression coefficient) and standardized regression coefficient (in parentheses)			
	Employed prior to 1925	Employed 1925 or after	Combined cohort	
			Four levels of exposure	Two levels of exposure
Exposure duration (years)				
Under 1	1.0	1.0	1.0	1.0
1–4	2.32 (2.69)	2.02 (3.40)	2.21 (4.37)	
5–14	1.98 (1.98)	1.59 (1.56)	1.74 (2.49)	2.07 (5.54)
15+	2.82 (4.20)	1.60 (1.21)	2.32 (4.22)	
Pre-1925 employment	—	—	1.54 (2.66)	1.56 (2.81)
Deviance (G^2)	47.0	48.6	104.8	106.0
Degrees of freedom	35	41	91	93
Tests of significance of exposure based on G^2				
Global	$\chi_3^2 = 20.6$	$\chi_3^2 = 12.2$	$\chi_3^2 = 31.0$	$\chi_1^2 = 29.8$
Trend	$\chi_1^2 = 18.9$	$\chi_1^2 = 6.4$	$\chi_1^2 = 23.5$	

that have no relation to the exposures. Prentice and Breslow (1978) make the same observation in deriving the analogous relationship for continuous data.

In order to carry out the proportional mortality analysis, we treat the d_{jk} as independent binomial random variables with denominators t_{jk} and probabilities p_{jk} of 'being a case' that satisfy the linear logistic model (4.20). Techniques of maximum likelihood estimation are applied exactly as described in Chapter 6 of Volume 1. Provided that the other causes of death are unrelated to the exposures, the regression coefficients may be interpreted as log relative risks in the usual fashion.

Example 4.4

The data in Appendix V include the total numbers of deaths observed in each of the 114 categories defined by the cross-classification in the Montana smelter workers study. These were analysed using the logistic regression model (4.20) with covariables $\mathbf{x}_{jk}$ defined just as in the earlier cohort analyses to represent the effects of period of hire and duration of moderate to heavy arsenic exposure. Table 4.14 presents the results in the same format as for the parallel cohort analyses (Table 4.10). The significance of the estimated exposure effects is somewhat reduced in comparison, as might be expected since more restricted data are being used. The deviances measuring the goodness-of-fit of the models to the proportional data are considerably higher. Note that three degrees of freedom have been lost in comparison with Table 4.10, due to the fact that there was no death at all ($t_{jk} = 0$) in three cells. Nevertheless, the estimated regression coefficients for the proportional mortality analysis are quite comparable to those for the full cohort analysis. There is a slight reduction in the estimated effects for period of hire and for 15 or more years of arsenic exposure, indicating that these two factors may possibly have increased mortality rates from causes other than respiratory cancer.

(b) Incorporating standard rates into the proportional mortality analysis

Suppose now that external standard rates λ_j^* and ν_j^* are available for deaths due to specific and nonspecific causes in stratum j. We continue to rely on the basic multiplicative model (4.19), except that the unknown log background rates α_j and γ_j

are replaced by $\alpha + \log \lambda_j^*$ and $\gamma + \log \nu_j^*$, respectively. Defining $p_j^* = \lambda_j^*/(\lambda_j^* + \nu_j^*)$ to be the standard proportions of deaths due to the cause of interest in the jth stratum, it follows that the probability that a death is due to that cause may be written

$$\text{logit } p_{jk} = \text{logit } p_j^* + (\alpha - \gamma) + \mathbf{x}_{jk}(\boldsymbol{\beta} - \boldsymbol{\delta}). \qquad (4.21)$$

The probabilities of 'being a case' continue to satisfy the linear logistic model (4.20). Now, however, the known variable logit p_j^* 'offsets' the model equation, and there is a constant term with coefficient $(\alpha - \gamma)$. This coefficient may be interpreted as the logarithm of the standardized relative mortality ratio (SRMR) for unexposed members of the cohort ($\mathbf{x} = \mathbf{0}$), where the SRMR is defined as the ratio of SMRs for specific *versus* nonspecific causes (Breslow & Day, 1975). The proportional mortality ratio as usually defined, namely the ratio of the number of deaths observed to those 'expected' on the basis of the stratum-specific proportions p_j^*, is of lesser interest for reasons discussed in §3.7.

Example 4.5

Table 4.15 presents the standard proportions p_j^* for the 16 age × year strata used with the Montana smelter workers data. These were obtained by dividing the standard death rates from respiratory cancer (Table 3.2) by the corresponding standard death rates for all causes. The logistic transform of these standard proportions was used as an offset in a logistic regression analysis based on equation (4.21).

Table 4.16 presents the results in what has now become a standard format. Just as observed earlier for the full cohort analysis (Tables 4.10 and 4.13), the relative risk estimated for pre- *versus* post-1925 employment is greater when the standardized proportions are used as a basis of comparison than when these same proportions are estimated internally. This suggests that the association between the SMR (or SRMR) and period of employment is confounded by one or more of the stratification factors, an interpretation that is confirmed by more detailed analyses of data from the Montana cohort reported below. Otherwise, the agreement between the two types of proportional mortality analyses is quite good. The difference between the constant terms for the full cohort analysis (Table 4.13) and the proportional analysis (Table 4.16) suggests that the γ coefficient in equation (4.21) is nonzero. This implies simply that the SMR for nonrespiratory cancer deaths among cohort members with zero covariates is different from unity.

4.8 Further grouped data analyses of the Montana cohort

The preceding illustrative analyses of the Montana smelter workers study are limited in scope by the requirement that they be based on the relatively small data set presented in Appendix V. More realistic analyses were undertaken also by fitting multiplicative models to a more elaborate set of grouped data (Breslow, 1985a; Breslow & Day, 1985). Respiratory cancer deaths and person-years of exposure were

Table 4.15 Standard proportions of deaths due to respiratory cancer: US white males

Age group (years)	Calendar year			
	1938–1949	1950–1959	1960–1969	1970–1977
40–49	0.021515	0.038246	0.052288	0.070208
50–59	0.028478	0.055765	0.074081	0.095478
60–69	0.021247	0.047646	0.072328	0.095159
70–79	0.009894	0.024390	0.041900	0.064688

Table 4.16   Fitting of multiplicative models to grouped data from the Montana smelter workers study: proportional mortality analysis with external control

Variable fitted	Relative risk (exponentiated regression coefficient) and standardized regression coefficient (in parentheses)			
	Employed prior to 1925	Employed 1925 or after	Combined cohort	
			Four levels of exposure	Two levels of exposure
Constant (SRMR)	2.02 (4.77)	1.13 (1.16)	2.22 (6.54)	2.26 (6.83)
Exposure duration (years)				
Under 1	1.0	1.0	1.0	1.0
1–4	2.26 (2.64)	1.90 (3.14)	2.02 (4.11)	
5–14	2.15 (2.25)	1.49 (1.36)	1.72 (2.45)	2.03 (5.42)
15+	2.89 (4.37)	1.54 (1.11)	2.35 (4.31)	
Pre-1925 employment	—	—	2.07 (5.33)	2.13 (5.74)
Deviance (G)	55.9	65.6	123.8	125.2
Degrees of freedom	47	56	106	108
Tests of significance of exposure based on G				
Global	$\chi^2_3 = 21.8$	$\chi^2_3 = 10.3$	$\chi^2_3 = 29.8$	$\chi^2_1 = 28.4$
Trend	$\chi^2_1 = 19.6$	$\chi^2_1 = 5.3$	$\chi^2_1 = 23.7$	

classified in six dimensions: (i) age in four ten-year intervals; (ii) calendar year in four intervals; (iii) date of first employment (pre- *versus* post-1925); (iv) birthplace (US-*versus* foreign-born); (v) number of years worked in moderate arsenic areas (<1, 1–4, 5–14, 15+) and (vi) number of years worked in heavy arsenic areas (<1, 1–4, 5+). Of the $4 \times 4 \times 2 \times 2 \times 4 \times 3 = 768$ possible cells in this six-dimensional table, only 478 actually contained any person-years observation. The results obtained in this section will serve as a useful point of reference for those based on more complicated methods of analysis of continuous data that are considered in the next chapter.

(a) Preliminary analyses

Table 4.17 presents respiratory cancer SMRs according to a large number of possible risk variables, including several not mentioned above, and without regard to possible confounding effects. The time-dependent exposure variables were lagged two years in an attempt to estimate the exposure status at the time of disease onset, rather than at the time of death, and thus to avoid some of the healthy worker selection problem. Tests of significance were based on the heterogeneity statistic (3.11), or the trend test (3.12), as appropriate.

From this preliminary analysis, we conclude that period of first employment, birthplace, years since first employed and level of arsenic exposure may each have some effect on the age-specific rates. We also note a sharp decline in the SMR with calendar year, indicating that the respiratory cancer rates for the cohort as a whole have not increased in constant proportion with those for the general population, although they have remained consistently higher (see Example 2.4). This serves as a warning of a possible lack of comparability of the SMRs for the various exposure

Table 4.17 Variations in respiratory cancer SMRs among Montana smelter workers[a]

Factor analysed	Level	Number of deaths	SMR(×100)[b]	Test of significance[c]
Period of first employment	1885–1924	115	362	$\chi_1^2 = 39.5$
	1925–1955	161	164	$(p < 0.0001)$
Age at hire (years)	<24	69	255	$\chi_1^2 = 5.2$
	25–34	116	222	$(p = 0.07)$
	35+	91	184	
Birthplace	US	198	180	$\chi_1^2 = 28.5$
	Foreign	80	381	$(p < 0.0001)$
Time since first employed[d] (years)	1–14	101	165	$\chi_2^2 = 24.0$
	15–29	59	185	$(p < 0.0001)$
	30+	116	315	
Time since last employed[d] (years)	None	110	230	$\chi_2^2 = 3.2$
	0–9	84	227	$(p = 0.20)$
	10+	82	181	
Arsenic exposure[d]	Light only	153	160	$\chi_2^2 = 44.4$
	Moderate[e]	91	339	$(p < 0.0001)$
	Heavy[e]	32	434	
Age at follow-up (years)	40–49	21	166	$\chi_3^2 = 2.5$
	50–59	80	199	$(p = 0.48)$
	60–69	117	228	
	70–79	58	223	
Year at follow-up	1938–1949	34	403	$\chi_3^2 = 28.4$
	1950–1959	65	294	$(p < 0.0001)$
	1960–1969	94	211	
	1970–1977	83	151	

[a] From Breslow (1985a)
[b] Calculated with reference to US mortality rates for white males by age and calendar year
[c] Test for homogeneity of SMRs among categories shown based on equations (3.11) or (3.12)
[d] Time-dependent exposure variable lagged two years
[e] Worked in moderate or heavy arsenic exposure area for at least one year

classes due to confounding with calendar year. Additional confounding may result from the high correlation between certain exposure variables. For example, due to the fact that follow-up started only in 1938, virtually everyone employed before 1925 contributed person-years only to the last two categories of years since first employment.

Table 4.18 presents an analysis of variance of the log SMRs based on the model equation (4.18) and various indicator regression variables. This shows clearly that the effects of duration of employment are easily explained by the correlation with period of first employment, whereas those for arsenic exposure are not. Selection of the variables for the final analysis was based on such considerations.

(b) Regression analyses

Table 4.19 presents further multiple regression analyses based on equations (4.18) (first two columns) and (4.11) (last column). When calendar year is included in the

Table 4.18 Analysis of variance based on a multiplicative model for SMRs: respiratory cancer deaths in Montana smelter workers[a]

Source of variation[b]	Degrees of freedom	Chi-square
PERIOD of hire and TIME since first employment	3	41.0
PERIOD alone	1	39.5
TIME after PERIOD	2	1.5[c]
TIME alone	2	24.0
PERIOD after TIME	1	17.0
PERIOD and ARSENIC level	3	77.6
PERIOD alone	1	39.5
ARSENIC after PERIOD	2	38.1
ARSENIC alone	2	44.4
PERIOD after ARSENIC	1	33.2

[a] From Breslow (1985a)
[b] See Table 4.17 for definition of factor levels
[c] Not statistically significant; all others have $p < 0.0001$

SMR analysis, the regression coefficient for period of hire is much closer to that obtained when baseline rates are estimated internally. This confirms that part of the difference between the SMRs for those hired before and after 1925 is due to the confounding effects of calendar year on the ratios of cohort to standard death rates. Appropriate adjustment is made either by including calendar year as a covariable in

Table 4.19 Regression coefficients ± standard errors in the multiplicative model: two methods of analysis of grouped data from the Montana smelter workers study[a]

Regression variable	Method of analysis		Internal estimation of baseline rates by age and year
	External standard rates (SMR analysis)		
	Without calendar year effects	With calendar year effects	
Constant (α)	0.256 ± 0.092	0.581 ± 0.219	—
Hired before 1925	0.564 ± 0.133	0.441 ± 0.143	0.444 ± 0.151
Foreign born	0.492 ± 0.142	0.407 ± 0.147	0.445 ± 0.153
Heavy arsenic			
1–4 years	0.170 ± 0.310	0.199 ± 0.303	0.193 ± 0.305
5+ years	1.067 ± 0.230	1.076 ± 0.230	1.069 ± 0.230
Moderate arsenic			
1–4 years	0.587 ± 0.166	0.604 ± 0.166	0.600 ± 0.166
5–14 years	0.253 ± 0.242	0.262 ± 0.242	0.259 ± 0.242
15+ years	0.678 ± 0.204	0.683 ± 0.205	0.689 ± 0.206
Calendar period			
1950–1959		-0.075 ± 0.216	
1960–1969		-0.235 ± 0.215	
1970–1977		-0.480 ± 0.228	

[a] From Breslow and Day (1985)

the SMR analysis or else, and what is almost the same, by conducting a parallel internally controlled analysis in which background rates are estimated from the data. If age, year and age × year interactions are all included as covariables in the SMR analysis, the externally and internally controlled analyses yield identical results as far as the β coefficients are concerned. The difference in the coefficients for foreign-born between the second and third columns suggests some possible residual confounding by age.

4.9 More general models of relative risk

One possible drawback to the multiplicative model (4.10), at least when applied with quantitative exposure variables, is that it leads to relative risk functions that increase exponentially with increasing exposure: $RR(x) = \exp(x\beta)$. Apparently, some risks do increase this fast. For example, our analyses of the Ille-et-Vilaine case-control study in Volume 1 showed that alcohol had such an effect on the risk of oesophagael cancer. This example is atypical, however, and in most epidemiological studies the rate of increase would be less dramatic (see Chapter 6). In Ille-et-Vilaine, the relative risk of oesophageal cancer was approximately proportional to the square root of the daily dose of tobacco.

(a) Transformations of dose

Many of the quantitative dose-response relations actually observed in cancer epidemiology approximate a power relationship of the form

$$RR(x) = (x + x_0)^\beta. \tag{4.22}$$

Here $x_0 > 0$ is a small 'background' exposure level introduced to account for the spontaneous incidence of cancer among the unexposed. This relative risk function may be approximated by first transforming the dose to $z = \log(x + x_0)$ and then fitting the multiplicative model (4.10) in the form

$$\log \lambda_{jk} = \alpha_j + z_k\beta = \alpha_j + \{\log(x_k + x_0)\}\beta. \tag{4.23}$$

The choice $x_0 = 1$ is not uncommon as a 'starter' dose since it yields the usual $RR(x) = 1$ at the baseline level $x = 0$. x_0 may also be treated as an unknown parameter and the best fitting value found by trial and error or some other more systematic technique. However, the model is then no longer a log-linear one, and determination of the variances and covariances of the parameter estimates may be seriously complicated. There is a high degree of correlation between the estimates of x_0 and β, as might be expected from the fact that the slope of the relative risk function (4.22) at $x = 0$ is given by $RR'(0) = \beta x_0^{1-\beta}$. Since small variations in x_0 often have little effect on the overall goodness-of-fit, it is usually adequate simply to select a nominal background dose a priori and to proceed assuming that x_0 is fixed.

(b) Additive relative risk model

Certain formulations of multistage theory and other more general considerations lead to relative risk functions that are linear or quadratic in measured exposures, for example $RR(x) = 1 + \beta x$ or $RR(x) = 1 + \beta x + \gamma x^2$ (Berry, 1980; Thomas, D.C., 1981). These are special cases of a general class of models of the form

$$\lambda_{jk} = \exp(\alpha_j)\{1 + \mathbf{x}_{jk}\boldsymbol{\beta}\} \tag{4.24}$$

which we shall call the *additive relative risk model*. One drawback of these is that the range of the $\boldsymbol{\beta}$ parameters is necessarily restricted by the requirement that $\mathbf{x}_{jk}\boldsymbol{\beta} > -1$ for all values of $\mathbf{x}_{jk}$, since negative relative risks would otherwise result. This suggests that, wherever possible, the regression variables $\mathbf{x}_{jk}$ be coded so that they have positive coefficients. As usually happens for models in which there is a range restriction on the parameters, the log-likelihood function is skewed and not at all like the quadratic, symmetric log-likelihood of the approximating normal distribution. Estimates of the parameters may be unstable, and standard errors that are determined from the usual likelihood calculations may be unhelpful in assessing the degree of uncertainty. (This contrasts with additive models for absolute risk, where t statistics perform reasonably well. See Example 4.2.) Substantial differences may exist in practice between the observed and expected information measures, and score tests based on the former may give seriously misleading answers (Storer *et al.*, 1983). Irregularities in the likelihood surface may frustrate the search for maximum likelihood estimates. The usual iterative procedures can diverge unless starting values in the immediate vicinity of the maximum likelihood are available.

In view of these complications, we do not recommend the additive relative risk model for routine applications. It often suffices to transform the exposure variables and to approximate the additive relative risk model by a multiplicative model in the transformed variables. Nevertheless, one sometimes finds that the extra work involved in fitting the model (4.24) results in a substantially better fit to the data or is necessary in order that the regression coefficients have precisely the desired interpretation.

(c) Fitting general models to Poisson rates

The additive relative risk model (4.24) is a generalized linear model that involves a composite link function (Thompson & Baker, 1981): two separate linear functions (linear predictors) of the explanatory variables are related to the mean values $E(d_{jk}) = n_{jk}\lambda_{jk}$. Since it is a nonlinear regression model for Poisson rates, however, it still may be fitted using GLIM or other programs that facilitate iterated reweighted least-squares analyses (Frome, 1983). However, the implementation is more involved than for the multiplicative (4.16) or power (4.15) models considered earlier.

In their most general form Poisson regression models may be written

$$\lambda_{jk} = g(\mathbf{x}_{jk}^*; \boldsymbol{\beta}^*), \tag{4.25}$$

where the asterisks on $\boldsymbol{\beta}^*$ and $\mathbf{x}_{jk}^*$ indicate that these are the expanded vectors of length $J + p$ that involve the J stratum indicators and associated coefficients α_j in addition to the exposure variables. Maximum likelihood fitting of such models can be programmed as a series of weighted least-squares analyses involving dependent variables

$$y_{jk} = d_{jk} - n_{jk}\hat{\lambda}_{jk},$$

weights

$$w_{jk} = (n_{jk}\hat{\lambda}_{jk})^{-1}$$

and independent variables

$$z_{jk} = n_{jk}\frac{\partial g(\mathbf{x}_{jk}^*; \boldsymbol{\beta}^*)}{\partial \boldsymbol{\beta}^*}$$

that are recalculated at each stage of iteration using fitted rates

$$\hat{\lambda}_{jk} = g(\mathbf{x}_{jk}^*; \hat{\boldsymbol{\beta}}^*)$$

based on the current parameter estimates $\hat{\boldsymbol{\beta}}^*$. The change in the estimated coefficient going from one iteration to the next is given by

$$\Delta\hat{\boldsymbol{\beta}}^* = (\mathbf{Z}^T\mathbf{W}\mathbf{Z})^{-1}\mathbf{Z}^T\mathbf{W}y,$$

where $\mathbf{Z}$ is a matrix with rows z_{jk} and $\mathbf{W}$ is a diagonal matrix with diagonal elements w_{jk}.

Programming the likelihood calculations in this fashion leads to regression diagnostics that help evaluate the goodness-of-fit and stability of the model just as we saw earlier for the multiplicative model and the power family (4.16). The diagonal terms h_{jk} of the 'hat' matrix obtained at convergence of the iterative procedure,

$$\mathbf{H} = \mathbf{W}^{1/2}\mathbf{Z}(\mathbf{Z}^T\mathbf{W}\mathbf{Z})^{-1}\mathbf{Z}^T\mathbf{W}^{1/2}, \tag{4.26}$$

provide information about the general influence of the data in cell (j, k) on the fit. The specific changes in the estimated regression coefficients occasioned by deletion of those data are approximated by the vector

$$(\Delta\hat{\boldsymbol{\beta}}^*)_{-jk} \simeq -(\mathbf{Z}^T\mathbf{W}\mathbf{Z})^{-1}z_{jk}y_{jk}w_{jk}/(1 \quad h_{jk}). \tag{4.27}$$

A family of general relative risk models that is intermediate in generality between (4.24) and (4.25) is given by

$$\lambda_{jk} = \exp(\alpha_j)r(\mathbf{x}_{jk}; \boldsymbol{\beta}),$$

where the relative risk function is specified by the power relation

$$\log r(\mathbf{x}_{jk}; \boldsymbol{\beta}) = \begin{cases} \dfrac{(1 + \mathbf{x}_{jk}\boldsymbol{\beta})^\rho - 1}{\rho} & ,\rho \neq 0 \\ \log(1 + \mathbf{x}_{jk}\boldsymbol{\beta}) & ,\rho = 0. \end{cases} \tag{4.28}$$

This yields the additive relative risk model (4.24) at $\rho = 0$ and the standard multiplicative model (4.10) at $\rho = 1$. Thomas, D.C. (1981) proposed another family $RR(\mathbf{x}) = \exp(\rho\mathbf{x}\boldsymbol{\beta})\{1 + \mathbf{x}\boldsymbol{\beta}\}^{1-\rho}$, which also contains both additive and multiplicative forms. These two families, which specify how the exposure effects combine to yield a factor $r(\mathbf{x}; \boldsymbol{\beta})$, which then multiplies background, should be contrasted with the family (4.16),

BRESLOW AND DAY

Table 4.20   GLIM macros for fitting the relative risk model specified by equation (4.28) to grouped cohort data

```
$sub porr ! macros for power transform relative risks
!            MACRO PORR REQUIRES THE FOLLOWING INPUT DATA
!            r = NUMBER OF CASES (BINOMIAL NUMERATOR)
!            n = NUMBER OF CASES + CONTROLS (DENOMINATOR)
!            %l = POWER TRANSFORM USED IN RELATIVE RISK (%l = 0 FOR LOG)
!            strt = FACTOR WITH %i LEVELS THAT CONTAINS STRATUM INDICATORS
!            %i = NUMBER OF LEVELS FROM STRATUM INDICATOR STRT
!            b = INITIAL VALUES FOR PARAMETERS (LENGTH %l + 8)
!      x1 ... x8 = REGRESSION VARIABLES CODED TO HAVE POSITIVE RELATIVE RISK
!                  CODE XI = 0 FOR THOSE THAT ARE NOT TO BE FITTED.
!
!            ON EXIT THE FOLLOWING QUANTITIES ARE AVAILABLE
!
!            p = PREDICTED PROBABILITY OF 'BEING A CASE'
!            h = DIAGONAL TERMS FROM 'HAT' MATRIX
!            cs = STANDARDIZED RESIDUALS (CHI-SQUARE TYPE)
!            %vc = MATRIX OF VARIANCES AND COVARIANCES OF ESTIMATES
!
$mac ftnl ! macro to fit nonlinear relative risk model
$cal %k = 10 : %c = 0.0001 ! set convergence criteria
$err n !
$wei w $yvar y $while %k porr $dis e $ext %vl $cal h = %vl*w !
$cal cs = (r − n*p)/%sqrt(w) : %t = %cu(cs*cs) !
$cal %u = 2*%cu(r*%log(r/(n*p)) + (n − r)*%log((n − r)/(n*(1 − p)))) !
$pri 'chi-square' %t 'deviance' %u $ !
$del %pe y w %fv z1 z2 z3 z4 z5 z6 z7 z8 xb th db %vl $$endmac !
$mac porr ! rr(x) = ((1 + xb)**%l − 1)/%l
$cal xb = b(%i + 1)*x1 + b(%i + 2)*x2 + b(%i + 3)*x3 + b(%i + 4)*x4 + b(%i + 5)*x5
 + b(%i + 6)*x6 + b(%i + 7)*x7 + b(%i + 8)*x8 !
$cal xb = %if(%le(xb, 0), 0.0001, xb) !
$cal %a = 1 + %eq(%l, 0) $switch %a pow log $
$cal xb = (1 + xb)**(%l − 1) !
$cal p = %exp(th) : p = p/(1 + p) !
$cal w = n*p*(1 − p) : y = (r − n*p)/w !
$cal z1 = x1*xb : z2 = x2*xb : z3 = x3*xb : z4 = x4*xb : z5 = x5*xb : z6 = x6*xb !
$cal z7 = x7*xb : z8 = x8*xb !
$sca 1 !
$fit strt − %gm + z1 + z2 + z3 + z4 + z5 + z6 + z7 + z8 $ext %pe $cal db = %pe : b = b + db !
$pri %k 'estimates' b !
$use cchk ! check for convergence
$$endmac
$mac pow $cal th = b(strt) + ((1 + xb)**%l − 1)/%l $$endmac !
$mac log $cal th = b(strt) + %log(1 + xb) $$endmac !
$mac cchk ! convergence check
$cal db = %if(%le(db, 0), −db, db)/b !
$cal db = %if(%le(db, %c), 0, 1) : %t = %cu(db) !
$cal %k = %k − 1 : %k = %if(%le(%t, 0), 0, %k) $$endmac !
$return
```

which specifies how exposure and background effects combine. Table 4.20 contains a series of GLIM macros, based on the general iterated least-squares methodology just described, that were used to fit the class of models (4.28) in the illustrative examples. The multiplicative model with $\rho = 1$ is easily fitted using standard features of GLIM, and convergence is guaranteed. A recommended procedure is to fit this model to get starting values of $\boldsymbol{\beta}^* = (\alpha, \boldsymbol{\beta})$ for use with nearby values of ρ, say $\rho = 0.9$. One then uses the $\boldsymbol{\beta}^*$ values obtained at convergence with $\rho = 0.9$ to start the procedure with $\rho = 0.8$, and so on until the additive relative risk model $\rho = 0$. However, due to the general problems with additive and other nonmultiplicative relative risk models mentioned above, it may prove impossible to implement this procedure with some data sets once ρ decreases beyond a certain point. Comparison of deviances for various values of ρ allows one to judge which (if either) of the additive or multiplicative relative risk models provides a reasonable description of the data, just as in Example 4.2. Thompson and Baker (1981) describe an alternative methodology for fitting models with composite link functions, which may be implemented using the OWN feature of GLIM to fit (4.28). Pierce *et al.* (1985) have developed a flexible program to fit models in which the rates are expressed as a sum of products of multiplicative and additive terms.

Example 4.6

In order to illustrate the fitting of the additive relative risk model, we consider another set of data from the British doctors study (Doll & Peto, 1978). Table 4.21 presents numbers of lung cancer deaths and

Table 4.21 Numbers of lung cancers (O) and person–years of observation (P–Y) by age and smoking level among British male doctors[a]

No. of cigarettes smoked per day	Average number smoked		Age in years							
			40–44	45–49	50–54	55–59	60–64	65–69	70–74	75–79
0	0	O	0	0	1	2	0	0	1	2
		P–Y	17846.5	15832.5	12226	8905.5	6248	4351	2723.5	1772
1–4	2.7	O	0	0	0	1	1	0	1	0
		P–Y	1216.0	1000.5	853.5	625	509.5	392.5	242.0	208.5
5–9	6.6	O	0	0	0	0	1	1	2	0
		P–Y	2041.5	1745	1562.5	1355	1068	843.5	696.5	517.5
10–14	11.3	O	1	1	2	1	1	2	4	4
		P–Y	3795.5	3205	2727	2288	1714	1214	862	547
15–19	16.0	O	0	1	4	0	2	2	4	5
		P–Y	4824	3995	3278.5	2466.5	1829.5	1237	683.5	370.5
20–24	20.4	O	1	1	6	8	13	12	10	7
		P–Y	7046	6460.5	5583	4357.5	2863.5	1930	1055	512
25–29	25.4	O	0	2	3	5	4	5	7	4
		P–Y	2523	2565.5	2620	2108.5	1508.5	974.5	527	209.5
30–34	30.2	O	1	2	3	6	11	9	2	2
		P–Y	1715.5	2123	2226.5	1923	1362	763.5	317.5	130
35–40	38.0	O	0	0	3	4	7	9	5	2
		P–Y	892.5	1150	1281	1063	826	515	233	88.5

[a] From Doll and Peto (1978)

Table 4.22 Results of fitting several relative risk models to the data on lung cancer in British doctors: internal estimation of age effects[a]

Model no.	Equation for relative risk (RR) or excess risk (ER) as a function of daily no. of cigarettes (x)	Degrees of freedom	Deviance	Parameter estimate	Standard error
1	Separate RR each dose group	56	45.74	(see Fig. 4.6)	
2	$RR = \exp(\beta x)$	63	68.91	0.0853	0.0063
3	$RR = \exp(\beta x + \gamma x^2)$	62	51.87	0.1801	0.0263 (β)
				−0.00226	0.00059 (γ)
4	$RR = (1 + x)^\beta$	63	55.87	1.187	0.123
5	$RR = 1 + \beta x$	63	58.36	1.130	0.510
6	$RR = 1 + \beta x + \gamma x^2$	62	51.03	0.4105	0.2880 (β)
				0.0237	0.0116 (γ)
7	Separate ER each dose group	56	184.7		
8	$ER = \beta x$	63	205.8	4.4×10^{-5}	0.6×10^{-5}

[a] From Breslow (1985b)

approximate person-years denominators classified by age and number of cigarettes smoked per day. Data for ages 80 and above were excluded from consideration, since the diagnosis is often uncertain at such advanced ages, while data for persons who reported smoking more than 40 cigarettes per day were excluded on the grounds of being unreliable and uncharacteristic. This latter exclusion, made also by Doll and Peto (1978), has a substantial impact on the dose-response analyses and has been the subject of some controversy.

Table 4.22 presents the results of fitting a variety of models to these data. In addition to the smoking parameters, estimates of which are shown in the table, each requires estimation of eight α_j parameters to represent the effects of age. The first four models are multiplicative. Smoking is treated qualitatively in model 1, with a separate relative risk being estimated for each smoking level. In models 2 and 3, the quantitative dose variable $x =$ 'average number of cigarettes smoked per day' and then its square are introduced into the exponential term. Model 4 is the power relative risk model specified by equation (4.23), and models 5 and 6 are additive relative risk models as specified by (4.24).

Except for model 2, all the relative risk models (models 1–6) fit the observed data reasonably well. Model 4 fits best among those that require only a single parameter to describe the relative risk. The fact that a quadratic term significantly improves the fit of the additive relative risk model ($\chi^2_1 = 58.36 - 51.03 = 5.35$; $p = 0.02$) was interpreted by Doll and Peto (1978) as consistent with the notion that both an early and a late stage in the carcinogenic process are affected by cigarette smoke (see Chapter 6).

Figure 4.6 shows the relative risks estimated from four of the models. By definition, all relative risks are constrained to equal unity at zero dose. However, since most lung cancer deaths occur among smokers, the regression coefficients are largely determined by a comparison of rates for different classes of smokers, rather than by a comparison of smokers with nonsmokers. The fact that nonsmokers form the baseline category thus explains the apparently aberrant behaviour of the estimated relative risk curve for the power model. Were a more typical category used as a baseline, say, smoking of 20 cigarettes per day, all the curves would pass through unity at that point and would appear to be in better harmony. See the parallel discussion in §6.9 of Volume 1.

Certain drawbacks of the additive relative risk model are evident from Table 4.22. The standard errors for the regression coefficients are quite large in comparison with those for the multiplicative model, to the extent that t statistics of the form $t = \hat{\beta}/\text{SE}(\hat{\beta})$ seriously understate the true statistical significance of the smoking effect. The t statistics for the multiplicative models 2 and 4 are $t = 0.0853/0.0063 = 13.5$ and $t = 1.187/0.123 = 9.7$, each highly significant, while that for model 5 is only $t = 1.130/0.510 = 2.2$. The contrast

Fig. 4.6 Three relative risk (RR) functions fitted to data on lung cancer rates from the British doctors study

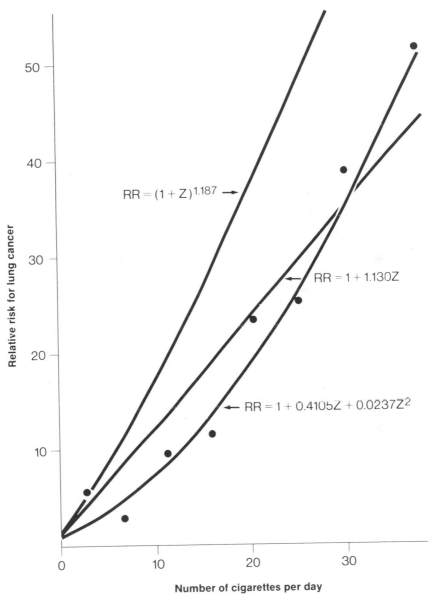

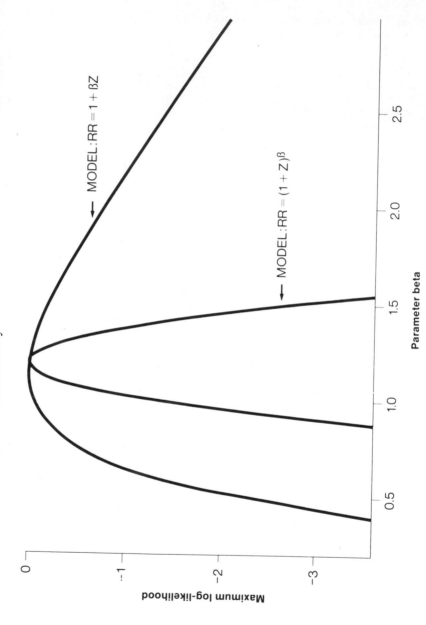

Fig. 4.7   Maximum (profile) log-likelihood functions for the additive and multiplicative relative risk (RR) models fitted to lung cancer rates from the British doctors study

between the maximum log-likelihood functions for the multiplicative and additive relative risk models (Fig. 4.7) is also striking. The β parameter in the additive relative risk model is less well determined, as indicated by the flatter log-likelihood, and there is substantial skewness. These problems may be largely overcome, however, by reparametrizing the model as $\lambda_{jk} = \alpha_j(1 + e^{\beta}x_k)$ (Thomas, D.C., 1981), or as discussed by Barlow (1986).

The last two models in Table 4.21 are additive models. Model 7 has the form $\lambda_{jk} = \alpha_j + \beta_k$, where a separate excess risk β_k is estimated for each dose category. Model 8 is $\lambda_{jk} = \alpha_j + \beta x_k$, where the excess risk is assumed to be linear in dose. Neither fits the observed data at all well. In fact, as soon as one moves much away from the relative risk models 1–6, for example, by considering the power family (4.16) with ρ departing slightly from 0, the goodness-of-fit declines substantially. Thus, although there may be some doubt about the specific form of relative risk as a function of dose, smoking does appear to act multiplicatively on the age-specific rates.

(d) Incorporating external standard rates

External standard rates λ_j^* are incorporated into the additive relative risk model by writing it in the form

$$\lambda_{jk} = \theta\lambda_j^*\{1 + \mathbf{x}_{jk}\boldsymbol{\beta}\}$$
$$= \theta\lambda_j^* + \lambda_j^*\mathbf{x}_{jk}\boldsymbol{\psi}, \qquad (4.29)$$

where $\boldsymbol{\beta} = \boldsymbol{\psi}/\theta$ is the parameter of interest. This is formally equivalent to the additive model (equation (4.16) with $\rho = 1$), except that there is only one stratum parameter θ and all the regression variables are pre-multiplied by the known rates λ_j^*. Thus, it may be fitted directly in GLIM without recourse to the specialized macros given in Table 4.20.

Although there are fewer parameters to estimate, (4.29) has the same drawbacks as (4.24) with regard to instability of the β coefficients. Indeed, it is clear from the relation $\beta = \psi/\theta$ that much of the instability in this model is due to the extremely high dependence between the estimated relative risks and the estimates of the baseline rates, or between the relative risks and the scale factor θ used to adjust those rates.

Example 4.7

The same series of models considered in Example 4.6 was fitted to the British doctors data shown in Table 4.21, except that the baseline age-specific rates were assumed to be proportional to $\lambda_j^* = (t_j - 22.5)^{4.5} \times 10^{-11}$, where t_j is the midpoint of the jth age interval. Here, $t_j - 22.5$ represents the approximate duration of exposure to the putative carcinogen in the jth age group and the exponent 4.5 represents a compromise between five and six stages in the multistage theory of carcinogenesis (Doll & Peto, 1978). Thus, the external 'standard' rates are based on theoretical concepts, rather than on national vital statistics as in some earlier examples.

The results, shown in Table 4.23, are little different from those in Table 4.22, where the age effects were estimated directly from the data. One would expect that the standard errors of the regression coefficients of the smoking variables might be reduced somewhat, reflecting an increase in precision stemming from the stronger assumptions made about the background rates. Theoretical calculations (Stewart & Pierce, 1982; Breslow, 1985b) indicate that such an increase would be expected if age were a strong confounder, in the sense that average smoking levels changed markedly from one age group to the other. While there is some evidence for such confounding in these data, it is evidently not strong enough that knowledge of the background rates, at least up to a constant of proportionality, would contribute a significant advantage in terms of increased precision.

If the additive relative risk model is expressed in terms of the parameters θ and ψ, as in (4.29), we estimate $\hat{\theta} = 0.837 \pm 0.356$, $\hat{\psi} = 0.954 \pm 0.741$ and $\text{Cov}(\hat{\theta}, \hat{\psi}) = -0.00686$. A test of the smoking effect is

Table 4.23 Results of fitting several relative risk models to the data on lung cancer in British doctors; age effects assumed proportional to $(\text{age}-22.5)^{4.5} \times 10^{-11}$

Model no.	Equation for relative risk (RR) or excess risk (ER) as a function of daily no. of cigarettes (x)	Degrees of freedom	Deviance	Parameter estimate	Standard error
1	Separate RR each dose group	63	47.13		
2	$RR = \exp(\beta x)$	70	70.29	0.0854	0.0063
3	$RR = \exp(\beta x + \gamma x^2)$	69	53.26	0.1802	0.0261 (β)
				-0.00226	0.00059 (γ)
4	$RR = (1 + x)^\beta$	70	57.35	1.192	0.122
5	$RR = 1 + \beta x$	70	60.00	1.141	0.516
6	$RR = 1 + \beta x + \gamma x^2$	69	52.43	0.409	0.286 (β)
				0.0239	0.0116 (γ)
7	Separate RR each dose group	63	200.0		
8	$ER = \beta x$	70	225.2	4.2×10^{-5}	0.6×10^{-5}

From Breslow (1985b)

thus given by $t = \hat{\psi}/\text{SE}(\hat{\psi}) = 12.9$, of the same order of magnitude as with the multiplicative models. However, the test based on $\hat{\beta} = \hat{\psi}/\hat{\theta} = 1.141$ divided by its standard error $\{\text{Var}(\hat{\theta})\hat{\beta}^2 - 2\,\text{Cov}(\hat{\theta}, \hat{\psi})\hat{\beta} + \text{Var}(\hat{\psi})\}^{1/2}/\hat{\theta} = 0.516$ yields a t statistic of only 2.2. This suggests that a large part of the instability in $\hat{\beta}$ in the additive relative risk model is its high correlation with parameter estimates (here $\hat{\theta}$) that represent the background rates. Further confirmation of this interpretation is given in Figure 4.8, which shows contour plots of the deviances obtained by varying the two parameters in the model equation (4.29). Although the minimum deviance of 60.0 occurs at $\hat{\beta} = 1.141$ (Table 4.23, model 5), nearly identical fits are obtained for a wide combination of parameter values (θ, β). The corresponding Figure 4.9 for the multiplicative model (Table 4.12, model 4) shows that, while there is still a strong dependence between the parameters representing relative risk and background, it is not so extreme as to lead to serious instability.

(e) General risk functions for proportional mortality

The relative risk models considered for proportional mortality analyses in §4.7 may also be generalized using the techniques of this section. In place of (4.19) we suppose

$$\lambda_{jk} = \exp(\alpha_j) r(\mathbf{x}_{jk}; \boldsymbol{\beta})$$
$$\nu_{jk} = \exp(\gamma_j), \tag{4.30}$$

where $r(x; \beta)$ denotes the general relative risk function for the cause of interest and where we have explicitly assumed that death rates for other causes are not affected by the exposures. The probabilities p_{jk} of 'being a case' then satisfy

$$\text{logit } p_{jk} = (\alpha_j - \gamma_j) + \log r(\mathbf{x}_{jk}; \boldsymbol{\beta}). \tag{4.31}$$

As shown above, a flexible and convenient family of models for the log relative risks (although by no means the only one that could be suggested for this purpose) is the

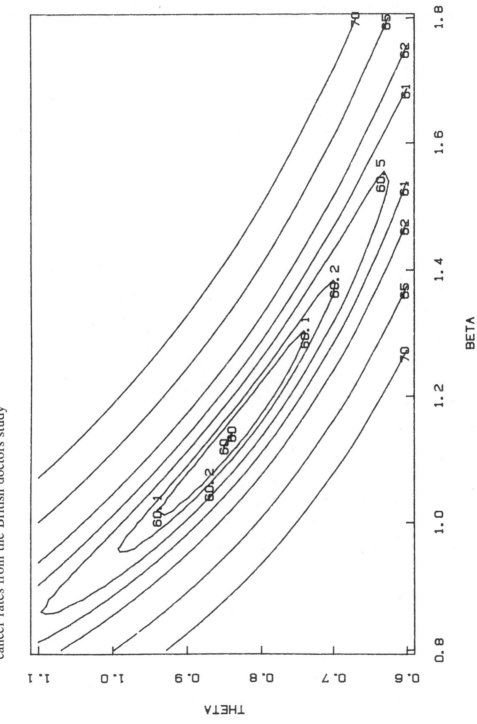

Fig. 4.8   Contour plot of deviances (G^2) when fitting the additive relative risk model with external standard rates to lung cancer rates from the British doctors study

Fig. 4.9 Contour plot of deviances (G^2) when fitting the multiplicative model with external standard rates and log transform of smoking to lung cancer rates from the British doctors study

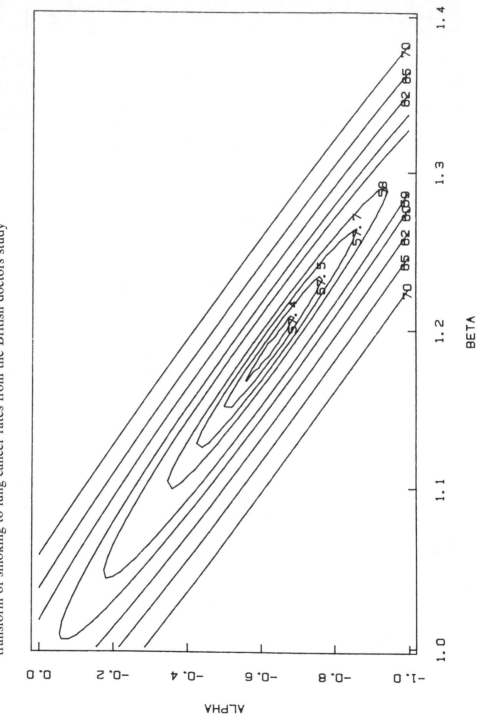

family

$$\log r(\mathbf{x}; \boldsymbol{\beta}) = \frac{(1 + \mathbf{x}\boldsymbol{\beta})^{\rho} - 1}{\rho},$$

which contains both additive ($\rho \to 0$) and multiplicative ($\rho = 1$) relative risk functions as special cases. Breslow and Storer (1985) illustrate the fitting of such general relative risk functions to grouped data from actual case-control studies. The same techniques can be used in proportional mortality analyses.

4.10 Fitting relative and excess risk models to grouped data on lung cancer deaths among Welsh nickel refiners

Appendix ID presents a detailed discussion of the background and design of the study of Welsh nickel refinery workers. Summary data on nasal sinus cancer deaths (Appendix VI) were considered briefly in Example 4.1 in order to illustrate some features of the fitting of multiplicative models to grouped data. Published data from this study provided us in Chapter 3 with examples of the use of internal standardization. With the approval of Kaldor *et al.* (1986), we undertake in this section a more comprehensive analysis of grouped data on lung cancer deaths in order to contrast the results obtained with relative and excess risk models. In the next chapter, continuous variable modelling techniques are applied to the study of rates of nasal sinus cancer deaths that occurred among these same workers.

(a) Basic data and summary statistics

Table 4.24 was compiled by Peto, J. *et al.* (1984) to summarize the mortality experience through 1981. The excess mortality was due largely to nasal sinus and lung cancers and was essentially confined to the 679 men employed before 1925, to whom attention is henceforth confined. Appendix VIII lists basic data for each of the 679 men that were used for all the grouped and continuous variable analyses reported in this

Table 4.24 Mortality experiences (O, observed; E, expected) of Welsh nickel refiners[a]

Period first employed	Number of men		Cancers			Other causes			All causes
			Lung	Nasal sinus	Other	Circulatory disease	Respiratory disease	Other	
Before 1925	679	O	137	56	67	220[b]	63	60	603
		E	26.86	0.21	59.44	194.76	62.39	75.74	419.38
1925–1929	97	O	11	0	11	26[b]	13	14	75
		E	5.48	0.03	8.08	26.19	8.46	9.04	57.28
1930–1944	192	O	11	0	16	58	13	12	110
		E	9.13	0.05	12.90	42.43	12.92	11.70	89.12

[a] From Peto, J. *et al.* (1984)
[b] Including one death in which nasal sinus cancer was an underlying cause

monograph. There are slight differences between this data set and that analysed by Peto, J. *et al.* (1984), Kaldor *et al.* (1986) and others, due to the continual process of data editing. Thus, the person-years of observation, expected numbers of deaths and relative risks shown in Tables 4.24 and 6.8 and in our own summaries (e.g., Table 4.25) differ very slightly. However, these differences have no material effect on the results or interpretation.

Six basic pieces of information are available for each subject: (i) ICD (7th revision) cause of death; (ii) exposure, defined as the number of years worked in one of seven 'high-risk' job categories prior to the start of follow-up (see below); (iii) date of birth; (iv) age at initial employment; (v) age at start of follow-up; and (vi) age at death for those who died, age last seen for those lost to observation, or age at end of study for those withdrawn alive. Nasal sinus cancer deaths are coded 160 under the 7th ICD revision, and lung cancer deaths are 162 or 163. Further dates of interest, such as date entered follow-up and date of initial employment, are obtained by adding the corresponding ages to the date of birth.

The nasal sinus cancer, lung cancer and total (all causes) death rates for England and Wales by five-year intervals of age and calendar time, listed in Appendix IX, were used to compute the expected numbers of deaths and the values of an age-dependent covariable, consisting of the standard death rate for each subject, at specified points in time.

(b) Construction of the exposure index

Company records were used to classify each year of an individual's employment into one of ten categories, depending on the area of the plant in which he worked on 1 April of that year. Such data were available for 82% of the 9354 calendar years during which the 679 subjects were employed prior to 1925. Kaldor *et al.* (1986) used a synthetic case-control approach to analyse the relation between work area and respiratory (nasal sinus and lung) cancer risk. They identified five exposure categories that appeared to be significantly related to the risk of both cancers: calcining I, calcining II, copper sulphate, nickel sulphate and furnaces. (See Table 6.7.) On this basis, they developed an exposure index equal to the number of calendar years employed in these categories. A contribution of a half rather than a full year was given for the first and last calendar year of such employment. In contrast to the Montana study, there was no overlap of exposure and follow-up periods and hence no change in the exposure index with follow-up. This simplified the analysis considerably.

Due to the circularity involved in construction of the exposure index, the excess risks may be overstated slightly. Another possible deficiency is that the index does not account for the time or age at which 'high-risk' exposures were received. Any difference between high-risk exposures received during 1905–1909 and those received between 1920 and 1924 is ignored. Furthermore, the use of date of initial employment to represent the start of exposure may obscure the fact that relevant exposures were primarily received in high-risk areas. One might consider an analysis of two exposure duration variables – years since initial employment *and* years since initial employment in a high-risk area. However, due to the undoubtedly high correlation between them, estimation of their separate effects would be problematic. Hence, time since first employment is used as the only time-dependent variable in the ensuing analyses.

(c) Grouping of data for analysis

From the data in Appendix VIII we constructed a four-dimensional table of observed numbers of lung cancer deaths, person-years of observation, and expected numbers of lung cancer deaths, and likewise for nasal sinus cancer. The dimensions were (i) age at first employment (AFE) in four levels; (ii) calendar year of first employment (YFE) in four levels; (iii) the exposure index (EXP) in five levels; and (iv) time since first employment (TFE) in five levels. The calculation used Clayton's algorithm (Appendix IV) to combine the 679 original records with the national death rates for England and Wales. At one point it was necessary to add two more dimensions to the table, namely, current age and calendar year in the quinquinquennia for which the national rates were available. Person-years in each cell were multiplied by the corresponding standard rate and then summed to give expected numbers of lung cancer deaths. Only 242 of the $4 \times 4 \times 5 \times 5 = 400$ cells in the four-dimensional table had some person-years of observation time available. The data for these 242 cells are presented in Appendix VII so that the reader can more easily verify our results.

(d) Fitting the relative risk model

Table 4.25 shows the person-years and observed and expected numbers accumulated for each factor level. The sixth column of the table presents estimated relative risks (ratios of SMRs) for each factor, adjusted for the remaining three factors. These were estimated from a multiplicative model (equation (4.18)) that incorporated the standard rates and 14 binary regression variables to represent the simultaneous effects of the four factors. An overall SMR of 8.92 was estimated for the baseline category, namely for the period up to 20 years since date of hire for workers hired under 20 years of age before 1910 with no time spent in a high-risk job. The lung cancer relative risk increased fourfold with increasing exposure, but declined markedly as TFE advanced beyond 20 years. The smaller changes in the SMR with age and year of initial employment were not statistically significant (Table 4.26).

(e) Fitting the excess risk model

Due to the ageing of the cohort and the secular increase in cigarette smoking, the national rates used to determine the SMRs were themselves climbing rapidly with increasing follow-up. Thus, it is unclear from the decline in the SMRs with TFE what the temporal evolution of absolute excess risk may be. In order to investigate this question, Kaldor et al. (1986) employed a model for excess risk that had been proposed earlier by Brown and Chu (1983), namely,

$$\lambda_{jk} = \lambda_j^* + \exp(\alpha + \mathbf{x}_k \boldsymbol{\beta}). \tag{4.32}$$

Here, $\exp(\alpha)$ represents the excess mortality rate for someone with a standard set of

Table 4.25 Fitting of relative and excess risk models to data on lung cancer mortality among Welsh nickel refiners

Risk factor	Level	Person–years at risk	No. of lung cancer deaths		Relative risk (ratio of SMRs)	Excess mortality ratio (EMR)
			Observed	Expected[a]		
Age at	<20 years	3089.2	13	5.58	1.0	1.0
first	20–27.5	7064.9	72	13.30	1.43	2.78
employment	27.5–35.0	3711.9	41	6.25	1.23	2.86
(AFE)	35.0+	1364.9	11	1.75	0.91	2.64
Year of	1900–1909	1951.0	23	2.84	1.0	1.0
first	1910–1914	2904.5	39	4.52	1.08	1.37
employment	1915–1919	2294.0	13	4.12	0.62	0.99
(YFE)	1920–1924	8081.3	62	15.39	0.73	1.70
Exposure	0–	7738.8	42	14.91	1.0	1.0
index	0.5–4.0	4905.1	50	8.32	1.83	2.41
(EXP)	4.5–8.0	1716.9	27	2.47	2.95	4.19
	8.5–12.0	601.2	12	0.85	3.54	5.04
	12.5+	269.9	6	0.34	4.03	5.87
Time since	0–19 years	2586.1	6	0.56	1.0	1.0
first	20–29	4777.5	35	3.15	0.76	2.87
employment	30–39	4329.4	55	7.60	0.48	5.02
(TFE)	40–49	2461.4	31	9.20	0.22	4.77
	50+	1076.4	10	6.37	0.11	2.11
Baseline SMR:					8.92	
Baseline excess mortality (per 100 000 person–years)						30.0
Chi-square goodness-of-fit (deviance; 227 degrees of freedom)					195.4	194.8

[a] Based on rates for England and Wales by age and calendar year (Appendix IX)

covariable values $(\mathbf{x}_k = \mathbf{0})$, and $\exp(\mathbf{x}_k \boldsymbol{\beta})$ represents the excess mortality ratio (EMR), i.e., the factor by which the specific exposures modify the excess rate.

The model defined by (4.32) may be fitted easily with the GLIM OWN facility for user-defined models, just as (4.18) is fitted using standard features of the program. Table 4.27 lists the GLIM commands needed to read the 242 data records from

Table 4.26 Evaluating the significance of variations in the SMR and EMR for each risk factor: lung cancer mortality among Welsh nickel refiners

Risk factor[a]	Degrees of freedom	Effect on relative mortality (SMR difference)		Effect on excess mortality (EMR difference)	
		Chi-square	p value	Chi-square	p value
AFE	3	2.96	0.40	7.35	0.06
YFE	3	3.77	0.29	3.34	0.34
EXP	4	21.25	0.0003	24.26	0.0001
TFE	4	42.42	<0.0001	17.25	0.002

[a] AFE, age at first employment; YFE, year of first employment; EXP, exposure index; TFE, time since first employment

Table 4.27 GLIM commands needed to produce the results shown in Table 4.25[a]

```
$UNITS 242 $DATA AFE YFE EXP TFE CASES PYR EXPT $
$FORMAT
(4(X, F2.0), 11X, F3.0, 8X, 2(X, F12.6)) 
$C READ IN DATA FROM FORTRAN UNIT 1 – APPENDIX VII
$DINPUT 1 80$
$C DECLARE OFFSET TO BE LOGARITHM OF EXPECTED NUMBERS OF CASES
$CAL EXPT = EXPT/1000 $
$CAL LEX = %LOG(EXPT) $OFF LEX $
$YVAR CASES $ERR P $
$FAC 242 AFE 4 YFE 4 EXP 5 TFE 5 $
$C FIT MULTIPLICATIVE MODEL
$FIT AFE + YFE + EXP + TFE $
$DIS M E $
$C EXTRACT PARAMETER ESTIMATES AND CONVERT INTO RELATIVE RISKS
$EXT %PE $CAL RR = %EXP(%PE) $LOOK RR $
$C NOW CONTINUE WITH EMR MODEL
$OFF $
$MAC M1 $CAL %FV = %EXP(%LP)*PYR + EXPT $$ENDMAC
$MAC M2 $CAL %DR = 1./(%FV – EXPT) $$ENDMAC
$MAC M3 $CAL %VA = %FV $$ENDMAC
$MAC M4 $CAL %YV = %IF(%LT(%YV, .5), .0000001, %YV) $
$CAL %DI = 2.*(%YV*%LOG(%YV/%FV) – (%YV – %FV)) $$ ENDMAC
$OWN M1 M2 M3 M4 $FIT . $REC 10 $FIT . $
$DIS M E $EXT %PE $CAL RR = %EXP(%PE) $LOOK RR $
$STOP
```

[a] Adapted from Kaldor et al. (1986)

Appendix VII and produce the SMR and EMR estimates shown in Table 4.25. The excess risk was estimated to be approximately 30 lung cancer cases per 100 000 person-years for workers in the baseline category. It also increased sharply with the exposure index. By contrast to the pattern in the relative risk, however, the excess risk increased to a maximum some 40 years from date of hire and subsequently declined.

Brown and Chu (1983) note that one will sometimes wish to adjust the standard rates λ_j^* used in modelling the excess risk in order to account for the healthy worker selection bias or other systematic departures of baseline mortality rates in the study group from the national averages. They suggest $\lambda_{jk} = \theta \lambda_j^* + \exp(\alpha + \mathbf{x}_k \boldsymbol{\beta})$ as a generalization of (4.32) and arbitrarily set $\theta = 0.8$ or $\theta = 1.2$ in order to gauge the sensitivity of the $\boldsymbol{\beta}$ parameter estimates to variation in the assumed background rates. We used the AMFIT program of Pierce et al. (1985) to estimate θ by maximum likelihood and found $\hat{\theta} = 1.087$. Since there was scarcely any improvement in fit over the model with $\theta = 1$, it appears that the national rates do a reasonable job of representing background lung cancer mortality for the Welsh cohort.

Although the SMR and EMR models happen to fit this particular set of data equally well, they lead to markedly different estimates of lifetime risk for typical workers. Kaldor et al. (1986) estimated the lifetime (to age 85) probability of lung cancer for light smokers who were born in 1900, who started work at the nickel refinery in 1920, and who accumulated an exposure index of 10. The probability was 0.27 under the multiplicative model and 0.58 under the additive one. For a heavy smoker, the estimated lifetime probability was 0.65 for the multiplicative model and 0.61 for the additive one.

Section 6.6 presents a further discussion of these results in terms of the multistage theory of carcinogenesis.

5. FITTING MODELS TO CONTINUOUS DATA

CHAPTER 5

FITTING MODELS TO CONTINUOUS DATA

Grouping of cohort data into a multidimensional classification of cases/deaths and person-years by categories of age, calendar period, cumulative exposures indices and other fixed or time-varying factors is a convenient way of reducing a frequently massive set of information into a form suitable for statistical analysis. It encourages the investigator to examine disease rates calculated within each cell of the cross-classification, making plots of rates against quantitative exposure measurements for purposes of model development. Inferences regarding disease mechanisms are made possible by examining the data for trends in excess or relative risk measures according to ordered categories of age at onset of exposure, duration of exposure, or time since cessation of exposure. By assigning average duration or dose levels to these categories, quantitative regression models may be fitted for purposes of risk assessment. Validation of the fitted models is facilitated by the calculation of standardized differences (residuals) between observed and fitted numbers of cases in each cell.

We believe that such grouped data analyses are generally the method of choice for cohort analysis. Given the inherent limitations of cohort data in terms of the number of cases and the accuracy of recorded exposure variables, more elaborate approaches such as those embodied in the continuous data analyses that we now describe are perhaps best limited to special situations. A possible exception is the use of the method of case-control within a cohort sampling (§5.4) to conduct preliminary exploratory analyses in order to select variables for a final analysis, which is carried out using either grouped or continuous data techniques.

Restrictions on grouped data analyses

A key assumption of the grouped data approach is that disease rates are constant within each cell of the multidimensional cross-classification. While clearly an approximation, this assumption can be made more plausible by refining the classification, for example, by using five-year rather than ten-year intervals of age and calendar time. However, there are obvious restrictions on the number of different variables that can be considered simultaneously and on the number of levels or categories into which each variable is factored. When most cells contain few, if any, cases, the previously cited measures of goodness-of-fit based on comparisons of observed and expected (fitted) numbers of cases have little if any value. Practical difficulties arise in coping with large numbers of cells and estimating large numbers of parameters.

Scope of Chapter 5

This chapter develops methods of continuous cohort data analysis that utilize age, time and exposure measurements in their original form rather than after partitioning the data into discrete categories. Many different explanatory variables may be considered simultaneously in the same analysis. To a large extent, the methods presented here are applications and refinements of survival analysis techniques originally proposed by Cox (1972) and developed further in texts by Kalbfleisch and Prentice (1980) and Cox and Oakes (1984), which should be consulted for a more detailed development. We first review, in §5.1, the fundamental concept of a disease incidence rate, considered as a continuous function of age and/or time. We describe how model equations already developed to express the effects of exposure on disease rates calculated from grouped data are adapted to the continuous case. Section 5.2 introduces the 'partial likelihood' methodology for estimating regression coefficients in models in which the exposure variables are assumed to act multiplicatively on the background rates. It contains a detailed, worked example for the simplest situation – that of a single, binary (but age-dependent) exposure variable. In §5.3 we develop nonparametric estimates of unknown baseline disease rates, both for homogeneous samples and for heterogeneous ones in which the heterogeneity is expressed by covariables in the multiplicative model. When the background rates are determined from vital statistics or are assumed to have a specific parametric form, the same techniques provide a nonparametric description of how relative mortality rates (SMRs) may vary continuously with time since first exposure, time since cessation of exposure, or with some other relevant time variable. Plots of baseline or relative mortality functions against one or more time-varying factors are shown to be quite useful as a means of informally examining model assumptions. In §5.4, we present details about the 'case-control within a cohort' or 'synthetic retrospective study' sampling technique that was introduced in Chapter 1 as a device for conducting efficient, exploratory analyses of continuous cohort data. This section also presents analytical methods for gauging the influence of individual cases or controls on the estimated regression coefficients. In sections 5.5 and 5.6 these methods are applied systematically to the studies of Montana smelter workers and Welsh nickel refinery workers, and comparisons are made with results of grouped analyses of these same data sets already presented in Chapter 4.

5.1 Fundamentals of continuous data analysis

Continuous data methods rest fundamentally on the concept of an instantaneous disease rate considered as a continuous function of a continuous time variable t (see Chapter 2 of Volume 1). Let $\lambda(t)$ denote the rate for a given subject at time t such that $\lambda(t)\,dt$ is the probability of disease diagnosis or death in the time interval $(t, t + dt)$, given that he was alive and/or disease-free at its start. We assume there is a background rate function $\lambda_0(t)$ that represents the degree of risk for someone with no exposure or, in some cases, a standard set of exposures. The object of the data analysis is to construct models that describe how the exposure variables $\mathbf{x}(t)$, which may themselves vary continuously and depend on time, act to modify the background rates $\lambda_0(t)$. Exposure effects are expressed parametrically in terms of a vector $\boldsymbol{\beta}$ of unknown parameters, and the statistical problem is one of estimating $\boldsymbol{\beta}$ in the presence of the unknown nuisance function $\lambda_0(t)$. The most widely studied of such semi-parametric structures is the proportional hazards model of Cox (1972), in which $\lambda(t) = \lambda_0(t) \exp \{\mathbf{x}(t)\boldsymbol{\beta}\}$.

An important generalization is to consider several background rate functions $\lambda_s(t)$, one for each of S strata ($s = 1, \ldots, S$). The strata may also be time-dependent, and we denote by $s(t)$ the stratum at which the subject finds himself at time t. The exposure variables are generally assumed to act in the same way (e.g., additively, multiplicatively) on each of the background rates, regardless of stratum, and a single set of β parameters is used to describe their effects. Further generalizations are possible to situations in which the background rates vary continuously with two or more continuous time variables, but these methods have not yet been fully developed and are not presented here.

(a) Choice of basic time variable

Substantial flexibility is available with the continuous variable models, since different choices can be made for the basic time variable t. Candidates for t include time on study, time since first employment, age and calendar year. Once t has been specified, its effects on the background mortality rates are estimated nonparametrically in $\lambda_0(t)$. The effects of the remaining time-dependent factors are then modelled in regression variables $x(t)$. Stratification of the sample into several subgroups, each with its own background mortality rate function, allows even greater flexibility. The choice of t is important, and the investigator will usually want to think carefully about the goals of the analysis before deciding which time variable to model nonparametrically and which to account for by means of regression coefficients.

Several of the analyses we have carried out have used $t = $ age as the fundamental time variable. Secular trends in the age-specific background rates are accommodated by stratification of the sample into five- or ten-year intervals of calendar year or birthdate. One rationale for this choice of t is the fact that age is generally the most critical determinant of cancer rates. This suggests that one allow the greatest possible flexibility in their age dependence. The effects of various exposure indices that change with time on study are accommodated in the regression variables.

In other examples, particularly those involving external standard rates or in which the background age-specific rates are known to have a simple parametric form, we have examined the evolution of excess or relative risk as a nonparametric function of $t = $ time since first exposure. Sometimes, one may wish to conduct several parallel analyses with different choices of t, in order to determine the most appropriate parametric form for each one prior to its inclusion in subsequent analyses as a time-dependent regression variable. However, some caution must be exercised in order that an inappropriate choice for t not obscure the very effects that one is looking for. For example, suppose that major attention is focused on a cumulative exposure variable $x(t)$ that is highly correlated with time on study. If time on study is selected as

t, some of the effects that rightfully should be quantified in the regression coefficient of the exposure variable will instead be hidden in the estimate of the baseline risk function $\lambda_0(t)$.

(b) Construction of exposure functions

One potential advantage of continuous variable methods is their ability, at least in principle, to make full use of the time history of exposures that may be recorded for each individual in the study. Estimates of annual exposure increments may be available from periodic readings of radiation dosimeters, from personal records on dates of transfer between job sites, or periodic examination of blood, urine or tissue specimens. A wide variety of exposure functions may be constructed from such data.

We first considered an approach that is of interest primarily for historical reasons. Suppose $z(u)\mathrm{d}u$ denotes the increment in exposure estimated to occur in the time or age interval $(u, u + \mathrm{d}u)$. Several investigators have constructed regression variables representing time-weighted cumulative or average exposures in the form

$$x(t) = \int_{t_0}^{t} z(u)w(t - u)\, \mathrm{d}u, \tag{5.1}$$

where t_0 is the age at entry to the study and $w(u)$ is a suitable weight function. If $w(u) = 0$ or 1, according to whether $u \leq L$ or $u > L$ years, $x(t)$ represents a lagged cumulative exposure such that increments received during the preceding L years have no effect on risk (e.g., Gilbert & Marks, 1979). By defining $w(u) = \min(1, u/L)$, exposures may be phased in linearly over a period of L years before taking maximum effect. Berry et al. (1979) set $w(u) = \{1 - \exp(-\lambda u)\}/\lambda$ as a method of time-weighting accumulating exposure to asbestos fibres that allows for their elimination from the lungs at rate λ. By taking $w(u)$ to be a probability density, one can express the concept of a biological latent interval as the random duration of time between an exposure increment and its effect on disease (Knox, 1973). A typical choice for w is the density function of a log-normal distribution, with mode and variance possibly estimated from the data. The 'working level month' used in the study of Rocky Mountain uranium miners is defined in precisely this way (Lundin et al., 1979). We explore this method in §5.5, using data from the Montana smelter workers study.

One cause for concern regarding the uncritical use of cumulative exposure measurements is that they may fail to separate intensity and duration of exposure adequately. For example, radiation risks are commonly assessed in terms of lifetime excess cancer cases per cGy of exposure per million population, without consideration of dose fractionation or timing (Committee on the Biological Effects of Ionizing Radiation, 1980). While this practice may have some empirical justification in radiation carcinogenesis, its widespread adoption in other situations is surely to be deplored. Consider, for example, the lung cancer risk at age 60 among two smokers – one who consumed 10 cigarettes per day since age 20 and the other 20 cigarettes per day since age 40. The total number of cigarettes is the same, namely 20 pack-years or $20 \times 20 \times 365 = 146\,000$ cigarettes. However, data from the British doctors study and elsewhere suggest that the lung cancer risk is approximately proportional to $dt^{4.5}$, where d is the number of cigarettes smoked per day and t is years of smoking (Doll & Peto, 1978; see also Example 4.7 above). This suggests that the 20-pack-year smoker who started at age 20 has $0.5(2)^{4.5} = 11.3$ times the lung cancer risk of the 20-pack-year smoker who started at age 40. Analysing the two individuals in the same category of 'cumulative dose' would be a serious error.

The choice of exposure variables used in continuous data analyses can have a major influence on the results and interpretation and on any quantitative risk assessments that are made. It is important, therefore, to demonstrate the goodness-of-fit of the resulting model and to evaluate its sensitivity to perturbations in the weight function or model equation. Even when analysing data using continuously varying baseline age rates, it is often prudent as a first step in the analysis to define the regression variables so that they represent discrete levels of intensity and duration of exposure, just as was done for grouped data. Examination of the results of such descriptive analyses can then suggest a possible role for a more quantitative approach.

We suggest that initial explorations of the data be conducted using categorical binary variables that represent different levels of each of the factors of primary interest: age at onset of exposure; intensity of exposure averaged over the period of accumulation; duration of exposure; fractionation; and time since last exposure. Trends in excess or relative risk measures according to each of these factors are of inherent interest and may help to elucidate possible underlying mechanisms. In Chapter 6, we consider how such descriptive analyses may be interpreted in terms of mathematical models of carcinogenesis. Some authors (Thomas, D.C., 1983; Brown & Chu, 1987) have successfully fitted biomathematical models directly to data from cohort studies, but, often, the quality of the data does not warrant the considerable effort that must be made to achieve a good fit, nor can competing models be clearly differentiated in terms of the weight of evidence to support them.

(c) Some model equations

Models are available to express the effect of regression variables $\mathbf{x}(t)$ on background rates $\lambda_0(t)$ that parallel those for the grouped data analyses considered in Chapter 4. Thus, one has

$$\lambda(t) = \lambda_0(t) + \mathbf{x}(t)\boldsymbol{\beta} \tag{5.2}$$

for an additive effect and

$$\lambda(t) = \lambda_0(t) \exp\{\mathbf{x}(t)\boldsymbol{\beta}\} \tag{5.3}$$

for a multiplicative one with multiplicative combination of risk variables (Cox, 1972). More general relative risk models may be written

$$\lambda(t) = \lambda_0(t) r\{\mathbf{x}(t)\boldsymbol{\beta}\}, \tag{5.4}$$

where, for example

$$\log r(z) = \frac{(1+z)^\rho - 1}{\rho},$$

as in (4.24). This yields the multiplicative model (5.3) at $\rho = 1$, whereas the additive relative risk model

$$\lambda(t) = \lambda_0(t)\{1 + \mathbf{x}(t)\boldsymbol{\beta}\} \tag{5.5}$$

occurs in the limit as ρ tends to 0. More general relative risk functions $r\{\mathbf{x}(t); \boldsymbol{\beta}\}$ may be constructed in which the explanatory variables $\mathbf{x}$ and the parameters $\boldsymbol{\beta}$ do not combine in the usual linear regression fashion. Frome (1983) considers models of the form

$$\lambda(t) = \lambda_0(t)\{1 + \exp(\beta_2 + x\beta_3)\}$$

for his analysis of grouped data on lung cancer and smoking from the British doctors study. He also estimates the baseline rates as a parametric function

$$\lambda_0(t) = e^{\beta_0}t^{\beta_1},$$

rather than leaving them unspecified, as suggested here.

An alternative to (5.2), in which the excess risk is a multiplicative function of the covariables, is given by

$$\lambda(t) = \lambda_0(t) + \exp\{\mathbf{x}(t)\boldsymbol{\beta}\}. \tag{5.6}$$

Pierce and Preston (1984) consider parametric models such that $\lambda(t)$ is expressed as a sum of products of linear and multiplicative terms,

$$\lambda(t) = \mathbf{x}_1(t)\boldsymbol{\beta}_1 e^{\mathbf{y}_1(t)\boldsymbol{\gamma}_1} + \mathbf{x}_2(t)\boldsymbol{\beta}_2 e^{\mathbf{y}_2(t)\boldsymbol{\gamma}_2} + \cdots,$$

where the explanatory and regression variables are partitioned $\mathbf{x} = (\mathbf{x}_1, \mathbf{y}_1, \mathbf{x}_2, \mathbf{y}_2, \ldots)$ and $\boldsymbol{\beta} = (\boldsymbol{\beta}_1, \boldsymbol{\gamma}_1, \boldsymbol{\beta}_2, \boldsymbol{\gamma}_2, \ldots)$. This includes (5.6) as a special case, provided that $\lambda_0(t)$ is modelled parametrically. They implement a similar generalization of the relative risk model (5.5).

(d) External standard rates

External standard rates are incorporated into each of these model equations just as they were for grouped data. One simply replaces the unknown functions $\lambda_0(t)$ in (5.2)–(5.6) by the quantity $\theta\lambda^*(t)$ where $\lambda^*(t)$ is the standard background rate at time t for a subject, depending upon his age and the calendar period, and $\theta = \exp(\alpha)$ is an unknown scale parameter used to adjust the standard rates so as to give the best fit to the background rates actually observed for the cohort. (Alternatively, especially in the context of (5.2), $\lambda_0(t)$ might be replaced by $\theta + \lambda^*(t)$ whereby an additive constant is used to adjust standard to background.) The known rates $\lambda^*(t)$ are typically obtained from national vital statistics, but occasionally they may come from theoretical models of the disease process, as in Example 4.7. Explicit equations for models analogous to (5.2), (5.3) and (5.5) are thus

$$\lambda(t) = \theta\lambda^*(t) + \mathbf{x}(t)\boldsymbol{\beta}, \tag{5.7}$$

$$\lambda(t) = \lambda^*(t) \exp\{\alpha + \mathbf{x}(t)\boldsymbol{\beta}\} \tag{5.8}$$

and

$$\lambda(t) = \theta\lambda^*(t)\{1 + \mathbf{x}(t)\boldsymbol{\beta}\}. \tag{5.9}$$

The continuous time version of the excess mortality ratio model considered in §4.10 is

$$\lambda(t) = \theta\lambda^*(t) + \exp\{\mathbf{x}(t)\boldsymbol{\beta}\}. \tag{5.10}$$

The availability of information on background rates is of particular importance when estimating excess risks using (5.7) or (5.10). We are unaware of any method that may exist for fitting (5.6) when $\lambda_0(t)$ is left completely unspecified. Such models may be fitted when the data are grouped, as we saw in the last chapter, or when $\lambda_0(t)$ is expressed in terms of a small number of unknown parameters, as suggested by Pierce and Preston (1984). A fully nonparametric treatment of background rates is currently limited to the multiplicative models.

In addition to the disease rates $\lambda(t)$ of primary interest, an important conceptual role is played in the sequel by a function $v(t)$ that represents the instantaneous rate at which subjects are lost from view during the study. Such loss may be caused by death due to 'competing' illnesses, emigration from the study area, or other reasons. We make the important assumption that v does not depend on $\boldsymbol{\beta}$, meaning that the timing and nature of deaths due to other diseases or the withdrawal of persons from the study carry no information on how exposures affect the disease of interest. The fitted statistical model represents a 'smoothing' of the observed variation in disease rates according to exposure and other explanatory variables, in the presence of competing causes of death. Conclusions about exposure effects apply only to the conditions that prevail in the particular study and should not be expected *a priori* to hold in a population subject to other types of intercurrent mortality (Prentice *et al.*, 1978). The question as to whether or not the results can be generalized must be argued on a broader basis. These caveats apply equally, of course, to results obtained with more elementary methods.

5.2   Likelihood inference

Just as was true for grouped data analyses, statistical inference about the parameters of interest in models for continuous data requires construction of an appropriate likelihood function. Denote by t_i the age (or time) at which the ith subject ends the study, and define δ_i as 1 or 0 according to whether death or diagnosis has or has not occurred at t_i. Also denote $Y_i(t) = 1$ or 0 according to whether he is or is not under observation at age t, and let $t_i^0 = \inf\{t: Y_i(t) = 1\}$ denote the age at entry. General considerations suggest that the contribution of the ith subject to the likelihood function is

$$\lambda_i^{\delta_i}(t_i)v_i^{1-\delta_i}(t_i)\exp\left\{-\int Y_i(u)\{\lambda_i(u) + v_i(u)\}\,\mathrm{d}u\right\}, \tag{5.11}$$

where subscripts i have been added to the rate functions λ and v defined earlier to indicate that they usually vary from one subject to another. The exponential term represents the probability of being disease-free between ages t_i^0 and t_i. For subjects who develop the disease of interest ($\delta_i = 1$), the leading term $\lambda_i(t_i)$ represents the conditional probability of death or diagnosis at t_i, given that it has not occurred earlier; for those who do not ($\delta_i = 0$), the leading term $v_i(t_i)$ represents the conditional probability of loss. A rigorous derivation of this result requires consideration of the product integral of the instantaneous probabilities of death or disease at each age, conditional on past history (Kalbfleisch & Prentice, 1980; Johansen, 1981). Since v_i is assumed to be free of $\boldsymbol{\beta}$, its contribution to the likelihood factor is usually ignored.

The only unknowns for models that incorporate standard rates are the scalar $\theta = \exp(\alpha)$ and the vector $\boldsymbol{\beta}$. In this case, the log-likelihood function for the entire set of cohort data may be written

$$L(\alpha, \boldsymbol{\beta}) = \sum_i \left\{ \delta_i \log \lambda_i(t_i; \alpha, \boldsymbol{\beta}) - \int Y_i(u)\lambda_i(u; \alpha, \boldsymbol{\beta}) \, du \right\}, \tag{5.12}$$

where $\lambda_i(t; \alpha, \boldsymbol{\beta})$ is specified by any one of the equations (5.7)–(5.10) or an analogous model formula. Formal proofs that maximum likelihood estimates based on this expression have the usual properties of consistency and asymptotic normality, with covariances estimable from the inverse information matrix, may be based on the large sample theory of counting processes (Borgan, 1984). Likelihood analyses based on (5.12) have been implemented for the multiplicative model (5.8) by Breslow *et al.* (1983), who approximate the integrals and their first and second derivatives by a summation in which the time-dependent covariables are evaluated annually for each subject. Some results of these analyses are presented in §5.5.

(a) Poisson models for grouped data

A formal justification for the Poisson model (4.7) used for grouped data analysis is obtained by specializing (5.11) to discrete time. Suppose that there are $J \times K$ cells or states and that $\lambda_i(t) = \lambda_{jk}$ if the ith subject is in state (j, k) at time t. This condition holds for grouped data models, in which the background rates are given by $\lambda_i(t) = \lambda_j$ and the regression variables by $\mathbf{x}_i(t) = \mathbf{x}_{jk}$ for subjects in state (j, k) at that time. Summing up the log-likelihood contributions from (5.11) over all subjects in the study leads to the total log-likelihood (Holford, 1980),

$$\sum_j \sum_k \{ d_{jk} \log(\lambda_{jk}) - n_{jk}\lambda_{jk} \},$$

where d_{jk} are the numbers of deaths that occur while a subject is in the (j, k)th state and n_{jk} is the total observation time (person-years) in that state. This is precisely the log-likelihood for the Poisson distribution on which the statistical methods of Chapter 4 were based, and each of the models (5.2)–(5.10) reduces to its discrete counterpart as considered there.

(b) Partial likelihood for multiplicative models

The likelihood for models (5.2)–(5.6) involves the unknown nuisance functions $\lambda_0(t)$, the presence of which considerably complicates estimation of $\boldsymbol{\beta}$. Cox (1972, 1975) solved this problem for the subgroup of multiplicative models (5.3)–(5.5) by constructing an appropriate 'partial likelihood', in which the contribution of the nuisance function is eliminated and only β remains. His approach is easily generalized to accommodate several background nuisance functions $\lambda_s(t)$ in a stratified analysis. Suppose, for example, that the ith individual is known to have died (or been diagnosed) at age t_i in calendar period (stratum) s_i. Denote by R_i the set of all subjects 'at risk' of death at that same age and period, meaning those who were alive and under observation just prior to age t_i and who were in calendar period s_i at that age. The conditional probability that the ith subject died, given that one death occurred among those in the risk set R_i, is thus

$$\lambda_i(t_i) \Big/ \Big\{ \sum_{j \in R_i} \lambda_j(t_i) \Big\}.$$

Summing up the logarithms of such contributions for all subjects who die or develop disease yields the log partial likelihood

$$L(\beta) = \sum_i \left[\log r\{\mathbf{x}_i(t_i); \beta\} - \log \sum_{j \in R_i} r\{\mathbf{x}_j(t_i); \beta\} \right], \tag{5.13}$$

where r denotes the relative risk function. If several deaths (or disease cases) occur in a given risk set R_i, each one contributes a term to (5.13). The expression then serves as an approximation to the log partial likelihood, which is adequate so long as the deaths form only a small fraction (e.g., under 5%) of the total number in each risk set (Peto, R., 1972; Breslow, 1974).

Other methods are needed when the times of death or diagnosis are grouped, so that a substantial number d_i of cases occurs among those in the risk set at a specified t_i. Cox (1972) also proposed a linear logistic model for discrete survival data, such that each risk set yields a partial likelihood contribution proportional to

$$\frac{\prod_{j=1}^{d_i} r\{\mathbf{x}_{ij}(t_i); \beta\}}{\sum_l \prod_{j=1}^{d_i} r\{\mathbf{x}_{il_j}(t_i); \beta\}}, \tag{5.14}$$

where the numerator is a product of relative risks over the d_i cases, and $\mathbf{x}_{ij}(t_i)$ denotes the covariable vector for the jth member of R_i. Assuming that the risk set also contains g_i noncases, the denominator is a summation over all $n_i \cdot Cd_i$ ways of selecting a 'control sample' containing d_i of the $n_i = d_i + g_i$ individuals in R_i. Each control sample is specified by a set of indices $l = \{l_1, l_2, \ldots, l_{d_i}\}$ chosen from the numbers $\{1, 2, \ldots, n_i\}$ that identify the 'risk set' members. The labels $\{1, 2, \ldots, d_i\}$ are assumed to correspond to cases. Although the large number of terms in the denominator sum renders its calculation unfeasible if both d_i and g_i are large, recursive algorithms developed by Gail et al. (1981) and Storer et al. (1983) permit this approach to be used when there is a moderate number of cases – say, no more than 20 or so – in each risk set.

For the special case $r(\mathbf{x}; \beta) = \exp(\mathbf{x}\beta)$, Andersen and Gill (1982) show that the usual likelihood calculations based on differentiation of (5.13) yield asymptotically normal estimates, the variances and covariances of which may be estimated from the observed information matrix. Prentice and Self (1983) derived analogous results for models (5.4) and (5.5), in which the relative risk function is given by $r(\mathbf{x}; \boldsymbol{\beta}) = 1 + \mathbf{x}\boldsymbol{\beta}$ or a more general expression. As already mentioned, satisfactory nonparametric methods of estimation for the additive models (5.2 and 5.6) have not yet been developed.

Example 5.1

Hutchinson and colleagues (1980) conducted a historical cohort study of nearly 1500 women treated for benign breast disease to determine their subsequent incidence of breast cancer. A later analysis of these data related each woman's history of treatment with hormones (oestrogens) to breast cancer risk (Thomas, D.B. et al., 1982). The data used here for illustrative purposes were compiled by Persing (1981) from 1353 cases with a histological confirmation of the initial benign lesion.

A simple tabulation of the data, shown in Table 5.1, leads to a relative risk estimate for hormone users *versus* nonusers of $(25 \times 499)/(33 \times 522) = 0.72$, and suggests a possible protective effect of the oestrogens. However, it ignores the person-years of observation denominators and, more importantly, the relationship between the age at which each woman started to take oestrogens and the age at which she developed, or was at risk of developing, breast cancer. Oestrogen use and age were strongly related, since the cohort had been assembled during a 35-year surgical practice over which time there were marked changes in the use of oestrogens for contraception or treatment of post-menopausal symptoms.

A partial likelihood analysis was undertaken with $t = $ age in order to account for the age dependence of both exposure and disease risk. Table 5.2 lists the integral ages t_i at which diagnoses of breast cancer were made and the composition of the risk sets for 1036 women for whom it was known whether or not and, if so, at what age, oestrogen use began. A woman contributed to the risk set R_i provided that her benign breast disease had been diagnosed before age t_i, so that she was under observation, and provided also that she had not yet died, been lost to follow-up or otherwise removed from risk of breast cancer, for example, by having a double mastectomy.

In this example, there is a single, age-dependent binary covariate $x_1(t)$ indicating whether or not a woman has received oestrogen. It is defined as 1 for all women in R_i who received hormone prior to t_i, i.e., for the women in columns labelled H1 in Table 5.2, and 0 for the remaining women. Note that a woman's covariable value may change from $x_1(t) = 0$ to $x_1(t) = 1$ as she is followed forward in the study. A parallel analysis in terms of a fixed (i.e., not age-dependent) covariable, taking values 1 or 0 according to whether a woman ever received oestrogen (columns H1 and H2), yields fallacious results, since some women are then analysed as 'exposed' at ages before the exposure actually began.

Suppose that the relative risk function is defined by $r(x; \beta) = \exp(x\beta)$, so that the relative risk is $\psi = \exp(\beta_1)$ for prior exposure $\{x_1(t) = 1\}$ and $1 = \exp(0)$ for no prior exposure $\{x_1(t) = 0\}$. The data in each risk set are conveniently arranged in a 2×2 table of exposed *versus* nonexposed and cases *versus*

Table 5.1 Distribution of 1353 women treated for benign breast disease according to history of oestrogen use and development of breast cancer[a]

Oestrogen use	Breast cancer		
	Yes	No	Total
Yes	25	522	547
No	33	499	532
Unknown	8	266	274
Total	66	1287	1353

[a] From Persing (1981), from data originally collected by Hutchinson *et al.* (1980)

Table 5.2 Composition of the risk sets at each age of diagnosis of breast cancer

Age = t_i	Total number in risk set R_i	Cancer cases[a]			Non-cancer cases[a]		
		H1	H2[b]	no H	H1	H2	no H
30	148	0	0	1	27	63	57
37	279	0	0	1	38	130	110
38	304	1	0	2	40	139	122
41	409	0	0	2	58	180	169
44	507	1	0	2	99	200	205
45	528	2	0	2	109	194	221
46	567	1	0	3	135	192	236
48	602	1	0	3	154	179	265
49	602	0	0	1	178	160	263
50	610	2	0	1	196	140	271
51	598	0	0	3	216	115	264
52	577	2	0	2	226	94	253
54	520	1	0	1	221	66	231
58	389	4	0	0	158	35	192
60	348	2	0	0	147	17	182
61	313	1	0	1	124	14	173
62	285	1	0	1	100	11	172
64	234	2	0	1	73	9	149
65	200	1	0	0	55	7	137
67	159	0	0	1	40	2	116
68	137	1	0	1	29	2	104
69	121	0	0	3	27	0	91
76	37	0	0	1	5	0	31

[a] H1, hormone (oestrogen) users at ages less than or equal to t_i; H2, hormone users at ages greater than t_i; no H, hormone nonusers
[b] This column contains only zeros, since women who developed breast cancer at age t_i were removed from further study

noncases. For example, at age $t_i = 52$ we have

	Exposed	Nonexposed	
Cases	2 (e_i)	2	4 (d_i)
Noncases	226 ($f_i - e_i$)	347	573 (g_i)
Total	228 (f_i)	349	577 (n_i)

The contribution to the numerator of the partial likelihood (5.14) for the risk set at age $t_i = 52$ is thus $\psi^2 1^2 = \psi^2$. More generally, if e_i of the d_i cases are exposed, the contribution is ψ^{e_i}. If a 'control' sample $\{l_1, \ldots, l_{d_i}\}$ in the denominator yields u exposed and $n_i - u$ nonexposed, its contribution to the denominator is ψ^u. Since the number of such samples with exactly u exposed is

$$\binom{d_i}{u}\binom{g_i}{f_i - u},$$

the total contribution of the risk set R_i to the partial likelihood is proportional to

$$\frac{\binom{d_i}{e_i}\binom{g_i}{f_i - e_i}\psi^{e_i}}{\sum_{u=0}^{d_i}\binom{d_i}{u}\binom{g_i}{f_i - u}\psi^u}. \tag{5.15}$$

For example, the risk set at age $t_i = 52$ years yields the contribution

$$\frac{\binom{4}{2}\binom{573}{226}\psi^2}{\binom{4}{0}\binom{573}{228}\psi^0 + \binom{4}{1}\binom{573}{227}\psi^1 + \binom{4}{2}\binom{573}{226}\psi^2 + \binom{4}{3}\binom{573}{225}\psi^3 + \binom{4}{4}\binom{573}{224}\psi^4}.$$

For this special case of a single binary exposure variable, the partial likelihood (5.15) is identical to the exact conditional likelihood used for estimation of relative risk in a series of 2×2 tables compiled from case-control data (§7.5 Volume 1; Breslow, 1976). The computer program LOGODDS, presented in Appendix VI of Volume 1, may be utilized for this special problem, although some modifications are needed to accommodate the large binomial coefficients that occur in (5.15).

The full partial likelihood is a product of terms of the form (5.15), one for each line in Table 5.2. Maximizing this, we find $\hat{\psi} = 1.80$. The Mantel–Haenszel test of the hypothesis H_0: $\psi = 1$ (§4.4, Volume 1), known also as the logrank test (Peto, R. & Peto, 1972), yields $\chi^2 = 4.41$ ($p = 0.02$). We conclude that oestrogen use significantly increased the breast cancer risk in this population of women with benign breast disease. However, part of the observed association might be related to the confounding effects of other risk factors that were increasing with calendar time. Both oestrogen use and breast cancer incidence were rising during the course of the study, and inclusion of year of birth as an additional covariate in the model reduced the estimated relative risk for oestrogen to $\hat{\psi} = 1.49$, $\chi^2 = 1.82$ (Thomas, D.B. et al., 1982).

Repeating the analysis in terms of the improper (fixed) exposure covariate yields $\hat{\psi} = 0.70$, $\chi^2 = 1.59$ (NS), a result rather close to that for the summary data in Table 5.1 where we ignored age altogether. Careful examination of Table 5.2 shows the reason for the discrepancy. When averaged over the 23 risk sets, with weights proportional to their size, the proportion of women who used oestrogen at any time (H1 + H2) is 0.38 for cases and 0.52 for noncases. However, the average proportions of women who had started using oestrogens previously are instead 0.38 and 0.29. In other words, when cases and noncases are compared in terms of whether or not they had a history of exposure *at the same age,* the cases are more likely to have used the hormone. More noncases were observed during the later ages and calendar periods, at which oestrogen treatment was more common.

We tested whether or not the relative risk for oestrogen use varied with age by including an age-dependent covariable $x_2(t) = x_1(t) \times (t - 55)$ in the model $\lambda(t) = \lambda_0(t) \exp\{\beta_1 x_1(t) + \beta_2 x_2(t)\}$. Here, $\psi = \exp(\beta_1)$ denotes the relative risk at age 55, while $\exp\{\beta_2(t - 55)\}$ is a multiplicative factor that measures the change in the relative risk for younger or older women. Alternatively, we could have set $x_2(t) = x_1(t) \times \log(t/55)$, in which case the relative risk would be modelled as a power function $\psi(t/55)^{\beta_2}$. With the addition of $x_2(t)$ to the model, the contributions to (5.15) become

$$\frac{\binom{n_i}{e_i}\binom{g_i}{f_i - e}\exp[e_i\{\beta_1 + \beta_2(t_i - 55)\}]}{\sum_{u=0}^{d_i}\binom{n_i}{u}\binom{g_i}{f_i - u}\exp[u\{\beta_1 + \beta_2(t_i - 55)\}]}.$$

Using once again a modification of the program LOGODDS, we find $\hat{\beta}_1 = 0.614 \pm 0.285$, $\hat{\beta}_2 = 0.017 \pm 0.029$ and a score statistic for testing $\beta_2 = 0$ of $\chi_1^2 = 0.32$ (NS). Thus, there is no evidence for a trend in the relative risk with age.

An explicit formula for the score statistic used to test $\beta_2 = 0$ was given in Volume 1, equation (4.31). Contrary to the assertion made there, however, the estimates $\hat{\psi}$ of relative risk inserted in equations 4.30 and 4.31 of Volume 1 must be maximum (partial) likelihood estimates in order that these statistics have asymptotic chi-square distributions under the null hypothesis. Modifications of the equations are needed when the Mantel-Haenszel estimate $\hat{\psi}_{\mathrm{MH}}$ is used in place of the maximum likelihood estimate. (See Breslow *et al.* (1984) for the modification needed in the test for trend, and Tarone (1985) for the corresponding global test of homogeneity of relative risk.)

(c) Goodness-of-fit

The goodness-of-fit of models fitted to grouped cohort data may be evaluated relatively easily by comparing the observed and fitted numbers of deaths in each cell of the cross-classification, by plotting the adjusted residuals (4.13) in various ways and by examining the summary chi-square (4.6) or deviance (4.12) goodness-of-fit statistics. Indeed, an advantage of this approach is that one is almost forced to examine how well the model predicts the outcome in each cell. Unfortunately, no such safeguard is built into the continuous data analysis, and extra steps are needed to determine whether or not the model provides a reasonable summary of the observed data.

One of the most important methods for examining the goodness-of-fit of the proportional hazards model was introduced in Example 5.1. It involves adding to the model age- or time-dependent covariables that represent the interaction of exposure effects with those of age or time. Such covariables typically take the form $y(t) = x(t) \log (t/c)$ or $y(t) = x(t)(t - c)$, where c is a constant representing a standard age and $x = x(t)$ represents an exposure that may or may not be time-dependent. The sign of the regression coefficient estimated for $y(t)$ indicates whether the trend in relative risk associated with a given amount of exposure is increasing or decreasing with age. Additional interaction variables with quadratic terms $(t - c)^2$ or $\log^2 (t/c)$ may be needed if the relative risk first rises and then declines with age.

An alternative approach that may be implemented without explicit recourse to age-dependent covariables is to carry out separate analyses for each of two or three age intervals by dividing the risk sets into groups depending on t_i. Comparison of regression coefficients for the same exposure variables in different age groups indicates the direction of any trend, and comparison of the maximized partial likelihood for the combined analysis with the sum of the maximized partial likelihoods for the separate analyses provides a formal test of the statistical significance of the differences in the coefficients.

A third approach that retains some of the features of the grouped data analysis is to define a partition of age into J intervals and exposure into K categories. Separate binary covariables are then defined for each of the JK cells in the cross-classification. The score test for the addition of these covariables to the regression models compares the observed and expected numbers of cases in each cell. However, since the expected values are based on the model fitted to continuous data, the simple $\sum (O - E)^2/E$ chi-square formula does not apply (Schoenfeld, 1980; Tsiatis, 1980). It is necessary to estimate the covariances of the $O - E$ differences in order to carry out the test.

A graphical approach to the evaluation of goodness-of-fit of proportional hazards is to partition the sample into a small number of (possibly time-dependent) categories of persons with similar exposure histories. Separate estimates of the age-specific disease incidence functions are modelled for each one. When plotted against age on a semilogarithmic scale, these curves should stay roughly a constant distance apart if the hypothesis of proportionality holds. This procedure is illustrated below with the benign breast disease data. (See especially Figure 5.2.)

A variation of this graphical analysis is helpful when the exposure variables are numerous, and estimation of a separate age incidence function within categories of exposure is not feasible. One defines a partition of the data into K subgroups on the basis of the estimated relative risk function $r\{x(t); \hat{\beta}\}$. If $x = x(t)$ depends on age, therefore, so will subgroup membership. Separate estimates of the age-incidence curves for each subgroup, say, $\hat{\lambda}_k(t)$ for $k = 1, \ldots, K$, are compared with the fitted age-incidence curves $r_k \hat{\lambda}_0(t)$, where r_k is the average relative risk in the kth subgroup and $\hat{\lambda}_0(t)$ is the background age incidence function estimated from the total cohort. Breslow (1979) gives an illustration using data from clinical trials.

The addition of exposure × age interaction variables to the basic equation is also applicable as a means of assessing goodness-of-fit when the background rates are assumed to be proportional to external standard rates or are modelled parametrically. A graphical method for evaluating the proportionality assumption is illustrated in Figures 5.4 to 5.6.

(d) Nonmultiplicative models

Partial likelihood unfortunately provides only a partial solution to the problem of fitting continuous models to cohort data. The approach is not applicable if the basic model is additive, for example, or has any other form in which the exposure effects do not act multiplicatively on the background rates. It is necessary in such circumstances to assume that the background rates are given by some formula that depends on parameters α and to base the inference on the general log-likelihood (5.12). This is precisely what one does when the background rates are assumed to be known up to a constant $\theta = \exp(\alpha)$ of proportionality, or when explicit parameters are used to represent background rates by age and year in grouped data analyses.

(e) Notes on computing

Example 5.1 is a very special case in that it involves only a single binary covariable. This allows the data to be represented as a series of 2×2 tables and allows use of programs for the regression analysis of log odds ratios in 2×2 tables in the analysis. Most problems, including analyses of the data on Montana smelter and on Welsh nickel workers, presented below, involve multiple discrete and continuous regression variables $x(t)$. Here, the computing problems are considerably more complex. One must either compute and store the covariable history $x(t)$ for each individual at times $t = t_i$ for *each* of the risk sets R_i in which he appears, or else supply a set of covariable function subroutines that calculate the requisite covariables, at different times, from basic data available for each subject. An exception is the additive relative risk model (5.5), for which only the covariable values for the cases and the *average* of the covariables for the other risk-set members need to be stored (Gilbert, 1983; Prentice & Mason, 1986). For large cohort studies, it is generally not possible to store all the data needed in the central memory of a computer. This means that a separate pass through the data files is made at each iteration of the procedure used to find the maximum partial likelihood estimate $\hat{\beta}$. The program must also be capable of accommodating time-dependent stratification, whereby the stratum index for each subject is available from stored data, or from function subprogram calculations, for each risk set in which he appears.[1]

5.3 Nonparametric estimation of background rates

Nonparametric estimates of cumulative disease incidence or death rates based on continuous data sampled from a homogeneous population were introduced in Volume 1 (§2.3) with an illustrative application to data on mouse skin tumours. Virtually identical techniques are used to estimate cumulative disease rates from cohort data. Suppose that the distinct times or ages at which deaths or cases occur are $0 < t_1 < t_2 < \cdots < t_I$. Denote by d_i the number of cases at t_i and by $n_i = d_i + g_i$ the total size of the risk set R_i, i.e., the number of cohort members under observation at t_i. Let $\Lambda(t) = \int_0^t \lambda(s) \, ds$ denote the unknown cumulative rate in the general population. The usual estimate of Λ, often ascribed to Nelson (1969), is

$$\hat{\Lambda}(t) = \sum_{t_i \leq t} \frac{d_i}{n_i}. \tag{5.16}$$

Some motivation for this formula is provided by the fact that the differentials

$$\frac{\hat{\Lambda}(t_i) - \hat{\Lambda}(t_{i-1})}{t_i - t_{i-1}} = \frac{d_i}{n_i(t_i - t_{i-1})},$$

which equal the observed number of deaths divided by the approximate person-years observation time in the age interval (t_{i-1}, t_i), are obvious estimates of the corresponding instantaneous rates.

The variance of $\hat{\Lambda}(t)$ is estimated using Greenwood's (1926) formula

$$\mathrm{Var}\, \hat{\Lambda}(t) = \sum_{t_i \leq t} \frac{d_i}{n_i(n_i - d_i)}. \tag{5.17}$$

This is the continuous data analogue of equation (2.2) for the standard error of a cumulative or directly standardized rate calculated from grouped data. When considered as a random function of t, $\hat{\Lambda}$ is approximately distributed as a Gaussian stochastic process with mean $\Lambda(t)$ and a covariance function $C(s, t) = \mathrm{Cov}\{\hat{\Lambda}(t), \hat{\Lambda}(s)\}$ that is estimated for $t \leq s$ by (5.17) (Breslow & Crowley, 1974). This fact has enabled statisticians to develop simultanous confidence bands for $\Lambda(t)$, or the corresponding 'survival' function $S(t) = \exp\{-\Lambda(t)\}$, over an interval of time or age (Gillespie & Fisher, 1979; Hall & Wellner, 1980).

The same approach may be used to obtain separate estimates of cumulative hazard

---

[1] Pat Marek of the Fred Hutchinson Cancer Research Center (see Peterson *et al.*, 1983) developed the program that we used for the illustrative analyses presented here. This program is currently being simplified and adapted to run on microcomputers.

or mortality within each of several subsets or strata. One simply classifies the d_i deaths and n_i risk-set members according to the particular stratum in which they appear at time t_i. As we noted earlier, plots of the estimated $\hat{\Lambda}_s(t)$ for different strata are useful for examining the consistency of the data with the assumption of proportional hazards. If the disease incidence rates $\lambda_1(t)$ and $\lambda_2(t)$ are in constant ratio $\lambda_2(t) = \theta\lambda_1(t)$, then so are the integrated hazards $\Lambda_2(t) = \theta\Lambda_1(t)$. Plots of $\hat{\Lambda}_1$ and $\hat{\Lambda}_2$ on a semilogarithmic scale should therefore be roughly a constant distance apart.

Example 5.2

From the data in Table 5.2 and equation (5.16), one may construct an estimate of cumulative breast cancer incidence for women who had no prior exposure to oestrogen and another for women with such exposure. For example, the cumulative incidence at age $t = 45$ for women without prior exposure is estimated to be

$$\hat{\Lambda}_1(45) = \frac{1}{121} + \frac{1}{241} + \frac{2}{263} + \frac{2}{351} + \frac{2}{407} + \frac{2}{417} = 0.0354,$$

whereas for women with an exposure history it is

$$\hat{\Lambda}_2(45) = \frac{1}{41} + \frac{1}{100} + \frac{2}{111} = 0.0524.$$

Figure 5.1 shows these two functions, plotted using arithmetic (Fig. 5.1A) and logarithmic (Fig. 5.1B) scales for $\hat{\Lambda}$. Although there is considerable instability in the estimates due to the small numbers, there is no evidence of a systematic trend in the difference between the two curves on the semilogarithmic plot. This confirms the results of the formal analysis of Example 5.1 in which we tested whether the ratio of rates for exposed *versus* unexposed showed a trend with age and concluded that the assumption of proportionality was justified.

Note that the estimated lifetime cumulative incidence for oestrogen nonusers in this cohort is approximately twice that of the general population rate of 7%. The rates for users are even higher. This illustrates the fact that a history of benign breast disease itself augments the subsequent breast cancer risk (Hutchinson *et al.*, 1980).

(a) Smoothed estimates of age- or time-specific rates

Estimates of cumulative incidence or mortality rates such as shown in Figure 5.1 are not as informative as they might appear at first sight. They tend to overemphasize the jumps that occur at very high ages, at which the estimate is least stable due to declining numbers at risk. Also, the age- or time-specific rates are usually of greater intrinsic interest than the cumulative rate. Recent work by Ramlau-Hansen (1983) and Yandell (1983) has validated kernel estimates of $\lambda(t)$ that have the form

$$\hat{\lambda}(t) = \frac{1}{b}\int_0^\infty K\left(\frac{t-s}{b}\right)\mathrm{d}\hat{\Lambda}(s) = \frac{1}{b}\sum_{i=1}^I K\left(\frac{t-t_i}{b}\right)\frac{d_i}{n_i}. \tag{5.18}$$

Here, $K(x)$ is a smooth, positive kernel function integrating to one, and b is a bandwidth that determines the degree of smoothness in the estimate. Thus, $\hat{\lambda}(t)$ is simply a weighted average of the increments d_i/n_i in $\hat{\Lambda}(t)$, with K defining the weights and b the size of the 'window' about t within which the estimates of the instantaneous rates are averaged. Its standard error is given by

$$\mathrm{SE}\{\hat{\lambda}(t)\} = \frac{1}{b}\left\{\sum_{i=1}^I K^2\left(\frac{t-t_i}{b}\right)\frac{d_i}{n_i^2}\right\}^{1/2}. \tag{5.19}$$

Fig. 5.1   Cumulative incidence of breast cancer for women with benign breast disease
with (solid line) and without (dotted line) prior exposure to oestrogen. (A)
Arithmetic scale; (B) log scale

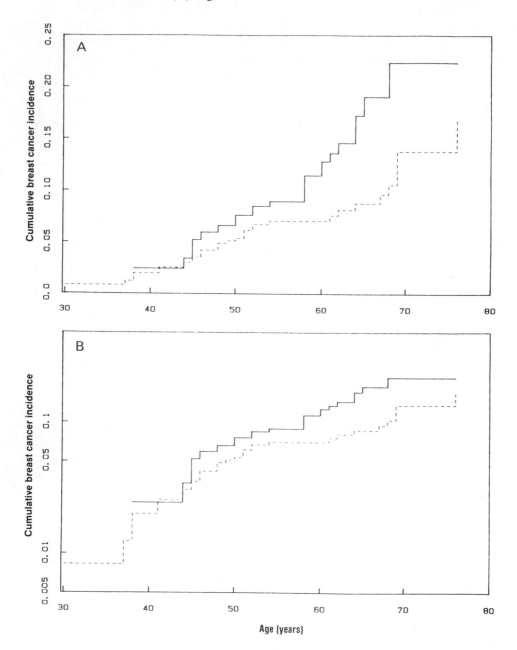

In the examples below we have used the kernel defined by $K(x) = (0.75)(1 - x^2)$ for $-1 \leqslant x \leqslant 1$, and $K(x) = 0$ elsewhere. Bandwidths are varied to achieve a compromise between too much random noise (small b) and too great a loss of structure in the estimated rates (large b). The final choice is based largely on visual appearance, although objective criteria are also available (Titterington, 1985). Note that $\hat{\lambda}(t)$ is defined only over the interval $(t_1 + b, t_I - b)$, where t_1 and t_I are the minimum and maximum times at which cases were observed to occur. In a refinement of this method, Tanner and Wong (1984) select the bandwidths depending on age, so that they are narrow when deaths are frequent and risk-set sizes are large, and wide elsewhere.

Example 5.3

Figure 5.2 graphs smoothed estimates of breast cancer incidence for the data on women with benign breast disease shown in Table 5.2. These were obtained from the cumulative incidence estimates $\hat{\Lambda}$ shown in Figure 5.1 by applying (5.18) with $K(x) = 0.75(1 - x^2)$ for $|x| \leqslant 1$ and two bandwidths $b = 10$ (Fig. 5.2A) and $b = 15$ years (Fig. 5.2B). Relatively large bandwidths were necessary to achieve statistical stability because of the small number of cases in this study, namely 23 among women with prior exposure to oestrogens and 34 among those not so exposed. Consequently, they may obscure somewhat the true variation in incidence with age. Note the greater degree of smoothing achieved with the larger bandwidth. Although the rate ratio for exposed *versus* unexposed seems to increase slightly over the 40–65-year age range, we already know from the partial likelihood analysis in Example 5.1 that this trend is not statistically significant.

The observation that the age-specific rates are nearly constant over the age range shown, especially for women with no prior exposure to oestrogen, is not surprising. As mentioned in the previous example, there was a strong birth cohort effect on the age-specific breast cancer rates in this particular population. Since the data are analysed here on a cross-sectional basis, ignoring birth cohort, the observed age-incidence curve is distorted (flattened) in comparison with the more typical pattern of rising incidence until the age of menopause with a change in slope thereafter. A similar phenomenon was observed in Volume 1 for breast cancer rates in Iceland that were analysed according to both calendar year and birth cohort. Compare Figures 2.3 and 2.4 in Volume 1, and also Figure 4.2.

(b) *Estimating baseline rates under the multiplicative model*

These techniques are easily extended to provide estimates of the cumulative baseline rate function

$$\Lambda_0(t) = \int_0^t \lambda_0(u) \, du$$

under the various multiplicative models proposed for heterogeneous samples. Using a heuristic argument to achieve joint maximum likelihood estimation of Λ_0 and β in Cox's (1972) model (5.3), Breslow (1974) derived the estimate

$$\hat{\Lambda}_0(t) = \sum_{t_i \leqslant t} \frac{d_i}{\sum_{j \in R_i} \exp\{\mathbf{x}_j(t_i)\hat{\boldsymbol{\beta}}\}}, \tag{5.20}$$

where $\hat{\boldsymbol{\beta}}$ is the maximum partial likelihood estimate from (5.13) or (5.14). The obvious

Fig. 5.2   Smoothed estimates of breast cancer incidence for women with benign breast disease with (solid line) and without (dotted line) prior exposure to oestrogen. (A) Ten-year bandwidth; (B) 15-year bandwidth

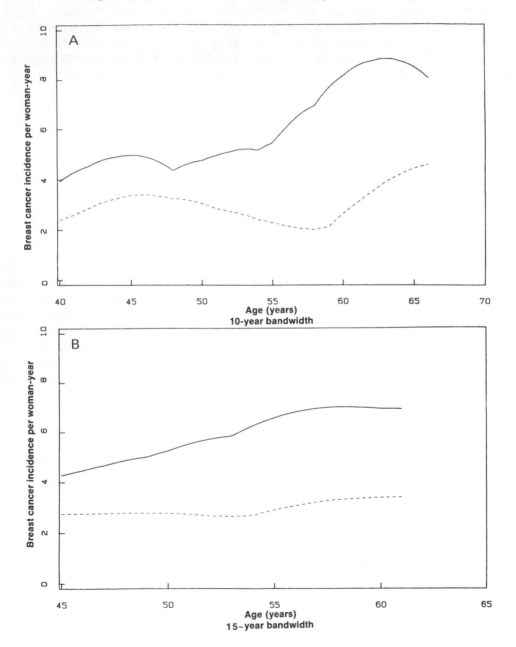

extension for the general multiplicative model is to

$$\hat{\Lambda}_0(t) = \sum_{t_i \leq t} \frac{d_i}{\sum_{j \in R_i} r\{\mathbf{x}_j(t_i); \hat{\boldsymbol{\beta}}\}}. \tag{5.21}$$

The main difference between (5.20) or (5.21) and the equation applicable to homogeneous samples is that the size of the risk set at t_i, which appears in the denominator of (5.16), is replaced by the total estimated relative risk for the risk set at that time. Tsiatis (1981) has shown that $\hat{\Lambda}_0(t)$ defined by (5.20) also has an asymptotic Gaussian distribution.

If the data are stratified, separate estimates of the background rates

$$\Lambda_s(t) = \int_0^t \lambda_s(u)\, du$$

are obtained for each stratum simply by restricting the deaths and risk sets in (5.20) or (5.21) to that stratum. Smoothed estimates of the age-specific baseline rates $\lambda_s(t)$ are available *via* (5.18). However, their standard errors are more complicated than that shown in (5.19) because of the need to account for the error in estimation of $\boldsymbol{\beta}$ (Andersen & Rasmussen, 1982). We present some illustrative examples in §§5.5 and 5.6 below.

(c) Nonparametric estimation of relative mortality functions

An extension of the multiplicative models, incorporating external standard rates, allows the equations and computer programs already developed for nonparametric estimation of cumulative baseline rates to be used also for nonparametric estimation of cumulative *relative* mortality functions (Andersen *et al.*, 1985). Consider first the simple model $\lambda(t) = \theta\lambda^*(t)$, whereby each subject's disease rate is assumed to be equal to a constant multiple of the standard rate for a person of the same age and sex. Maximization of the parametric likelihood (5.12) in this situation yields the usual ratio of observed to expected deaths, i.e., the SMR

$$\hat{\theta} = \frac{\sum_{i=1}^I d_i}{\sum_{i=1}^I \int Y_i(u)\lambda_i^*(u)\, du}, \tag{5.22}$$

as the 'optimal' estimate (Breslow, 1975). Here, Y_i is as defined in §5.2.

One way of looking for changes in the SMR that would invalidate its use as a single summary measure is to divide the age or time axis into a number of discrete intervals and to cumulate the deaths and integrated standard rates within each one. The methods developed for testing the homogeneity of such SMRs with grouped data (§3.4) continue to apply and indeed are strongly recommended. Formal justification is provided in terms of a generalization of the basic model to $\lambda(t) = \theta_k\lambda^*(t)$ for $t_{k-1} < t \leq t_k$.

A further generalization of this approach allows the SMR to be modelled as a continuous function of time, i.e., $\theta(t) = \lambda(t)/\lambda^*(t)$ or $\lambda(t) = \theta(t)\lambda^*(t)$. Comparing this formula with (5.3), we note that the two models are formally identical: $\theta(t)$ plays the role of the unknown baseline rate $\lambda_0(t)$, and $\log \lambda^*(t)$ is a time-dependent covariate with known regression coefficient $\beta = 1$. Just as we were earlier able to estimate the cumulative baseline rate

$$\Lambda_0(t) = \int_0^t \lambda_0(u)\, du$$

nonparametrically in terms of a step-function (equations 5.16, 5.20 and 5.21), here we are able to estimate the cumulative or integrated SMR

$$\Theta(t) = \int_0^t \theta(u)\, du.$$

Note that the cumulative SMR equals the average SMR over the time interval $(0, t)$ multiplied by the length of the interval. It is measured in units of time. $\Lambda(t)$, however, is the product of a rate with time and is thus dimensionless. These differences notwithstanding, an estimate of the integrated SMR is obtained from (5.20) as

$$\hat{\Theta}(t) = \sum_{t_i \leq t} \frac{d_i}{\sum_{j \in R_i} \lambda_j^*(t_i)}. \tag{5.23}$$

The estimate of the average SMR over the time interval (t_{i-1}, t_i) is thus given by the number of deaths or cases observed at time t_i divided by the total expected number among the risk-set members.

Introduction of explanatory variables $\mathbf{x}(t)$ into the model allows covariance adjustment of the nonparametric SMR estimates. In its most general form, the underlying model for the unknown disease rate is written

$$\lambda(t) = \theta(t)\lambda^*(t)r\{\mathbf{x}(t); \boldsymbol{\beta}\}.$$

The β parameters in the relative risk function are estimated by a generalization of the partial likelihood (5.14), namely

$$\prod_{i=1}^{I} \frac{\prod_{j=1}^{d_i} \lambda_j^*(t_i)r\{\mathbf{x}_{ij}(t_i); \boldsymbol{\beta}\}}{\sum_l \prod_{j=1}^{d_i} \lambda_{l_j}^*(t_i)r\{x_{il_j}(t_i); \boldsymbol{\beta}\}}. \tag{5.24}$$

In practice, $\lambda_j^*(t_i)$ or its logarithm is incorporated into the model as an 'offset' or covariable with known regression coefficient. Once $\boldsymbol{\beta}$ is obtained *via* maximization of (5.24), the integrated SMR is estimated as

$$\hat{\Theta}(t) = \sum_{t_i \leq t} \frac{d_i}{\sum_{j \in R_i} \lambda_j^*(t_i)r\{\mathbf{x}_{ij}(t_i); \hat{\boldsymbol{\beta}}\}}, \tag{5.25}$$

generalizing (5.21). Adjusted or unadjusted estimates $\hat{\Theta}(t)$ based on (5.25) and (5.23), respectively, are smoothed *via* the kernel method to yield nonparametric estimates of the SMR:

$$\hat{\theta}(t) = \frac{1}{b} \int_0^\infty K\left(\frac{t-s}{b}\right) d\hat{\Theta}(s) = \frac{1}{b} \sum_{i=1}^{I} K\left(\frac{t-t_i}{b}\right) \frac{d_i}{R_i^+}, \tag{5.26}$$

where R_i^+ is the total standard risk at t_i, either

$$R_i^+ = \sum_{j \in R_i} \lambda_j^*(t_i)$$

for the unadjusted estimate or

$$R_i^+ = \sum_{j \in R_i} \lambda_j^*(t_i) r\{\mathbf{x}_{ij}(t_i); \hat{\boldsymbol{\beta}}\}$$

for the adjusted one. The standard error of the unadjusted estimate is

$$\text{SE } \hat{\theta}(t) = \frac{1}{b} \left[\sum_{i=1}^{I} K^2\left(\frac{t-t_i}{b}\right) \frac{d_i}{(R_i^+)^2} \right]^{1/2}, \tag{5.27}$$

analogous to (5.19).

Sections 5.5 and 5.6 contain several illustrations of nonparametric estimation of baseline and relative disease mortality functions and the fitting of multiplicative models to continuous cohort data by partial likelihood. Flexible model structures are available even within the multiplicative environment by varying the fundamental time variable t, the definitions of the covariables $\mathbf{x}(t)$ and the relative risk function r. The choice should be made separately for each study, taking into account the goals of the investigation and the nature of the available data. If good a-priori information suggests that the background rates are of a simple parametric form, it may be preferable to model them by time-dependent covariables, rather than nonparametrically in the function $\lambda_0(t)$. For example, population data and multistage theory both suggest that cancer incidence rates are proportional to a power of age. Defining one of the covariables $x(t)$ to be the logarithm of age at 'time' t, this sort of age dependence is easily accommodated in relative risk functions of the form $r\{\mathbf{x}(t); \boldsymbol{\beta}\} = \exp\{\mathbf{x}(t)\boldsymbol{\beta}\}$. In this case, and also when the background rates are assumed to be proportional to standard rates $\lambda^*(t)$, one may want to set $t = $ 'time since onset of exposure' in order to have a nonparametric evaluation of the evolution of relative risk with continuing exposure. Alternatively, if we set $t = $ age and incorporate $x(t) = \log(t)$ into the exponential relative risk function, our nonparametric estimate of $\theta(t)$ *via* (5.26) provides a graphical evaluation of the goodness-of-fit of the assumed parametric model.[1]

5.4 Sampling from the risk sets

Implementation of the methods of analysis of continuous data outlined in the preceding sections is expensive and time-consuming in the case of data from large cohort studies. This is true whether one uses external standard rates and the log-likelihood (5.12) or adopts the partial likelihood approach based on (5.13) or (5.14). In the former instance, the basic data for each subject are needed to re-evaluate integrals of the form $\int Y_i(u)\lambda_i(u; \alpha, \boldsymbol{\beta}) \, du$ at each cycle of iteration. In the latter case, one must re-evaluate the relative risks $r\{\mathbf{x}_j(t_i); \boldsymbol{\beta}\}$ for each subject in every risk set in

---

[1] Recent work by F. O'Sullivan at the University of California, Berkeley, on spline-smoothed hazard estimates with cross-validation may offer some advantages over the kernel methods suggested here.

which he appears (except, as noted earlier, for the additive relative risk model). It is often possible to store some intermediate quantities, such as the covariable values $x_j(t_i)$ for each subject at each time of death, for use in subsequent iterations. However, this may not be advisable if it greatly increases the amount of reading the computer does from disk files.

(a) Complexity of partial likelihood analyses

Suppose that the basic time variable is in fact age and that birth cohort or calendar year is accounted for by stratification. Let R denote the risk set consisting of all persons being followed in the study at a given age t at some time during a specified calendar period s. In practice, we have found that integral ages and five- or ten-year calendar periods generally provide sufficient accuracy for construction of the risk sets. Because of ties in the recorded data, several deaths may occur in some of the risk sets. This would not happen if they were defined in terms of exact (continuous) ages at death. However, since the number of deaths or cases is generally much smaller than the total size of the risk set, which may well be of the order of hundreds or even thousands depending on the size of the original cohort, the approximation inherent in the use of (5.13) with such tied data is excellent.

Example 5.4

Table 5.3 shows the distribution by age and calendar period of 142 respiratory cancer deaths that occurred among the Montana smelter workers during the years 1938–1963, this being the period of follow-up of the initial study reported by Lee and Fraumeni (1969). When classified by integral age at death and by calendar year in six intervals of five years or less, they define 91 separate risk sets. Most risk sets contain a single respiratory cancer death, but the multiplicities range as high as $d_i = 4$, for example, among workers aged 51 or 67 during the period 1955–1959. Also shown for each risk set are the numbers of deaths from other causes, these being the matched 'controls' one would use in a proportional mortality analysis.

Table 5.4 presents the numbers of noncases (g_i) for each of the risk sets defined in Table 5.3. These range from 17 workers (in addition to the one case) under observation at age 84 during 1950–1954, to 880 workers on study at age 40 during 1955–1959. The mean risk-set size was 322, with a standard deviation of 215. Thus, each of the 8014 subjects appeared on average in 3.6 risk sets. Since the calculations needed for a partial likelihood analysis treat each such risk-set appearance as a separate observation, the effective 'sample size' is of the order of 30 000 observations, of which 142 are cases. This gives some feeling for the magnitude of the computing problem.

(b) Risk-set sampling

It is evident from equations (5.13) and (5.14) that the information about relative risks associated with the exposure variables is provided by a comparison of the exposures of the case(s) with the exposures of the remainder of the cohort members in each risk set. Since most risk sets are very large in comparison with the number of cases, little information would be lost if the comparison were made between the cases and a small sample of 'controls' drawn randomly from among the other cohort members in the risk set. This is the idea of matched 'case-control within a cohort' sampling proposed by Thomas, D.C. (1977) for efficient analyses of continuous cohort data. Mantel (1973) earlier suggested a similar strategy for stratified analyses under the label 'synthetic retrospective study'. As emphasized in Volume 1, the idea of sampling controls from an on-going but unobserved (and possibly only conceptual) cohort

Table 5.3 Respiratory cancer deaths (d) and deaths from other causes (t−d) for the Montana cohort by age and year; construction of the risk sets[a]

Age (years)	1938–1939		1940–1944		1945–1949		1950–1954		1955–1959		1960–1963	
	d	t−d	d	t−d	d	t−d	d	t−d	d	t−d	d	t−d
40									1	4		
45			1	2								
46			3	5							1	6
47							1	5				
48			1	5								
49							1	5	2	3		
50			1	0					1	10	1	4
51									4	10		
52					1	3			1	6		
53			2	3			1	16	1	13	1	10
54							2	6	2	13		
55									3	11	1	6
56											2	9
57			1	5	1	8	1	7	3	15	1	14
58			1	7	3	4			1	13	4	12
59					1	3					1	13
60							2	6	3	5	1	12
61							2	8	2	7	3	11
62			2	5			1	7	2	11	3	11
63			1	6	1	10			1	12	3	11
64			1	6	1	5			1	12		
65					1	4	1	4	2	9	2	9
66	2	1	1	2			1	11			1	10
67			1	3	1	10	1	9	4	7	1	8
68			1	4			3	6	1	9	3	5
69			1	5			1	11	1	9	1	3
70							2	9	1	9	1	8
71	1	1									1	10
72											1	7
73					1	8	1	7	1	13	1	6
74					1	7			3	16		
76					2	8			3	10		
79							1	4				
80											1	6
81											1	4
83							3	4				
84							1	1				

[a] Entries appear for a given age/calendar year only if one or more respiratory cancer deaths occurred.

Table 5.4 Numbers of Montana smelter workers alive and under observation at particular ages and calendar periods; sizes of the risk sets with cases excluded

Age (years)	Calendar year					
	1938–1939	1940–1944	1945–1949	1950–1954	1955–1959	1960–1963
40					880	
45		344				
46			504			762
47				688		
48		309				
49				644	745	
50		279			726	722
51					726	
52			374		722	
53		252		516	707	645
54				484	663	
55					635	587
56						607
57		241	289	374	538	583
58		258	264		484	569
59			270			511
60				290	398	487
61				284	358	441
62		200		266	337	400
63		167	254		312	371
64		151	238		282	
65			209	240	248	299
66	56	143		229		261
67		146	168	208	217	246
68		137		211	195	230
69		125		193	201	195
70				167	192	184
71	37					163
72						144
73			102	102	163	136
74			85		138	
76			61		87	
79				46		
80						53
81						37
83				25		
84				17		

investigation is one of the main justifications for the validity of inferences made in actual case-control investigations.

(c) Likelihood analysis

Under the general multiplicative model, the contribution to the likelihood from a risk set containing d cases with exposure variables $\mathbf{x}_1(t), \ldots, \mathbf{x}_d(t)$, and m randomly sampled 'controls' with exposure variables $\mathbf{x}_{d+1}(t), \ldots, \mathbf{x}_{d+m}$, is proportional to

(Prentice & Breslow, 1978)

$$\frac{\prod_{j=1}^{d} r(\mathbf{x}_j(t); \boldsymbol{\beta})}{\sum_{\mathbf{l}} \prod_{j=1}^{d} r(\mathbf{x}_{l_j}(t); \boldsymbol{\beta})}. \tag{5.28}$$

The numerator of this expression is the product of the relative risks for the actual cases. The denominator summation is over all possible subsets $\ell = (\ell_1, \ldots, \ell_d)$ of size d drawn from the $d + m$ members of the risk set, there being $\binom{d+m}{d}$ such subsets in all. Each may be thought of as representing a possible set of d cases that might have been observed to die from the cause of interest at time t and whose relative risk product is compared to that for the actual cases. Precisely the same likelihood is used for the matched analysis of actual case-control studies. However, in Volume 1 (equation 7.1), we restricted consideration to multiplicative relative risk functions of the form $r(\mathbf{x}; \boldsymbol{\beta}) = \exp(\mathbf{x}\boldsymbol{\beta})$. The same expression is used also for the full partial likelihood analysis (5.14), except that there the denominator sum is taken over the much larger number $\binom{n}{d}$ of subsamples drawn from the full risk set.

An important feature of the case-control within a cohort method of analysis is that the time-dependent covariables for the controls need be evaluated only at the particular age t for which they are sampled. Once calculated, they are easily stored in a rectangular data array in central memory for efficient computer processing. In a partial likelihood analysis, the time-dependent covariables for each cohort member must usually be re-evaluated for each risk set in which he appears.

(d) Model selection and regression diagnostics

The primary advantage of the risk-set sampling methodology is that it reduces the effective number of observations to a reasonable size for efficient computer processing. This encourages the investigator sitting at a computer terminal to fit a variety of models involving different exposure variables to the sampled data and select those that fit well for further examination. Such interactive data analysis is often not possible with a full partial likelihood approach. Depending on the size of the data set and the available computer, one may have to wait several hours or even overnight before seeing the results of a particular fit.

Regression diagnostics for matched case-control and partial likelihood analyses, analogous to those considered in §4.3 for grouped data, have recently become available as a result of work by Pregibon (1984), Moolgavkar et al. (1984) and Storer and Crowley (1985). For the most part, these are developed in terms of approximate changes in estimated regression coefficients or test statistics that would accompany deletion of individual observations (cases or controls), or deletion of entire risk sets. As shown earlier, such diagnostics are helpful in evaluating the stability of the fitted model and the extent to which the results depend on data for only one or a few individuals. An illustration of their use in case-control within a cohort analyses appears in §5.6. One may also use the predicted within-risk set 'probability of being a case' as a guide to goodness-of-fit. This is defined for each subject as his estimated relative risk divided by the sum of relative risks for the entire risk set (assuming one case per set). Such predicted probabilities are usefully summed across individuals when there are particular covariate values for comparison with the corresponding observed numbers. They may also be used to define 'residuals' for case-control studies.

(e) Estimating background and relative rates from the case-control samples

An examination of equations (5.20), (5.21), (5.23) and (5.25), used to estimate the cumulative background rates $\Lambda(t)$ or the cumulative relative rates $\Theta(t)$, suggests how they may be adapted to serve also for case-control samples. The essential requirement is that one know the sampling fractions used to select controls within each risk set, i.e., the total size of the risk set from which the controls are sampled. This requirement is met for the 'synthetic' case-control technique suggested here, where one explicitly constructs the risk sets using the cohort data base and then carries out the control sampling by computer. It usually will not be met for case-control studies conducted outside the context of a cohort study. One then needs supplementary data in order to estimate absolute risks.

Denote by $\mu_i = \mu_i(\hat{\boldsymbol{\beta}})$ the average of the estimated relative risk factors associated with the $n_i = d_i + g_i$ subjects in the ith risk set. Thus,

$$\mu_i = \frac{1}{n_i} \sum_{j \in R_i} r_{ij},$$

where r_{ij} is the estimated relative risk $r\{\mathbf{x}_j(t_i); \hat{\boldsymbol{\beta}}\}$, or estimated absolute risk $\lambda_j^*(t_i) r\{\mathbf{x}_j(t_i); \hat{\boldsymbol{\beta}}\}$, depending upon whether Λ or Θ is under consideration. The estimates $\hat{\Lambda}$ and $\hat{\Theta}$ may both be expressed in the general form

$$\sum_{t_i \leq t} (d_i / n_i \mu_i).$$

If we lack data for the entire risk set but do have available a sample of m_i controls drawn without replacement from the g_i noncases in R_i, we could estimate μ_i by the sample mean

$$\bar{r}_i = \frac{1}{m_i} \sum_{j=1}^{m_i} r_{ij}.$$

A refinement would be to substitute $n_i^{-1}\{d_i \bar{s}_i + g_i \bar{r}_i\}$ for $\bar{r}_i$, where $\bar{s}_i$ denotes the average (relative) risk for the d_i cases. However, this should make little difference unless the cases constitute a large fraction of the risk set. Substituting $\bar{r}_i$ for μ_i in (5.21) thus yields

$$\hat{\Lambda}_0(t) = \sum_{t_i \leq t} \frac{d_i}{n_i \bar{r}_i} \tag{5.29}$$

as our approximation to $\hat{\Lambda}$, and a similar substitution in (5.25) gives an approximation to $\hat{\Theta}$.

The main drawback to this approach is the fact that the reciprocal of a sample mean is a biased estimator of the mean. The problem is acute for the small control sample sizes typically used, with m_i in the range from 1 to 20. Breslow and Langholz (1987) suggest two possible ways of correcting the bias in (5.29) to yield a better estimate. The most promising, based on a Taylor series expansion of $\bar{r}^{-1}$ about μ^{-1}, leads to the equation

$$\hat{\Lambda}_T(t) = \sum_{t_i \leq t} \frac{d_i}{n_i \bar{r}_i} \left\{ 1 - \frac{\hat{\sigma}_i^2}{m_i \bar{r}_i^2} \right\}, \tag{5.30}$$

where $\hat{\sigma}_i^2 = (m_i - 1)^{-1} \sum_j (r_{ij} - \bar{r}_i)^2$ is the within-risk-set variance. The other, derived from the jackknife principle of Quenouille (1949), leads to

$$\hat{\Lambda}_J(t) = \sum_{t_i \leq t} \frac{d_i}{n_i \bar{r}_i} \left\{ m_i - \frac{(m_i - 1)^2}{m_i} \sum_{j=1}^{m_i} \frac{1}{(m_i - r_{ij}/\bar{r}_i)} \right\}. \tag{5.31}$$

Note that (5.30) and (5.31) both reduce to (5.29) if $r_{ij} = \bar{r}_i$ for all of the sampled controls.

Section 5.5 illustrates the application of these equations to data from the Montana cohort (see especially Figure 5.8). Neither applies very well for $m_i = 5$, but both perform satisfactorily for $m_i = 20$. If only five controls or fewer are available from each risk set, it is probably wise to pool the controls sampled from each R_i with those from neighbouring risk sets R_j, i.e., those with $|t_j - t_i| < b$ where b is a designated bandwidth, in order to increase the effective number of controls for each. The rationale for this procedure is that the average (relative) risk μ_i should be reasonably constant over risk sets within a narrow time interval, since their membership will change little.

(f) Selection of controls

The procedure recommended here for construction of the matched sets of cases and controls that will actually be used in the analysis is as follows: First select from the risk set R_i all d_i cases that develop or die from the disease of interest at time t_i. Then select m_i controls, *at random and without replacement*, from among the g_i members of R_i who do *not* develop the disease at that time. The total of d_i cases and m_i sampled controls then constitutes a reduced risk set R_i^*.

Early theoretical arguments given in support of this procedure (Prentice & Breslow, 1978) assumed that the number g_i of potential controls was effectively infinite. This meant that there would be no overlap between the controls sampled from different risk sets, nor would a subject who later developed disease be sampled as a control. In practice, of course, this assumption is not met. Indeed, the risks sets corresponding to advanced ages are often quite small (see Table 5.4), and it may be desirable to sample all available controls from them. It is then quite conceivable that an individual sampled as a control at one age will turn out to be a case later on or be sampled again as a control at that time. With the methodology employed here, therefore, the R_i^* can and do overlap, at least on occasion.

The fact that the reduced risk sets R_i^* may not be disjoint in finite cohorts has caused some concern about the validity of the inference procedure implicit in the use of (5.28), since this approach combines statistical information from each of them as if they were statistically independent. For example, Lubin and Gail (1984) mentioned the possibility of excluding previously chosen controls from consideration as future controls, yet including them as cases if and when they developed the disease. If the original risk sets R_i are small, however, this latter procedure is biased (Robins *et al.*, 1986a). Prentice *et al.* (1986) propose a rather more elaborate sampling procedure in which the controls sampled along with a case from R_i are also considered as controls in *each* of the risk sets in which that case previously appeared. This increases the amount of information available in the case-control sample by increasing the sizes of the sampled risk sets. However, it also introduces correlations between the partial likelihood contributions from different risk sets which then need to be accounted for in the analysis. In order to avoid these complications, and also to keep the effective sample size small enough to permit interactive analyses, we prefer the procedure outlined above in the context of case-control analysis of assembled cohort data. Oakes (1981) and Cox and Oakes (1984, section 8.8) have shown that the product of terms (5.28) is still a partial likelihood (Cox, 1975) and that estimates and standard errors derived from them have the same asymptotic validity as those based on all the data.

The question of the number of controls that should be sampled from each risk set is considered in §7.6.

(g) Computer programs

Appendix IV of Volume 1 contained the source code for a computer program that implemented matched case-control analyses based on the conditional likelihood (5.28) with $r(\mathbf{x}; \boldsymbol{\beta}) = \exp(\mathbf{x}\boldsymbol{\beta})$, $d = 1$ and variable m. Another program, given in Appendix V of Volume 1 (Smith *et al.*, 1981) permitted arbitrary numbers of cases and controls in each stratum or risk set. However, since the relative risk function was restricted to the log-linear form and since the program used an inefficient method of evaluating the denominator of (5.28) and related expressions, it is now outmoded. Gail *et al.* (1981) developed a more efficient algorithm for the log-linear model using a recursive method of calculation. This approach was developed further by Storer *et al.* (1983) so as to permit additive and other more general relative risk functions. The latest version of their program, known as PECAN, mimics the GLIM syntax for specifying terms in the model, allows for variable factoring and offsets to the regression equation, and provides an option for calculation of regression diagnostics in the manner of Storer and Crowley (1985).

5.5   Analyses of continuous data from the Montana smelter workers cohort

From descriptions of the Montana smelter workers study and the grouped data analyses presented earlier, especially in Examples 2.1 and 2.2 and in §§3.2, 4.5 and 4.8, the reader should already have a good understanding of how the occurrence of respiratory cancer in this cohort is related to date of hire, birthplace and duration of work in moderate or high arsenic exposure areas. In this section, we elaborate by reporting the results of fitting of continuous models to the original data set, consisting of 8014 individual data records containing details of exposure history and follow-up. Due to the complexity of the partial likelihood calculations, fitting each model generally required an overnight computer run in batch mode. In spite of this effort, the results serve mostly to confirm what has already been learned from the more economical grouped data analyses. They do not provide any really new insights.

(a) Respiratory cancer SMR and years since first employed

The simple ratios of observed to expected numbers of respiratory cancer deaths shown in Table 4.17 increased markedly about 30 years or so after date of initial employment. Here, we take a more detailed look at this change in relative risk using the nonparametric estimate (5.23) of the cumulative SMR, defining $t =$ 'years since initial employment'. Using all 288 respiratory cancer deaths, including 12 at 80 years of age or older that were excluded from most previous analyses, we obtained the results shown in Figure 5.3. The first case occurred at 4.07 years from date of hire and the last at 62.25 years. The cumulative SMR climbs steeply for the first few years, rises more gradually until about 35 years, and then steepens again. However, just as is true for estimates of the cumulative mortality function, it is hard to get a good visual impression of the SMR itself from this graph alone.

A much better representation of the temporal changes in the SMR is provided in Figure 5.4, where we graph the smoothed SMRs calculated from (5.26) using bandwidths of five and ten years. The ten-year bandwidth results in a substantially smoother curve, but also restricts the range over which the estimate is available. The sharp rise in the SMR appears to begin at about 30 years using the ten-year bandwidth and a little later with the shorter width. Such details may be obscured with a grouped analysis.

Figure 5.5 presents 90% confidence bands for the SMR estimated using a five-year

Fig. 5.3   Cumulative standardized mortality ratio (SMR) for respiratory cancer, by number of years since initial employment for Montana smelter workers

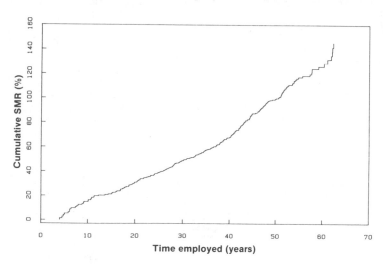

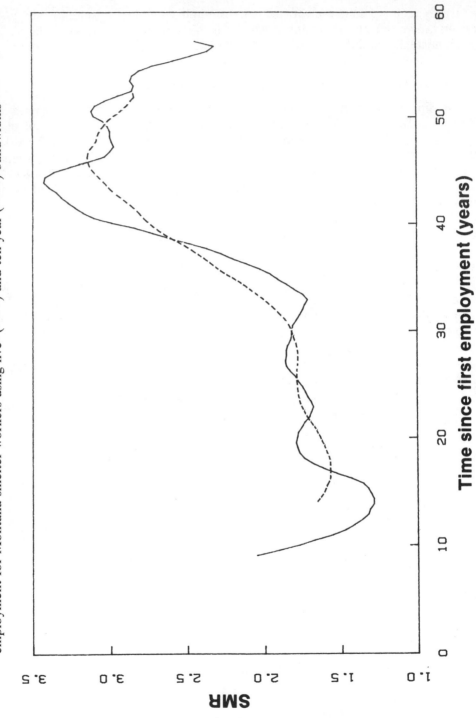

Fig. 5.4   Smoothed estimates of the standardized mortality ratio (SMR) for respiratory cancer, by years since initial employment for Montana smelter workers using five- (———) and ten-year (– – –) bandwidths

Fig. 5.5   Ninety percent confidence bands (–––) for the smoothed standardized mortality ratio (SMR) for respiratory cancer (——), Montana smelter workers

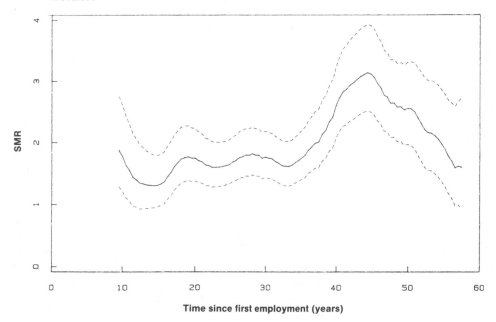

bandwidth. The confidence bands were derived on the log scale in order to approximate more closely a normal error distribution. Specifically, we used the formula

$$\log \hat{\theta}(t) \pm 1.645 \times \{SE(\hat{\theta}(t))\}/\hat{\theta}(t)$$

where $SE(\hat{\theta}(t))$ is given by (5.27).

One possible interpretation of the results depicted in Figure 5.4 would be that the Montana cohort as a whole had somewhat elevated rates of respiratory cancer in comparison with the US population, perhaps because of a higher prevalence of cigarette smokers, but that the specific effects of the arsenic exposure did not become manifest until after a latent period of some 30 years. However, we already know from our analyses in Table 4.18 that this interpretation is probably fallacious. Because of the study design, namely the fact that follow-up began no earlier than 1938 whereas the first employees were hired before the turn of the century, most of the person-years of observation for those hired before 1925 occurred in the interval from 25 to 63 years from date of hire. Since we already know that the SMR for those hired before 1925 is much greater than for those hired later, it seems likely that the apparent rise at 30 years from date of hire is an artefact caused by confounding with period of hire.

In order to confirm this latter interpretation, we conducted a proportional hazards regression analysis based on equation (5.3) with t = 'years since first employment'. In addition to the log standard rates $x_0(t) = \log \{\lambda^*(t)\}$, the covariables were x_1, a binary indicator of date hired coded 1 for 1885–1924; x_2 a binary indicator of birthplace coded 1 for foreigh born; $x_3(t)$ a lagged, continuous, time-dependent covariable giving the number of years worked in moderate arsenic exposure areas at time $t − 2$; and $x_4(t)$, as for x_3 for years worked in a heavy arsenic exposure area. There were 280 distinct times at which cases occurred (for eight pairs of cases, the recorded values of years for employment to death were tied), and thus 280 separate risk sets containing as many as 5000 members each. Even on a large computer system, the partial likelihood fitting of the model with four covariables would have been prohibitively expensive and time-consuming. For this reason, we rounded time since initial employment to the midpoint of the corresponding year, and also excluded the 12 deaths that occurred at age 80 and above, thereby reducing the number of risk sets from 280 to 57 for the adjusted analysis.

The regression coefficients (± standard errors) estimated with this approach for the four covariables were: $\hat{\beta}_1 = 0.70 \pm 0.18$, $\hat{\beta}_2 = 0.47 \pm 0.14$, $\hat{\beta}_3 = 0.017 \pm 0.007$ and $\hat{\beta}_4 = 0.041 \pm 0.010$. Two smoothed estimates of the SMR were constructed using a five-year bandwidth – one with and one without covariable adjustment. The difference is striking (Fig. 5.6). The curve calculated without covariable adjustment closely resembles that in Figure 5.4 but is a bit smoother due to the fact that some averaging took place by consolidating the number of risk sets from 280 to 57. The adjusted curve has a shape that closely resembles the unadjusted one for the first 30 years, but remains roughly constant thereafter and even starts to decline to values below 1.0. The sharp peak noted in the unadjusted SMR is thus entirely explained by the four covariables and mostly, as we have previously noted, by the first one. What appears from Figure 5.4 to be evidence for a 'latent interval' turns out on closer examination to be an artefact caused by the confounding effects of year of first employment.

Fig. 5.6   Smoothed estimates of the standardized mortality ratio (SMR) for respiratory cancer, by years since first employment for Montana smelter workers, with (– – –) and without (——) adjustment for covariable effects

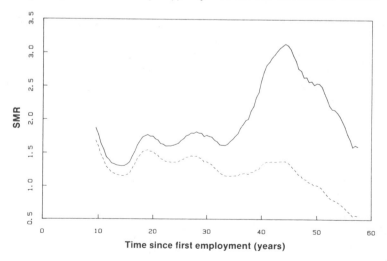

The adjusted curve in Figure 5.6 represents the SMR for a baseline category of US-born smelter workers hired in 1925 or after who spent their entire work history in 'light' arsenic exposure areas. If the model is reasonably correct, such workers had respiratory cancer rates that were only slightly elevated over those of the US population. There is no suggestion that the relative risk increased with time since initial employment once account is taken of the covariables. If anything, it declined!

(b) Comparison of grouped and continuous data analyses

Similar conclusions regarding the cohort to national rate ratio and its evolution in time may be drawn from the grouped data results presented in Table 4.19. See especially the middle column of that table, in which variations in the SMR with calendar year of follow-up (rather than time since initial exposure) are investigated. We estimated a rate ratio for US-born workers hired after 1924 with 'light' arsenic exposure of $\exp(0.581) = 1.79$ for the first calendar period of follow-up (1938–1949), but this declines to $\exp(0.581 - 0.480) = 1.11$ during the last period (1970–1977).

Table 5.5 compares the results of a grouped analysis of the Montana data (Table 4.19, column 3) with the results from a partial likelihood analysis of the full data set.

Table 5.5 Regression coefficients and standard errors from multiplicative models fitted to grouped and continuous data from the Montana smelter workers study: 1938–1977[a]

Regression variables	Method of analysis	
	Grouped	Continuous (partial likelihood)
All covariables binary (0/1)		
Employed before 1925	0.444 ± 0.151	0.405 ± 0.153
Foreign-born	0.445 ± 0.153	0.484 ± 0.154
Moderate arsenic[b]		
1–4 years	0.600 ± 0.166	0.601 ± 0.166
5–14 years	0.259 ± 0.242	0.261 ± 0.243
15+ years	0.684 ± 0.206	0.674 ± 0.207
Heavy arsenic[b]		
1–4 years	0.193 ± 0.305	0.170 ± 0.312
5+ years	1.069 ± 0.230	1.088 ± 0.232
Deviance	282.1	−3167.0[c]
Continuous arsenic variables		
Employed before 1925	0.441 ± 0.151	0.403 ± 0.153
Foreign-born	0.432 ± 0.153	0.473 ± 0.153
Years moderate arsenic[a] (×10)	0.222 ± 0.067	0.218 ± 0.068
Years heavy arsenic[a] (×10)	0.662 ± 0.138	0.664 ± 0.139
Deviance	292.1	−3177.0[c]

[a] From Breslow (1985a)
[b] Lagged two years
[c] Twice log-likelihood

Exposure variables for the partial likelihood analysis first were defined with discrete values that indexed the same categories of exposure that were used earlier to group the data. The results in the first part of the table indicate an excellent agreement between the two methods. This is not surprising in view of the fact that precisely the same model structures were used for relative risk. The grouped data analysis accounted for age and year effects by stratification into 16 age × year cells (four ten-year intervals for each) and explicit estimation of the corresponding parameters. The partial likelihood analysis accounted for age and year by stratification of the 276 respiratory cancer deaths into 167 risk sets on the basis of integral age at death and five-year calendar period. Evidently the age and year effects have been dealt with adequately by the broad categories used for grouping the data. There is little point in carrying out the costly and time-consuming partial likelihood analysis in this case.

The second part of Table 5.5 presents results for a partial likelihood analysis that incorporates the continuously changing arsenic variables defined by numbers of years of work in moderate or heavy exposure areas. A rather crude approximation to this continuous analysis can be obtained with the grouped data by assigning quantitative exposure values to each level of the two factors for arsenic exposure duration. From a sample consisting of 20 controls drawn from each risk set, we estimated that the average number of years of moderate arsenic exposure in the <1-year category was 0.05775 years, in the 1–4 category 2.272 years, in the 5–14 category 8.746 years and for the 15+ category 29.74 years. The corresponding averages for the three categories of heavy arsenic exposure were 0.0205, 2.219 and 16.69 years, respectively. These values were used to define the two quantitative variables for the grouped analysis. In spite of the rather approximate nature of their definition, the agreement between the grouped and continuous data analyses is still remarkably good.

Some information regarding the adequacy of the relative risk function $\exp(x\beta)$ proposed for the continuous exposure variable analyses is available by comparing the goodness-of-fit measures in the two parts of Table 5.5. Whether obtained from grouped or continuous analyses, there is a difference of 10.0 between the two measures of fit. Although the justification is approximate for the continuous analysis (due to the fact that the continuous exposure variables cannot be exactly represented as linear combinations of the corresponding discrete exposure variables), we referred this value to tables of chi-square on three degrees of freedom to gauge the relative merits of each fit and found $p = 0.02$. Thus, the assumption of a linear increase in log relative risk with increasing duration of exposure does *not* appear to be a tenable one. The separate coefficients for moderate arsenic exposure suggest that a plateau is reached after one year of exposure, whereas with heavy arsenic exposure the main effect is not seen until five or more years following exposure. See also Example 3.6.

(c) External standard rates versus partial likelihood

Breslow et al. (1983) conducted a partial likelihood analysis of continuous data from the Montana cohort and a parallel analysis based on the parametric likelihood (5.12) using US death rates for white males in five-year intervals of age and calendar year as a standard. These analyses, which were based on follow-up through 1963 only and ignored date of hire, are not comparable with those presented elsewhere in this monograph. The results are reproduced here because we did not wish to undertake the cumbersome job of reanalysing the 1938–1977 data using the fully parametric model. The sizes of the risk sets used in this analysis are those shown in Tables 5.3 and 5.4.

There were three exposure variables: x_1, a binary indicator of birthplace, coded 1 for foreign born; $x_2(t)$, a continuous, age-dependent variable specifying the number of years employed in one or more of the areas said to have moderate levels of arsenic exposure; and $x_3(t)$, defined analogously to x_2 for heavy arsenic exposure. The latter two variables were constructed from personnel records that allowed determination of the number of years a worker spent at moderate or high arsenic exposure levels for each of the seven calendar periods pre-1938, 1938–1939, 1940–1944, . . . , 1960–1963. The relative risk function that related these variables to the age- and year-specific background rates was $RR = \exp\{\beta_1 x_1 + \beta_2 x_2(t) + \beta_3 x_3(t)\}$ for the partial likelihood and $RR = \exp\{\alpha + \beta_1 x_1 + \beta_2 x_2(t) + \beta_3 x_3(t)\}$ for the parametric analysis.

The parametric analysis entailed approximation of the integral expression (5.12) and its first and second partial derivatives by a summation over years of calendar time. Functions of the covariable values evaluated at annual intervals were multiplied by each subject's contribution to the expected number of deaths (i.e., standard death rate × time on study during the year), and these products were summed over all calendar years that the subject was in the study.

The first two columns of Table 5.6 contrast the parameter estimates and standard errors obtained using these two very different approaches. There is again substantial agreement between the estimated regression coefficients. The parametric model, incorporating the external standard rates, also allows estimation of the constant term $\hat{\theta} = \exp(\hat{\alpha})$, which represents the SMR for cohort members with zero covariable values, relative to the national population. Since $\hat{\theta} = \exp(0.61) = 1.84$, one would interpret the results as saying that US-born workers who remained in light exposure

Table 5.6 Parameter estimates (± standard errors) obtained by fitting a variety of multiplicative models to continuous data from the Montana study: 1938–1963[a]

Regression variable		Method of analysis					Proportionate mortality (other deaths as controls)
		Parametric based on standard rates	Partial likelihood	Case and m controls			
				$m = 20$	$m = 10$	$m = 5$	
Constant	α	0.61 ± 0.12	—	—	—	—	—
Foreign-born	β_1	0.76 ± 0.18	0.72 ± 0.20	0.70 ± 0.21	0.66 ± 0.23	0.75 ± 0.25	0.72 ± 0.23
Moderate arsenic (×10)	β_2	0.22 ± 0.07	0.22 ± 0.07	0.21 ± 0.08	0.29 ± 0.10	0.35 ± 0.11	0.22 ± 0.10
Heavy arsenic (×10)	β_3	0.58 ± 0.13	0.60 ± 0.13	0.69 ± 0.16	0.74 ± 0.18	0.85 ± 0.23	0.53 ± 0.18

[a] From Breslow et al. (1983)

areas had respiratory cancer rates approximately 84% in excess of those of US white males of the same age. Foreign-born workers experienced mortality rates approximately $\exp(0.76) = 2.1$ times higher than this. For each year spent in a moderate or heavy arsenic exposure area, these rates were increased roughly by another 2% (moderate exposure) or 6% (heavy exposure). Of course, from our earlier analyses of grouped data for 1938–1977 (see especially Table 4.19), we know that these results are confounded to some extent with the effect of period of hire and that the change in relative risk with additional arsenic exposure, especially at moderate levels, does not increase smoothly as assumed by the model.

The excellent agreement between the results of the two analyses indicates that variations in the SMR by age and calendar year do not seriously confound the comparisons of SMRs for foreign- *versus* US-born or those with different degrees of arsenic exposure. Furthermore, when interaction terms were added to the partial likelihood model, there was no indication that the effects of the exposure variables changed systematically with age or year. This provides some mild evidence in support of the multiplicative model. However, with the grouped analysis of the data for 1938–1977 (Table 4.19), we noticed some confounding between calendar year of follow-up and period of hire, a variable that had been ignored in the analysis of the data for 1938–1963.

(d) Efficiency gains from use of an external standard

Perhaps just as striking as the agreement between the regression coefficients is the agreement in their standard errors as estimated by parametric and semiparametric (partial likelihood) analyses (Table 5.6, columns 1 and 2). According to the results of Oakes (1977, 1981), one would expect a substantial gain in efficiency from the use of external standard rates only if exposures varied between risk sets, that is to say with age and year. Consider a single exposure X considered as a random variable sampled from the risk sets. The relative efficiency of β estimation for the partial likelihood analysis, under the null hypothesis $\beta = 0$, is given by $E\{\text{Var}(X \mid R)\}/\text{Var}(X)$ where $\text{Var}(X)$ denotes the total and $\text{Var}(X \mid R)$ the conditional (within risk set) variance. A similar result holds for the alternative hypothesis $\beta \neq 0$, provided that the sampling probabilities for drawing subjects from risk sets are made proportional to their relative risks of death under the model.

In order to evaluate this result empirically, we estimated the within (σ_W^2) and between (σ_B^2) risk-set components of variance for each of the three exposure variables used in the analysis. We found ratios $\sigma_B^2/(\sigma_B^2 + \sigma_W^2)$ of 15.9% for birthplace, 4.5% for moderate arsenic exposure and 1.7% for heavy arsenic exposure. This is consistent with the small increases observed in estimated standard errors between parametric and partial likelihood analyses, these being about 10% for birthplace and smaller for the coefficients of the arsenic exposure duration variables.

(e) Results of sampling from the risk sets

Table 5.6 also shows the regression coefficients estimated by applying the conditional likelihood analysis, based on equation (5.28) with $r(\mathbf{x}; \boldsymbol{\beta}) = \exp(\mathbf{x}\boldsymbol{\beta})$, to case-control samples drawn from the 91 risk sets depicted in Tables 5.3 and 5.4. Twenty controls were sampled from each risk set, except that at age 84 (period 1955–1959) all 17 available controls were used. Subsamples of ten and five were then drawn from the 20. Thus, the errors in the estimated coefficients resulting from the post-hoc sampling are not statistically independent. Comparison of the case-control results with those of the full partial likelihood or parametric analyses shows that the standard errors of the estimated coefficients, especially for heavy arsenic exposure, increase sharply as m (the number of controls) decreases. This reflects the loss in information as fewer members of each risk set are utilized in the analysis. Twenty controls per case seems none too large a number if one wants estimates that are reasonably close to those obtained from the full partial likelihood analysis.

Table 5.7 presents the results of a similar set of case-control analyses, including data for the additional follow-up through 1977, for comparison with the partial likelihood results in Table 5.5. Sets of five, ten and 20 controls were drawn from each of 167 risk sets. The number of data records that were analysed thus approached 3600 when using the maximum number (20) of controls. This limited somewhat the number of exposure variables that could be accommodated, interfered with the interactive nature of the analysis, and thus reduced the advantages of the methodology. The increase in the estimated standard errors as one goes from the full partial likelihood analysis (Table 5.5) to $m = 5$ controls is in the range of 23% to 32% for the regression variables in the

Table 5.7   Regression coefficients and standard errors from case-control analyses of the Montana cohort: 1938–1977

Regression variable	Number of controls (m)			Proportionate mortality (other deaths as controls)
	m = 20	m = 10	m = 5	
All covariables binary (0/1)				
Employed before 1925	0.410 ± 0.163	0.527 ± 0.172	0.349 ± 0.189	0.368 ± 0.169
Foreign-born	0.539 ± 0.168	0.590 ± 0.183	0.452 ± 0.205	0.564 ± 0.181
Moderate arsenic				
1–4 years	0.639 ± 0.181	0.585 ± 0.193	0.594 ± 0.216	0.762 ± 0.198
5–14 years	0.211 ± 0.258	0.192 ± 0.271	0.187 ± 0.292	0.525 ± 0.275
15+ years	0.611 ± 0.227	0.495 ± 0.243	0.585 ± 0.269	0.583 ± 0.249
Heavy arsenic				
1–4 years	0.411 ± 0.337	0.552 ± 0.370	0.482 ± 0.405	0.065 ± 0.353
5+ years	1.228 ± 0.262	1.193 ± 0.288	1.303 ± 0.346	0.867 ± 0.280
−2 × log-likelihood	1432.82	1092.61	794.79	1076.37
Continuous arsenic exposure variables				
Employed before 1925	0.378 ± 0.164	0.502 ± 0.172	0.379 ± 0.188	0.359 ± 0.168
Foreign-born	0.554 ± 0.167	0.589 ± 0.182	0.430 ± 0.202	0.588 ± 0.180
Years moderate arsenic (×10)	0.159 ± 0.075	0.131 ± 0.081	0.140 ± 0.089	0.169 ± 0.082
Years heavy arsenic (×10)	0.538 ± 0.189	0.599 ± 0.256	0.489 ± 0.275	0.417 ± 0.138
−2 × log-likelihood	1448.78	1104.40	809.43	1090.97

second part of the table. The percentage increases in Table 5.6 were larger (25–77%). Theoretical calculations (see §7.6) suggest that the largest increases in standard error should occur with exposures that are relatively infrequent and that have large relative risks. This effect is seen in Table 5.6 but is not so obvious with the updated analysis in Table 5.7.

There is reasonably good agreement between the coefficients of the continuous arsenic exposure variables shown in Table 5.6 and those shown in the second part of Table 5.5, in spite of the fact that the number of respiratory cancer deaths used in the latter analysis was nearly twice that used in the former. However, the relative risk estimated for foreign birth has declined considerably from the earlier analysis. This is due to confounding with date of hire, which is not considered in Table 5.6.

(f) Proportional mortality analyses

The final columns of Tables 5.6 and 5.7 present results of parallel case-control analyses for the 1938–1963 and 1938–1977 data, respectively, in which the controls consist of all deaths from causes other than respiratory cancer in the 91 or 167 risk sets. These are reasonably comparable with the results of the other case-control analyses. However, the coefficients associated with heavy arsenic exposure generally appear to be smaller, which suggests that heavy arsenic exposure may have adverse effects on mortality from causes other than lung cancer.

(g) Estimating the 'latent interval'

One of the ways of constructing cumulative exposure functions from a time record of exposure levels is as a time-weighted average (see §5.1). This means selecting the weight function $w(u)$ in equation (5.1) to be a probability density. Several authors have proposed that the log-normal distribution has an intuitively reasonable shape in this context. They assume that there is a random interval of time T between each exposure increment and its effect on the probability of cancer development, and that log T has a normal distribution with mean μ and σ^2. The corresponding distribution of T has a mode at $\exp(\mu - \sigma)^2$, and its coefficient of variation is $\{\exp(\sigma^2) - 1\}^{1/2}$. Figure 5.7 graphs log-normal density functions with modes at 20 years and various coefficients of variation.

While this manner of constructing exposure functions has a strong intuitive rationale, it is not suggested by any particular biological theory of carcinogenesis, and its use in cancer epidemiology could well be questioned. Nevertheless, largely out of curiosity, we fit a number of models analogous to those shown in the second part of Table 5.7 but in which the cumulative exposure variables were calculated as time-weighted average exposures with log-normal densities. Table 5.8 presents the results. Comparing the goodness-of-fit measures and considering the curves in Figure 5.7, it is clear that strikingly different densities give very similar fits and that precise estimation of the 'latent interval' is simply not possible with this model and these data. The best fit is obtained with a rather peaked distribution (coefficient of variation = 0.1) and a mode at 20 years, but the interpretation of this result is unclear for the reasons already mentioned.

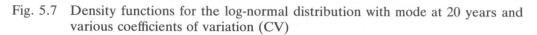

Fig. 5.7   Density functions for the log-normal distribution with mode at 20 years and various coefficients of variation (CV)

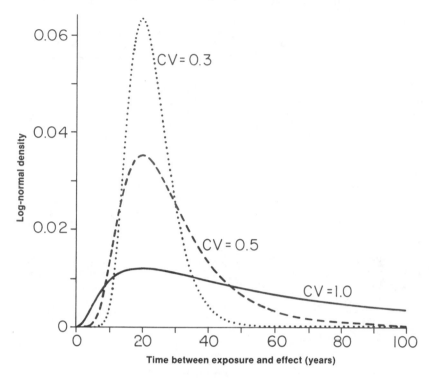

This approach is not, of course, limited to the log-normal distribution. Parameters in the other weight functions considered following equation (5.1) could also be varied, to see which gave the best fit.

(h) SMR by years since first employed: case-control approach

We now return to the analyses depicted in Figures 5.3–5.6, in which we studied the evolution in the respiratory cancer SMR as a function of years since initial employment. The object is to determine empirically how well we can reproduce these results, which required lengthy calculations involving the entire cohort data set, from the samples of the cases in each of the 57 risk sets plus five or 20 controls drawn from the noncases. The illustrative analyses are restricted to estimation of the SMR without covariate adjustment, since this curve had a more distinctive shape than the adjusted curve, even if it was misleading. The results shown are averages of those obtained with 25 separate samplings of five controls per risk set and 15 separate samplings of 20 controls. Elsewhere in this section we have considered results obtained from only a single sampling (as would be done in practice).

Table 5.8 Regression coefficients and standard errors for a series of log-normally time-weighted average exposure models fitted to the Montana cohort data; case-control (m = 20) analysis

Regression variable	Coefficient of variation			
	0.5	0.1	0.05	0.0[a]
A. Mode = 15 years				
Foreign-born	0.53 ± 0.16	0.54 ± 0.16	0.54 ± 0.16	0.53 ± 0.16
Moderate arsenic[b]	0.72 ± 0.28	0.52 ± 0.22	0.52 ± 0.22	0.54 ± 0.21
Heavy arsenic[b]	2.12 ± 0.45	1.51 ± 0.35	1.44 ± 0.34	1.42 ± 0.34
−2 × log-likelihood	1519.68	1523.36	1524.04	1523.53
B. Mode = 20 years				
Foreign-born	0.52 ± 0.16	0.53 ± 0.16	0.53 ± 0.16	0.52 ± 0.16
Moderate arsenic	0.88 ± 0.32	0.67 ± 0.24	0.67 ± 0.23	0.70 ± 0.22
Heavy arsenic	2.40 ± 0.53	1.83 ± 0.36	1.75 ± 0.35	1.67 ± 0.35
−2 × log-likelihood	1519.44	1515.44	1515.99	1516.43
C. Mode = 25 years				
Foreign-born	0.52 ± 0.16	0.53 ± 0.16	0.53 ± 0.16	0.52 ± 0.16
Moderate arsenic	1.05 ± 0.37	0.70 ± 0.25	0.68 ± 0.25	0.64 ± 0.23
Heavy arsenic	2.88 ± 0.66	1.86 ± 0.41	1.75 ± 0.38	1.61 ± 0.37
−2 × log-likelihood	1521.32	1519.68	1520.13	1521.26

[a] Exposure effect concentrated on a one-year period 15, 20 or 25 years later
[b] Lagged two years

Figure 5.8A contrasts the curve obtained using all the available data (also shown in Figure 5.6) with the average curves obtained by applying the Taylor series (5.30) and jackknife (5.31) estimates to case-control samples with five controls per risk set. The bias is clearly unacceptable, the Taylor series estimate overestimating the SMR and the jackknife underestimating it for the first 20–30 years. A much more satisfactory result is obtained by using 20 controls per risk set (Fig. 5.8B) or by pooling the five risk sets containing five controls each for which the t_i are within 2.5 years of the target value (Fig. 5.8C). The latter procedures both provide a reasonably faithful reproduction of the original result.

5.6 Continuous variable analysis of nasal sinus cancer deaths among Welsh nickel refiners

We continue our analyses of cohort data from the Welsh nickel refiners study in order to illustrate some further features of continuous variable modelling. These data have already been considered in Example 4.1 and §4.10.

Table 5.9 presents observed and expected numbers of nasal sinus cancer deaths according to the four risk variables of primary interest: age at first employment, year of employment, exposure index and time since first employment. Many of the essential features of the data are already evident from these simple descriptive statistics. The

Fig. 5.8 Smoothed estimates of the standardized mortality ratio (SMR) for respiratory cancer for Montana smelter workers estimated from 15 case-control samples. (A) Five controls per risk set, no pooling; (B) 20 controls per risk set, no pooling; (C) five controls per risk set with pooling of five neighbouring risk sets. ———, all controls; – – –, jackknife; —·—, Taylor series

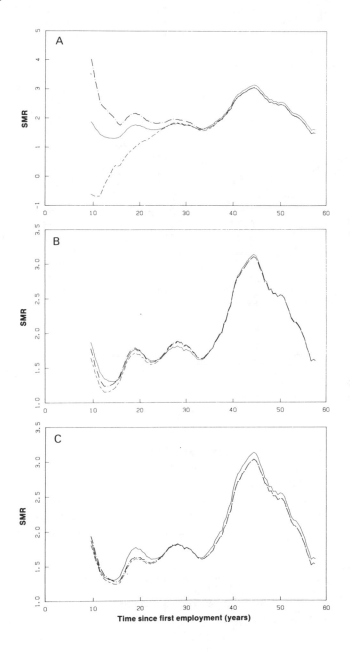

Table 5.9   Summary data on deaths from nasal sinus cancer among Welsh nickel refiners[a]

Variable	Category	Person-years	Nasal sinus cancer		
			Observed	Expected	Rate[b]
Age at first	15–19	3 089.2	2	0.029	0.6
employment	20–24	4 773.9	11	0.057	2.3
(years)	25–29	4 186.5	18	0.065	4.3
	30–34	1 816.3	11	0.031	6.1
	35–39	986.1	12	0.018	12.2
	40–44	233.9	1	0.006	4.3
	45+	144.9	1	0.003	6.9
Year of first	1900–1904	277.4	2	0.007	7.2
employment	1905–1909	1 673.6	9	0.033	5.4
	1910–1914	2 904.5	26	0.045	9.0
	1915–1919	2 294.0	9	0.030	3.9
	1920–1924	8 081.3	10	0.095	1.2
Exposure	0.0	7 738.8	10	0.102	1.3
category (years)	0.5–4.0	4 905.1	17	0.065	3.5
	4.5–8.0	1 716.9	12	0.027	7.0
	8.5–12.0	601.1	10	0.010	16.6
	12.5+	268.9	7	0.004	26.0
Time since first	15–19	2 586.1	1	0.011	0.4
employed (years)	20–24	2 194.3	3	0.016	1.4
	25–29	2 583.2	16	0.028	6.2
	30–34	2 379.3	10	0.033	4.2
	35–39	1 950.0	7	0.032	3.6
	40–44	1 426.2	5	0.028	3.5
	45–49	1 035.2	8	0.027	7.7
	50–54	652.9	5	0.020	7.7
	55+	423.5	1	0.014	2.4
Totals		15 230.8	56	0.210	3.7

[a] Determined from data shown in Appendix VIII. There are slight differences between Tables 4.23 and 5.9 in the totals of expected numbers of deaths due to the use of slightly different data.
[b] Nasal sinus cancer death rate per 1000 person–years of observation

nasal sinus cancer rates increase dramatically with duration of 'exposure': they seem to have one peak about 25–29 years from date of hire and another at about 50 years. However, both exposure and time since employment are correlated with age and year of employment. A major goal of our analysis will be to try to separate the effects of each of the explanatory variables using an appropriate regression model. Results for nasal sinus cancer are analysed without reference to standard rates since the 'background' is so inconsequential.

(a) *Analysis of nasal sinus cancer risk by time since first employment*

Figure 5.9A graphs the cumulative nasal sinus cancer death rate for the entire cohort as a function of time since initial employment (equation 5.16). We estimate the

Fig. 5.9   Death rate from nasal sinus cancer by years since initial employment, Welsh nickel refiners. (A) Cumulative rate; (B) smoothed instantaneous rate

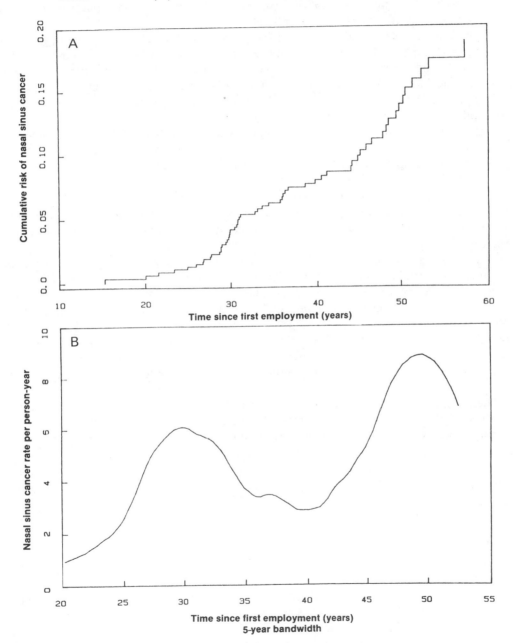

cumulative 'lifetime' risk (to age 85) to be about 15–20%, a striking figure when one considers how rare the disease is in the general population. The smoothed estimate of the annual death rates shown in part B of the figure, obtained from equation (5.18) with a five-year bandwidth, confirms the possibility of a bimodal pattern that was already evident in the grouped data of Table 5.9.

Our initial analysis of these data used the proportional hazards model with log-linear relative risk function (equation 5.3) and considered $t =$ 'time since first employment' (TFE) as the basic time variable. We define a number of indicator variables to identify levels of the factors age at first employment (AFE), year of first employment (YFE) and exposure (EXP). Recall that AFE, YFE and TFE were investigated jointly in the grouped data analysis of Example 4.1.

Since ages were recorded to two-decimal accuracy, and we retained this level of detail in the analysis, each of the 56 cases of nasal sinus cancer occurred at a unique time since first employment and generated a separate risk set. The first case occurred at 15.23 years from initial hire, at which time there were 284 individuals under observation. Risk-set sizes increased gradually to a maximum of 531 men at risk at 28.72 years since date of hire and then declined. The smallest risk set, with 73 subjects, was at 57.48 years since date of hire, the maximum number of years at which a case was observed.

Table 5.10 summarizes the results of fitting the model with categorical regression variables by partial likelihood. Each of the factors AFE, YFE and EXP is seen to have a strong, independent effect on risk. The rise in relative risk with age at first employment is a particularly striking and unusual observation (Peto, J. et al., 1984). While an increase in risk with AFE is evident in the summary data of Table 5.9, its magnitude is obscured by the fact that those hired at later ages generally did not survive to the point 45–50 years from date of employment at which the nasal sinus cancer rates are highest. Once this confounding is accounted for in the regression analyses, the role of AFE appears to be even more dramatic.

The baseline cumulative death rate is shown graphically in Figure 5.10A; a smoothed estimate of the instantaneous death rate, using a five-year bandwidth, appears in part B of the figure, and for a ten-year bandwidth in part C. Because of the coding of the covariables, this baseline risk is estimated for a (fictitious) subject who was under 20 years at hire, first worked before 1910 and was never assigned to high-risk categories. The estimated cumulative lifetime risk for this category does not exceed 1%, whereas for the cohort as a whole it approaches 15–20%. Furthermore, the peak in the nasal sinus cancer death rate at 30 years past employment that was suggested by the crude analysis (Fig. 5.9B) essentially dissappears when adjustment is made for the covariable effects.

The second part of Table 5.10 reports the fit of a model with continuous rather than discrete covariables. The definitions of the covariables used in this fit were determined after considering the results in the first part of the table and after conducting some exploratory analyses using the case-control technique (see below). Comparing the maximized partial likelihoods obtained from the grouped and continuous analyses, we conclude that the fit with four continuous covariables is almost as good as that with the larger number of binary variables that identified categories of risk.

Table 5.10 Results of fitting the multiplicative model by maximum likelihood to data on nasal sinus cancer deaths; 'time' = years since first employed

Variable[a]	Level	Parameter estimate ± standard error	p value	Relative risk
All covariables discrete				
AFE (years)	15–19			1.0
	20–27.5	1.48 ± 0.75	0.05	4.4
	27.5–35	2.21 ± 0.76	0.004	9.1
	35+	3.64 ± 0.79	0.00004	38.0
YFE	1900–1909			1.0
	1910–1914	1.03 ± 0.38	0.007	2.8
	1915–1919	1.11 ± 0.51	0.03	3.0
	1920–1924	0.01 ± 0.53	0.98	1.0
EXP (years)	0			1.0
	0.5–4.0	0.88 ± 0.40	0.03	2.4
	4.5–8.0	1.19 ± 0.47	0.01	3.3
	8.5–12.0	2.30 ± 0.52	0.001	10.0
	12.5+	2.84 ± 0.57	0.0001	17.2
	$-2 \times$ log-likelihood = 561.2			
All covariables continuous				
log(AFE-10)		2.22 ± 0.44	<0.00001	
(YFE-1915)/10		−0.09 ± 0.32	0.76	
(YFE-1915)^2/100		−1.26 ± 0.51	0.01	
log(EXP + 1)		0.77 ± 0.17	0.00001	
	$-2 \times$ log-likelihood = 568.9			

[a] AFE, age at first employment; YFE, year of first employment; EXP, duration of 'exposure' in designated job categories

One goal of constructing appropriate continuous covariables was to lay the foundation for assessing the goodness-of-fit of the multiplicative model by incorporating cross-product or interaction terms in the regression equation. Such analyses are more sensitive if the interactions can be expressed in a quantitative rather than a qualitative manner so that the chi-square statistics for testing their significance have at most a few degrees of freedom (see Volume 1, §6.6 and 6.7). For reasons of economy and convenience, however, these explorations for interaction effects were restricted to the case-control analyses reported below.

(b) Analysis of nasal sinus cancer risk by attained age

We did not choose attained age as the basic time variable in our initial partial likelihood analysis of the nasal sinus cancer deaths. Since it is obvious that all or nearly all such cases were caused by the specific nickel exposure rather than by general environmental exposures, the usual reasons for regarding age as the key explanatory variable were absent. Most persons concerned with the analysis of these data have considered duration of time since onset of exposure to the causal agent to be the most relevant time scale.

Fig. 5.10   Baseline death rate from nasal sinus cancer by years since initial employ-
ment for Welsh nickel refiners, estimated by the multiplicative model. (A)
Cumulative rate; (B) smoothed instantaneous rate (five-year bandwidth);
(C) smoothed instantaneous rate (ten-year bandwidth)

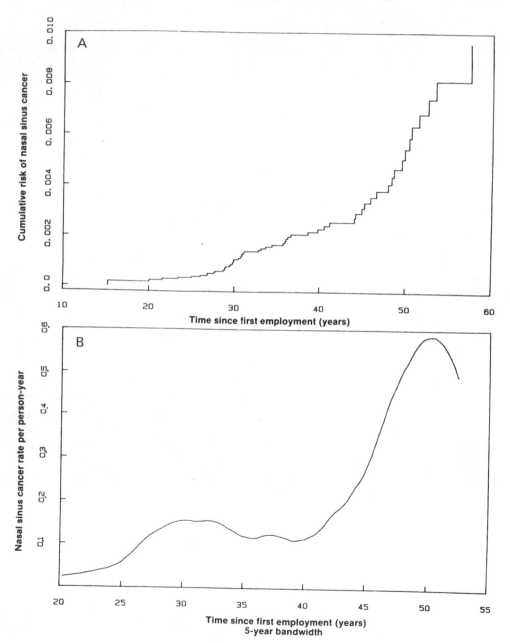

Fig. 5.10   (*contd*)

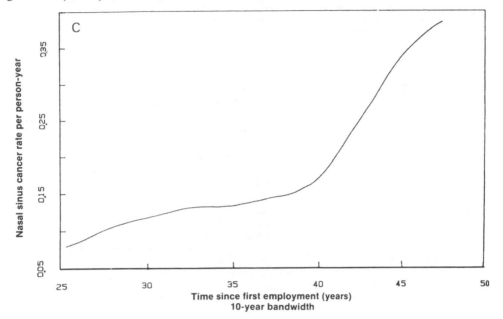

One might ask whether attained age should be included as an additional variable in the analysis to see whether it carries some explanatory value after accounting for age at onset and time since first exposure. However, since attained age is the sum of these latter two variables, it is clear that such an analysis cannot separate the (linear) effects of the three factors. The basic problem is the same as that which occurs also with age-period-cohort analyses.

Nevertheless, largely out of curiosity, we did conduct an alternative partial likelihood analysis with attained age *replacing* time since first employment as the basic time variable. Table 5.11 reports the regression coefficients for the discrete levels of the factors AFE, YFE and EXP obtained with this approach, and Figure 5.11 shows the smoothed estimate of the baseline death rate as a function of age. The relative risks associated with YFE and EXP depend little on whether the baseline risk is expressed as a function of age or of time since onset of exposure. The increase in relative risk with AFE, however, is substantially less when age is used as the basic time variable. Correspondingly, the baseline risk increases more smoothly and sharply as a function of age than as a function of time since onset of exposure. (Compare Figures 5.10B and 5.11.)

(c) Nasal sinus cancer deaths: sampling from the risk set

In order to reduce the volume of data so as to explore different ways of constructing continuous regression variables and to search for significant interactions, we carried out

Table 5.11 Results of fitting the multiplicative model by maximum partial likelihood to data on nasal sinus cancer deaths; 'time' = age

Variable[a]	Level	Parameter estimate ± standard error	p value	Relative risk
AFE (years)	15–19			1.0
	20–27.5	1.03 ± 0.75	0.17	2.8
	27.5–35	1.30 ± 0.75	0.08	3.7
	35+	2.08 ± 0.77	0.007	8.0
YFE	1900–1909			1.0
	1910–1914	0.93 ± 0.38	0.01	2.5
	1915–1919	0.93 ± 0.51	0.07	2.5
	1920–1924	−0.12 ± 0.52	0.82	0.9
EXP (years)	0			1.0
	0.5–4.0	0.82 ± 0.40	0.04	2.3
	4.5–8.0	1.10 ± 0.47	0.02	3.0
	8.5–12.0	2.24 ± 0.51	0.0001	9.4
	12.5+	2.77 ± 0.57	0.00001	16.1
	−2 × log-likelihood = 573.36			

[a] See legend to Table 5.10

Fig. 5.11   Adjusted nasal sinus cancer rates by age, smoothed using five- (———) and ten-year (– – –) bandwidths

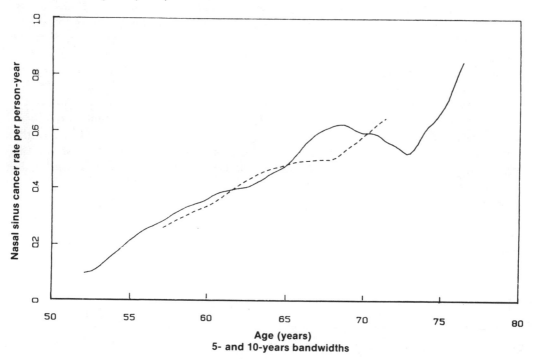

Age (years)
5- and 10-years bandwidths

Table 5.12 Results of fitting the multiplicative models by conditional maximum likelihood to matched sets of a nasal sinus cancer case and 20 controls; 'time' = years since first employed

Variable[a]	Level	Parameter estimate ± standard error	p value	Relative risk
All covariables discrete				
AFE (years)	15–19			1.0
	20–27.5	1.52 ± 0.76	0.048	4.5
	27.5–35	2.12 ± 0.78	0.006	8.2
	35+	3.60 ± 0.83	<0.001	36.7
YFE	1900–1909			1.0
	1910–1914	0.74 ± 0.40	0.064	2.1
	1915–1919	0.85 ± 0.53	0.127	2.3
	1920–1924	−0.30 ± 0.53	0.571	0.7
EXP (years)	0			1.0
	0.5–4.0	0.83 ± 0.42	0.049	2.3
	4.5–8.0	0.93 ± 0.48	0.049	2.5
	8.5–12.0	2.45 ± 0.56	<0.001	11.6
	12.5+	2.56 ± 0.63	<0.001	13.0
	Deviance = 259.80			
All covariables continuous				
$\log(\text{AFE-10})$		2.09 ± 0.46	<0.001	
$(\text{YFE-1915})/10$		−0.23 ± 0.32	0.438	
$(\text{YFE-1915})^2/100$		−1.01 ± 0.53	0.057	
$\log(\text{EXP} + 1)$		0.72 ± 0.18	<0.001	
	Deviance = 267.67			

[a] See legend to Table 5.10

Table 5.13 Deviances for various interaction terms when fitting the multiplicative model to matched sets of a nasal sinus cancer case and 20 controls; 'time' = years since first employed

Interaction variables included in equation[a]	Deviance
None	267.67
$\log(\text{AFE-10}) \times (\text{YFE-1915})/10 + \log(\text{AFE-10}) \times (\text{YFE-1915})^2/10$	267.22
$\log(\text{AFE-10}) \times \log(\text{EXP} + 1)$	267.51
$(\text{YFE-1915})/10 \times \log(\text{EXP} + 1) + (\text{YFE-1915})^2/100 \times \log(\text{EXP} + 1)$	267.04
$\log(\text{AFE-10}) \times \log(\text{AFE-10})$	267.62
$\log(\text{EXP} + 1) \times \log(\text{EXP} + 1)$	266.78
$\log(\text{AFE-10}) \times \text{TFE}$	266.92
$(\text{YFE-1915})/10 \times \text{TFE} + (\text{YFE-1915})^2/100 \times \text{TFE}$	265.41
$\log(\text{EXP} + 1) \times \text{TFE}$	267.66

[a] In addition to four continuous variables shown in the second part of Table 5.12; see legend to Table 5.10

the risk-set sampling procedure, selecting 20 controls from each of the 56 risk sets. This yielded a data file containing $21 \times 56 = 1176$ records that could be analysed with relative ease. Table 5.12 shows the results of fitting the same models to the case-control data as had been fitted earlier to the entire data set (Table 5.11). While there is reasonably good agreement, the relative risks associated with the highest exposure category and employment in the 1910–1919 period are underestimated with the case-control data. Just as we found for the full analysis, however, a summary of the data in terms of the four continuous variables is quite adequate in comparison with a summary in terms of the corresponding discrete factors.

Fig. 5.12   Deletion diagnostics for the model shown in the second part of Table 5.12; approximate effect on the standardized regression coefficients from deletion of individual cases. AFE, age at first employment; YFE, year of first employment; EXP, duration of 'exposure' in designated job categories

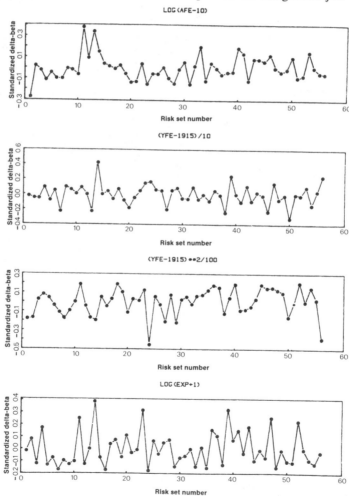

The question of possible interactions between the continuous variables which, if present, would tend to invalidate the results obtained with the simple multiplicative model is examined in Table 5.13. For no risk variable was there any indication of a (linear) dependence of its multiplicative effect on values of another risk variable or on time since first employment, nor was there strong evidence of curvature in the dependence of log relative risk on log $(AFE - 10)$ or log $(EXP + 1)$. Had there been, it would suggest that some other transformation of these variables be used instead.

One last check on the adequacy of the fitted model was to examine the approximate change in the regression coefficients estimated for each of the four continuous variables that would accompany the deletion of any one of the 56 cases from the analysis. Since each risk set contained a single case, deletion of a case has the same effect as deleting the entire risk set for these data. Results obtained using the procedure of Storer and Crowley (1985) are shown in Figure 5.12. The risk sets are numbered according to time since first employment so that number 1 corresponds to the case diagnosed at 15.23 years and number 56 to the case diagnosed at 57.48 years. For none of the four variables does deletion of a risk set change the estimated value of the β regression coefficient by more than half its standard error. The linear and square terms in YFE are correlated, so that the deletion of certain risk sets (e.g., numbers 14, 24, 56) causes the coefficient of (YFE-1915)/10 to increase and that for (YFE-1915)^2/100 to decrease, and *vice versa*.

6. MODELLING THE RELATIONSHIP BETWEEN RISK, DOSE AND TIME

CHAPTER 6

MODELLING THE RELATIONSHIP BETWEEN RISK, DOSE AND TIME

6.1 Introduction and rationale

The previous two chapters developed the statistical methods now available for fitting models to data from cohort studies. It was emphasized that the association between excess risk for disease and the temporal record of exposure may depend on many features of the exposure history, and that a misleading picture may emerge from the analysis if a relevant variable is omitted. An example is given in Figure 5.6, where much of the apparently powerful effect of time since first exposure is shown to result from a major change in exposure at the Montana smelter in 1925. The purpose of this chapter is to describe the types of variable that one might expect to be important, either from the behaviour of excess risk observed in previous studies, or from models of carcinogenesis derived theoretically but supported by both experimental and epidemiological results. Attention will also be given to the forms of dose-response curve that past experience or theoretical considerations would suggest might be appropriate. It is important, furthermore, that, however excess risk is modelled, the results of the analysis respond to the basic aims of the study. The underlying purposes of the investigation need to be kept firmly in view. These aims are essentially of two types – first, to provide a scientific basis for public health and, second, to contribute to the understanding of the biology of human disease. The former requires accurate assessment and prediction of risk, the latter requires an understanding of the role in the disease process played by different exposures over time.

In the area of public health, epidemiology is expected to assist in resolving such questions as:

(i) In early detection programmes for breast cancer, the breasts of women aged over 40 years might be exposed every year, or every two years, to a low dose of radiation, perhaps 0.2 rads per examination. Does this dose, cumulated over time, represent an appreciable hazard for inducing breast cancer? Is the hazard comparable in magnitude to the reduction in breast cancer mortality attributable to screening?

(ii) Do the materials used to replace asbestos represent a carcinogenic hazard? Are the data currently available sufficient to assess whether the risk is appreciably less than that associated with asbestos?

(iii) The carrier state for hepatitis B virus is a major risk factor for primary liver cancer. Given the dynamics of infection with this virus in a population, what long-term effect on liver cancer rates would be predicted by a mass vaccination programme?

To answer questions of this type, models are required relating risk to exposure, both in terms of the degree of exposure and the time during which exposure occurred. These models should provide a reasonable basis for extrapolation from the observed range of exposure to the levels of interest. Examination of the currently available data on a range of exposures should indicate what type of behaviour is observed epidemiologically, thus suggesting which models have empirical support (see §6.2).

To assist in understanding the biology of human disease, biological models of disease causation and development are helpful. These models come mainly from experimental or in-vitro work, in which the process of carcinogenesis is observed at the cellular level. To translate models constructed to describe cellular events into models that can describe events at the population level, i.e., incidence rates, requires a degree of abstraction that is best handled by mathematics. For this reason, mathematical models of the carcinogenic process have received considerable attention, since they have the potential for describing in a unified way a wide variety of phenomena. Use of these models for interpretation of epidemiological data may assist in understanding the mode of action of agents carcinogenic to man. Section 6.3 outlines some of the models of carcinogenesis that have been proposed, with the implication of these models for the behaviour of incidence rates. In §6.4, we attempt to describe the data of §6.2 in terms of these models.

The material of §§6.2 to 6.4 highlights the variables that appear to be the most concise predictors of future risk. These variables would therefore appear to be those of greatest value to incorporate in analyses of epidemiological studies.

In §6.5, we consider further the data from the South Wales cohort of nickel refiners to illustrate how multistage concepts may be used to aid in the interpretation of epidemiological results.

6.2 Dose-time relationships observed in epidemiological studies

In this section we examine the metameters of dose or exposure that have been used in a number of situations, the relationship of these metameters to excess risk and the influence of different time variables. The latter include duration of exposure, time since first exposure, time since exposure stopped and age at first exposure. The effect of these factors on incidence rates differs for different exposures, presumably in a manner determined by the mode of action of the exposure. This topic is considered in §§6.3 and 6.4.

As observed in Chapter 1, most of the data that provide quantitative information on the relationships of both time and dose with excess risk come from cohort studies, and we limit our discussion mainly to data of this type. The main factor thus excluded, for which quantitative data relating dose and risk are available, is alcohol. Quantitative data relating alcohol consumption to cancer come predominantly from case-control studies, some of which were described extensively in Volume 1.

(a) *Lung cancer and cigarette smoking*

The cohort study for which the most extensive follow-up results have been reported is that of the British doctors. In the publication (Doll & Peto, 1978) that considered specifically the quantitative association of amount smoked and duration of smoking with lung cancer risk, attention was confined to lifelong nonsmokers or men who reported a regular smoking pattern in response to the three questionnaires (i.e., men who started smoking between ages 16 and 25 years, and who never reported stopping, changing by more than five cigarettes/day, or smoking any form of tobacco other than cigarettes). The purpose of these restrictions was to obtain the most accurate estimate of the dose-response curve by limiting the analysis to individuals with the most stable and most accurately recorded smoking histories. A summary of the basic data has been given in Table 4.21, where person-years and numbers of observed lung cancer deaths are tabulated by current age and amount smoked. The analysis investigating the relationship between dose and risk used as a measure of dose the average number of cigarettes smoked per day. A two-factor multiplicative model was fitted (expression 4.2), with one set of parameters giving age effects and the second set of parameters giving dose effects. The ratio of these latter parameters can be interpreted as relative risks. The results of a similar analysis by the original authors are displayed in Figure 6.1. The exclusion from the formal analysis of those men smoking more than 40 cigarettes a day has aroused some discussion, but is defended at length by them. The functional form used by the authors to fit the curve of Figure 6.1 is

$$\text{Relative risk} = 0.0278(\text{Dose} + 6)^2, \tag{6.1}$$

the baseline being taken as nonsmokers. As described in Tables 4.22 and 4.23, other functional forms could be used to fit the observed curve, such as:

$$\text{Relative risk} = (1 + \text{dose})^k$$

or

$$\text{Relative risk} = 1 + b\ \text{dose} + c\ (\text{dose})^2,$$

which may yield a sightly better fit than the curve given in Figure 6.1. All three, however, indicate significant upward curvature.

This analysis has used data in which within-individual variation in smoking habits has been reduced to a minimum. In other studies, in which individuals with varying smoking habits were not excluded from the published analyses, the dose-response relationship appears almost linear. The main point at issue here, however, is not the existence of some upward curvature, but the metameter of exposure that was used – average number of cigarettes smoked per day.

The age parameters obtained from the preceding analysis were normalized to be interpretable as age-specific rates, standardized for dose. The logarithm of the rate was plotted against the logarithm of the age and against the logarithm of the duration of smoking before onset of disease (taken as age − 22.5). Both gave a reasonably straight line, although with a different slope, reflecting the high correlation between the

Fig. 6.1   Relative risk of lung cancer in terms of number of cigarettes smoked per day. The numbers of onsets in each group are given, and 90% confidence intervals are plotted. The point for those smoking more than 40 cigarettes/day is omitted. From Doll and Peto (1978)

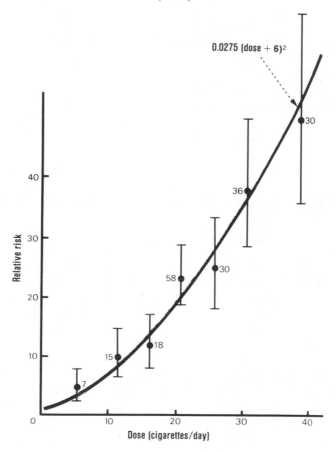

resulting estimates of k and w when fitting models of the form

$$\text{Mortality rate} \propto (\text{Age} - w)^k, \tag{6.2}$$

where $\propto$ denotes proportionality.

The choice between age or duration of smoking as the time variable to use to describe the mortality rates among smokers cannot be made on statistical grounds from these data. However, the exponent of 4.5 for duration of smoking is similar to the exponent for the power curve describing age-specific lung cancer rates among nonsmokers. Testing for interaction with dose gave no indication that the relationship of mortality with duration of smoking varied with amount smoked. Mortality rates for lung cancer among continuing smokers in the British doctors study could therefore be

Table 6.1   Evolution of mortality from lung cancer among ex-cigarette smokers[a]

	Time since smoking stopped (years)				
	0	<5	5–9	11–14	>15
No. of deaths among ex-smokers[b]		10	12	8	7
No. of deaths as percentage of no. expected among continuing smokers	100	68	35	25	11
No. of deaths divided by no. expected among lifelong non-smokers (i.e., relative risk)	15.8	10.7	5.9	4.7	2.0

[a] From Doll and Peto (1976)
[b] Excluding those who stopped smoking after developing lung cancer

succinctly summarized by a single expression incorporating both amount smoked and duration of smoking, as follows:

$$\text{Mortality rate} \propto (\text{cigarettes/day} + 6)^2 (\text{Age} - 22.5)^{4.5}. \tag{6.3}$$

In an earlier paper reporting on the same study, data were also given for ex-smokers (Doll & Peto, 1976). Within a few years of quitting smoking, lung cancer rates fell away from the rates seen in continuing smokers and after 15 years or more approached levels seen in nonsmokers of the same age. Table 6.1 gives the falling relative risks. The evolving risks after quitting smoking are displayed in Figure 6.2, from which it appears that the absolute rate for lung cancer freezes at the level reached when smoking stopped. Thus, for an ex-smoker, lung cancer rates can also be expressed in terms of duration of smoking and average amount smoked per day, as in expression (6.3). Duration of smoking could clearly be replaced by time since smoking started minus time since smoking stopped; the choice of which two of these three variables to use in expressing the effect of time is somewhat arbitrary. In the present situation, duration of smoking and time since stopped appear the most appealing. In a later example, time since first exposure is of particular importance.

In the British doctors study, the age at which cohort members started to smoke showed insufficient variation for it to be adequately studied. The preceding description of risk applies to individuals who started to smoke around the age of 20 years. The effect of age at which smoking started can be examined from other studies. Some results are given in Table 6.2, taken from the Dorn study of US military veterans (Kahn, 1966). Although the range of ages at starting to smoke is not large, it is broad enough to see that the mortality rates, given the duration of smoking, are independent of the age at starting. Thus, equation (6.3) above, expressing mortality as a function of dose and time, holds irrespective of the age at starting, provided that (age − 22.5) is replaced by duration of smoking. Thus, lung cancer rates among current smokers or ex-smokers can be expressed accurately just in terms of duration of smoking and of average number of cigarettes smoked per day.

Fig. 6.2 Mortality rates (logarithmic scale) of lung cancer in ex-smokers (●), expressed as a proportion of the rates expected in regular cigarette smokers at the ages at which smoking was stopped; by time since smoking was stopped. For comparison, similar proportions are shown for regular cigarette smokers of the same age (×) and for lifelong nonsmokers of the same age (○). From Doll (1978)

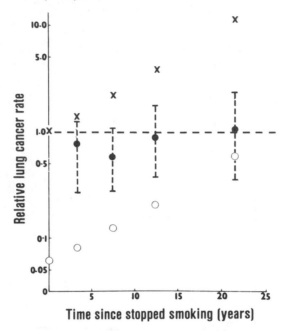

(b) *Asbestos and mesothelioma*

The high risk of cancer, mainly lung cancer and mesothelioma, following asbestos exposure has been extensively studied. A recent review (Peto, J. *et al.*, 1982) has examined in detail the risk of mesothelioma as a function of time, using the results of the five studies for which mesothelioma rates were available by time since first

Table 6.2 The effect of age at starting to smoke on mortality from lung cancer[a]

Age at starting to smoke (years)	Annual mortality rate per 100 000 population (age in years)	
	55–64	65–74
<15	251	
15–19	168	
20–24		241
25+		162

[a] From Appendix Table D of Kahn (1966)

exposure. The effect of age at first exposure was investigated in the cohort of North American insulation workers, which contributed two-thirds of the mesothelioma cases recorded in the five studies. Mesothelioma is rare among the general population, so that cases unrelated to asbestos in the study population would be unlikely. Thus, as in the analysis of the nasal sinus cancers in §5.6, mortality rates from mesothelioma among the exposed can be examined without the need for reference to a background rate. Mortality rates are shown in Figures 6.3A and 6.3B by age at death and by age at

Fig. 6.3   Cumulative risk of dying of mesothelioma in the absence of other causes of death among North American insulation workers first exposed to asbestos at age 15–25 (· – · –), 25–34 (——) or over 35 (· · ·), against age (A) and against years since first exposure (B). From Peto, J. *et al.* (1982)

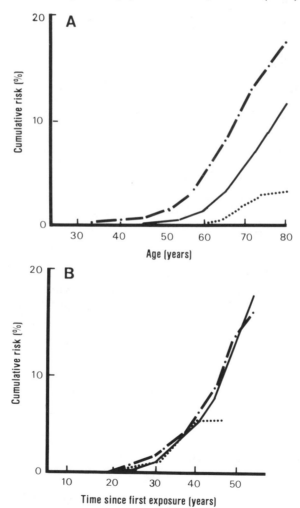

first exposure. As for lung cancer and cigarette smoking, age at first exposure does not affect the rates. The superposition of the curves in Figure 6.3B is striking.

Since age at first exposure can be ignored, curves of similar form can be used to relate time since first exposure to mesothelioma rates for each cohort without need for a stratification by age. Figure 6.4, displaying data for US insulation workers, indicates that mesothelioma rates increase with a power of age since first exposure:

$$\text{Mesothelioma mortality rate} = b(\text{time since first exposure})^k. \qquad (6.4)$$

One might interpret the parameter b to represent in some way the intensity of the exposure, and the parameter k to represent an inherent characteristic of the process of mesothelioma development. k might be similar in different cohorts, whereas b would be expected to vary between cohorts. The results of fitting the above expression simultaneously to the data from all five cohorts, with the same value of k for each cohort but allowing b to vary, are given in Table 6.3. The fit is excellent, and holds equally well for either pleural or peritoneal tumours (with a value for k of 3.2). As in the preceding example with cigarette smoking, other models of the form:

$$\text{Rate} \propto (\text{time of exposure} - w)^k$$

fit the data equally well, and in fact the expression

$$\text{Mesothelioma rate} = b(\text{time since first exposure} - 10)^2$$

fits better than (6.4) in the first 15 years, and equally well thereafter. Subtracting ten years may reflect the length of time taken for a transformed cell to progress into a fatal tumour.

The preceding discussion has ignored both length of exposure and any effect of stopping exposure. Once asbestos exposure has taken place, however, fibres remain in the body, and the relationship between external exposure and the more relevant tissue exposure is unclear. The latter may well continue long after the former has been removed. For this reason, both duration of exposure and time since last exposure are ill-defined for asbestos. Furthermore, it is clear from Table 6.3 that an adequate description of mesothelioma rates can be given without taking account explicitly of exposure cessation.

The parameter b, which varies considerably between the cohorts given in Table 6.3, would represent effective dose, incorporating average length of exposure, intensity of exposure and the potency for mesothelioma induction of the specific type of fibre. No data currently available suggest that the parameter k differs between cohorts with long-term continuous exposure and those with short-term exposure.

Thus, rates for mesothelioma induced by asbestos can be well summarized in terms of time since first exposure, together with some measure of cumulative exposure, which combines duration with dose level. The contrast with the cigarette smoking–lung cancer relationship is marked, and will be discussed in §6.3 in terms of models of carcinogenesis.

Fig. 6.4   Mesothelioma mortality among North American insulation workers first
exposed 1922–1946, by time since first exposure. Bars indicate 95%
confidence intervals. From Peto, J. *et al.* (1982)

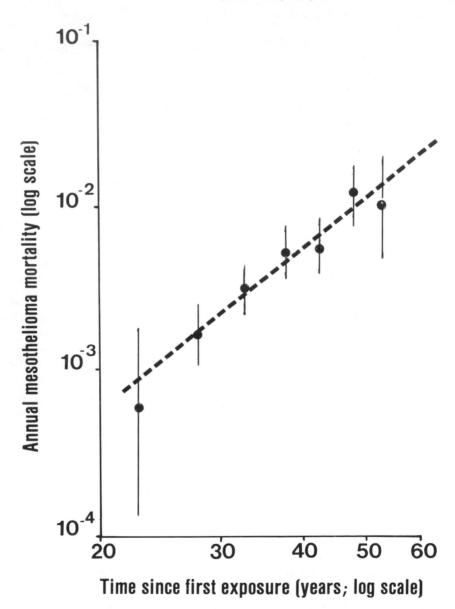

Table 6.3 Numbers of mesotheliomas (N), and man–years (M–Y) of observation in studies of asbestos workers. Expected numbers (E) are obtained by fitting death rate $= b$ (time since first exposure)$^{3.20}$, where b is constant[a]

Study		Years since first exposure									
		10–	15–	20–	25–	30–	35–	40–	45–	50+	Total
Selikoff et al. (1979) North American insulation workers (mixed exposure; $b = 4.37 \times 10^{-8}$)	N			3	22	47	46	25	28	9	180
	E			4.58	22.59	44.26	41.64	31.17	23.59	12.17	180.00
	M–Y			4939	12815	14711	8756	4391	2328	872	48812
Newhouse & Berry (1976) Factory workers (mixed exposure; $b = 4.95 \times 10^{-8}$)	N	1	6	15	11	12					45
	E	2.59	6.32	10.37	12.84	12.87[b]					45.00
	M–Y	16167	13438	9862	6423	3772					49662
Peto, J. (1980) Chrysotile textile workers ($b = 2.94 \times 10^{-8}$)	N	0	0	1	2	2	2	0			7
	E	0.16	0.52	1.10	1.77	1.69	1.32	0.44			7.00
	M–Y	1633	1800	1761	1496	837	414	92			8093
Hobbs et al. (1980) Australian crocidolite miners ($b = 2.94 \times 10^{-8}$)	N	1	12	13							26
	E	4.53	8.32	13.15[c]							26.00
	M–Y	27172	17012	12028							56212
Seidman et al. (1979) US amosite factory workers ($b = 4.91 \times 10^{-8}$)	N	0	0	2	5	7	0				14
	E	0.58	1.48	2.73	4.01	4.68	0.52				14.00
	M–Y	3628	3274	2618	2026	1383	98				12927

[a] From Peto, J. et al. (1982)
[b] 30 or more years; 32.5 assumed in calculating expected number
[c] 20 or more years; 22.5 assumed in calculating expected number

(c) *Asbestos and lung cancer*

Among cohorts exposed to asbestos, in which excesses of both mesothelioma and lung cancer are observed, the ratio of the excess number of lung cancers to the number of mesotheliomas decreases sharply with increasing time since first exposure. It increases, however, with increasing age at first exposure. It is clear, therefore, that the excess of lung cancer evolves with time in a different manner to the excess of mesothelioma.

A number of cohorts have been extensively studied, and a review of the major studies has been made by Acheson and Gardner (1980) to establish dose-response patterns. A linear relationship between cumulative dose and excess relative risk has been observed in several studies – for example, the study of Quebec asbestos miners (Fig. 6.5). Workers at an amosite asbestos factory in New Jersey during the Second World War were heavily exposed for short periods, and study of this cohort has provided a clear picture of a linear relationship between duration of exposure and excess relative risk (Fig. 6.6) (Seidman *et al.* 1979). In one study, little extra effect of reported asbestos exposure levels was seen after adjusting for duration of exposure (Peto, J., 1980). That is to say, duration of exposure may give a measure of cumulative dose which cannot be appreciably improved by measurement of dose level, given the relative imprecision of these latter measurements, at least in previous decades.

Fig. 6.5   Dose–response relationships for lung cancer following asbestos exposure in Quebec miners and millers. From Acheson and Gardner (1980)

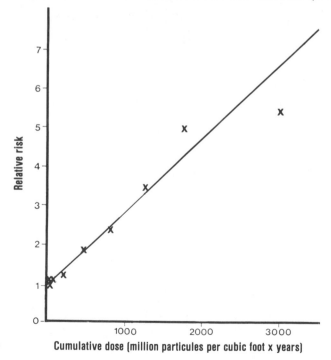

Cumulative dose (million particules per cubic foot x years)

Fig. 6.6   Relative risk of death from lung cancer in a group of amosite insulation workers, by duration of exposure (after Seidman *et al.*, 1979). From Acheson and Gardner (1980)

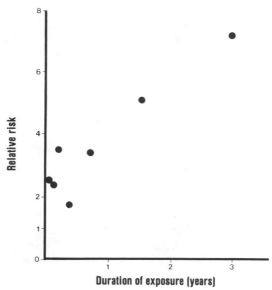

In the study of US insulators, follow-up has continued for 50 years since first exposure; the excess relative risk for lung cancer by year since first exposure is given in Table 3.10, and by age at first exposure in Table 6.4.

From Table 3.10 one can see that the relative risk reaches a plateau some 15 years after start of exposure, where it remains indefinitely. There is some indication that 40 years or more after exposure starts the relative risk begins to decrease. The significance of this fall is doubtful, however, since one might expect the attrition of smokers,

Table 6.4   Expected and observed numbers of deaths from lung cancer among 17 800 asbestos insulation workers, 1 January 1967–31 December 1971; distribution by age at onset of exposure[a]

Age at onset of exposure (years)	Deaths from lung cancer		
	Expected[b]	Observed	Ratio
<25	18.19	102	5.61
25–34	15.20	66	4.34
35–44	8.78	38	4.33
45+	2.25	7	3.11

[a] From Selikoff *et al.* (1973)
[b] Expected deaths are based upon age-specific death rate data of the US National Office of Vital Statistics. Rates for 1968–1971 were extrapolated from rates for 1961–1967.

particularly heavy smokers, to be even more rapid in this cohort than in the general population (see Chapter 3). This differential attrition would lead to an apparent fall of the excess relative risk of lung cancer with time, and contribute to the observed decrease. As mentioned earlier, the effect of stopping exposure is difficult to assess for asbestos. As seen in Table 6.4, the relative risk is roughly independent of age at first exposure, although a slight fall with increasing age is seen. Since lung cancer rates increase rapidly with age, the absolute excess risk rises rapidly with age at first exposure.

This overall behaviour has been summarized by saying that the excess relative risk of lung cancer increases linearly with duration of exposure and, for given duration of exposure, is independent of age at first exposure or time since first exposure. This behaviour should be contrasted with that seen for cigarette smoking, where the absolute rather than the relative excess risk was related to duration of exposure.

(d) Radiation and leukaemia

The association of leukaemia with radiation exposure was the original focus of several of the large cohort studies initiated in the 1950s, notably the study of patients with ankylosing spondylitis (Court Brown & Doll, 1965) and of women with cervical cancer (Hutchison, 1968). The study of atomic bomb survivors was, of course, much more broadly based, the Life-Span Study representing a systematic search for all mortality differentials associated with radiation, but the excess of leukaemia excited interest first.

In both the atomic bomb and the ankylosing spondylitis studies, the excess mortality from leukaemia was greater and occurred earlier than the excess mortality due to other malignancies. A joint analysis has been made of these two studies investigating the effects of age at exposure and time since exposure (Darby, 1984; Darby et al., 1985). The excess of leukaemia reaches a peak in the first five years after exposure, and then declines steadily. Little excess is seen among the ankylosing spondylitis patients more than ten years after exposure, whereas among the atomic bomb survivors, with a higher initial risk, an excess is still seen more than 20 years after exposure.

Little variation in relative risk is seen with age at exposure among the ankylosing spondylitis patients, nor among the atomic bomb survivors 15 years of age or more at exposure. Atomic bomb survivors less than 15 years of age at exposure, however, suffered a markedly higher risk. Among this latter group, the risk rose more rapidly, attained a higher peak, and then fell off more sharply (Beebe et al., 1977; Ishimaru et al., 1979; Committee on the Biological Effects of Ionizing Radiation, 1980).

The excess of leukaemia is confined to acute and nonlymphocytic leukaemia, none of the studies showing an excess of chronic lymphocytic leukaemia. In the study of ankylosing spondylitis patients, in which analyses have been based on death certificates and comparison with general population mortality rates, no formal analyses have been made by leukaemia subtype, since no population mortality rate is available. In the original analyses, however, none of the leukaemia deaths was attributed to the chronic lymphocytic type. Among the atomic bomb survivors, mortality rates for the subtypes of leukaemia can be studied since the comparison is with the lightly exposed (less than 10 rads) members of the cohort.

The follow-up of women irradiated for cancer of the cervix (Day & Boice, 1983) used cancer occurrence as an endpoint, and incidence rates from cancer registries as the basis for comparison. These data could therefore also be examined by subtype of leukaemia, illustrating the advantage of incidence rather than mortality as an endpoint, i.e., the ability of cancer registries to produce accurate population rates by finer disease categories. The results are shown in Figure 6.7. The excess risk reaches a peak in the first five years – although it is more modest than the peak seen in the ankylosing spondylitis series – then falls away to inappreciable levels ten years or more after exposure. The risk for chronic lymphocytic leukaemia is, if anything, below that of the general population.

Comparison of the excess risk seen in these three studies presents an apparent paradox. Both the cervical cancer patients and the ankylosing spondylitis patients received very high doses of radiation to part of the active bone marrow (several thousand rads). In contrast, the larger excess risk among the atomic bomb survivors was induced by a few hundred rads of whole-body irradiation, all the active bone marrow receiving similar exposure. The dose-response curve appeared approximately linear, as shown in Figure 6.8. [We shall leave aside in this discussion the different effects seen in Hiroshima and in Nagasaki, between sexes and between the neutron and gamma-ray components of the exposure. Resolution of these differences awaits new dose estimates (see, for example, Fujita, 1984) and may also depend on differential

Fig. 6.7   Observed to expected ratios of nonlymphocytic and acute leukaemia among patients with invasive cervical cancer treated with radiotherapy by time since diagnosis of cervical cancer; 80% confidence intervals presented. From Day and Boice (1983)

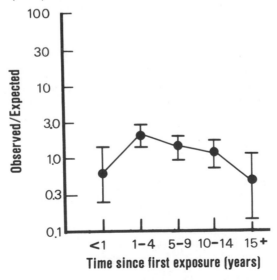

Fig. 6.8   Leukaemia deaths among Japanese survivors of the atomic bomb explosion, per 100 000 persons per year by (T65) dose and city. From Beebe *et al.* (1977)

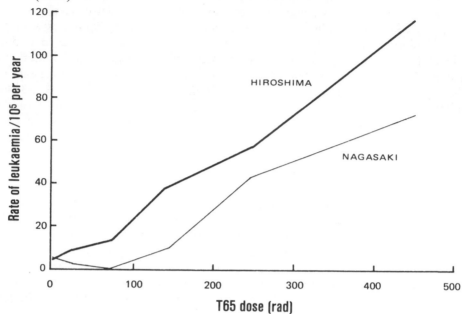

accuracy of the dose estimation (Gilbert, 1984)]. If this linear dose-response derived from the atomic bomb survivors could be extrapolated to higher dose levels, one might expect considerably larger risks in the two studies of irradiated patients. In the cervical cancer study, for example, one would have expected several hundred excess leukaemias rather than the 20 or so actually observed.

In the ankylosing spondylitis study, using as a measure of dose the mean exposure to the active bone marrow, no increase in risk with increasing dose is seen (Smith & Doll, 1982) (Fig. 6.9). The proposed explanation for the observed lack of linear increase in the dose-response curve is that radiation can sterilize cells as well as transform them, the sterilized cells having no potential for malignant growth. Sterilization is the major effect at high doses, transformation at lower doses. Incorporating cell sterilization into a dose-response model (see Brown, 1977) has led to expressions such as

$$\text{Excess relative risk} \propto \text{Dose} \cdot \exp\left(\alpha \text{Dose} - \beta \text{dose}^2\right). \tag{6.5}$$

Using this model with average dose to the active bone marrow gave a reasonable fit to the data of Figure 6.9. On occasion, however, it might be preferable to integrate expression (6.5) over the distribution of dose to the active bone marrow rather than to use simply the average dose. Such a calculation would, of course, require accurate determination of the dose distribution. One can see that this approach might be more suitable for the cervical cancer patients, among whom most of the active bone marrow received either a dose of which the major effect is cell sterilization, or a dose too low to

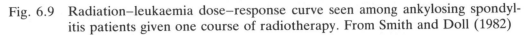

Fig. 6.9 Radiation–leukaemia dose–response curve seen among ankylosing spondylitis patients given one course of radiotherapy. From Smith and Doll (1982)

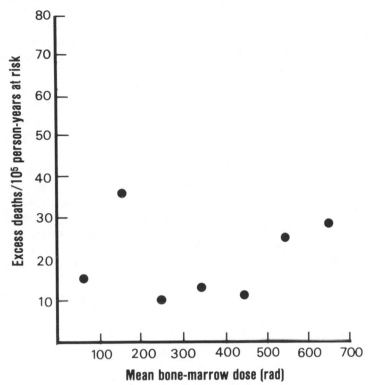

affect risk appreciably. Integrating expression (6.5) over a dose distribution of this type would clearly lead to a low predicted excess risk, as observed, whereas use of the average dose would predict considerably higher risk levels. [In fact, the results of a case-control study of leukaemia within the cervical cancer cohort indicate the importance of a cell-killing term in the dose-response relationship (M. Blettner, personal communication, 1986).]

These results demonstrate the importance of using available biological information to guide the choice of model that one uses. Uncritical use of models chosen for their statistical simplicity can lead to misleading or paradoxical results. To quote Pike (1985), 'At times, we may need to be more subtle in our approach.'

(e) Radiation and breast cancer

Several studies have examined the excess risk for breast cancer seen in groups of women exposed to radiation either for medical purposes or as a consequence of the atomic bomb explosion. The two largest studies are of the atomic bomb survivors and of Canadian women with tuberculosis examined by fluoroscopy (Howe, 1982). Two other widely quoted studies are of fluoroscopy-treated patients in Massachusetts (Boice

& Monson, 1977) and of radiation-treated mastitis patients in New York (Shore *et al.*, 1977). As described in Appendix IB, there has been an extensive effort to determine the dose received by each atomic bomb survivor, and for the cohorts of women irradiated for medical purposes considerable documentation of individual dose levels has been available. Although the duration of radiation treatment was relatively short when compared to the duration of some occupational exposures, being almost always less than five years, there were considerable differences in the degree of dose fractionation. In the atomic bomb survivors, the total dose was received from one explosion, whereas in the fluoroscopy series, a woman may have received several hundred fluoroscopies over a number of years, and in the mastitis series women may have received five to ten exposures over a period of weeks. No major difference has been seen in breast cancer risk attributable to the degree of fractionation, and analyses have been based on the total dose received. The three determinants of risk that have been studied in some detail are the total dose, the time since the dose was received, and the age at which the dose was received. Since the underlying breast cancer rates in the populations studied vary widely – for example, between Japan and the USA or between age groups – attention has also been given to the problem of which effect measure is more appropriate, relative excess risk or absolute excess risk. The two measures give estimates of lifetime risk which differ considerably, as discussed in Chapter 4.

The Massachusetts fluoroscopy study, the New York study of mastitis patients and the study of atomic bomb survivors have been analysed jointly (Land *et al.*, 1980). A number of models have been fitted, expressing the mortality rate of breast cancer, *I*, as a function of radiation dose, *D*, in particular

$$I(D) = \alpha_0 + \alpha_1 D \qquad\qquad\qquad \text{A.}$$
$$I(D) = \alpha_0 + \alpha_1 D + \alpha_2 D^2 \qquad\qquad \text{B.}$$
$$I(D) = (\alpha_0 + \alpha_1 D) \exp(-\beta_2 D^2) \qquad \text{C.}$$
$$I(D) = (\alpha_0 + \alpha_1 D + \alpha_2 D^2) \exp(-\beta_2 D^2) \qquad \text{D.}$$

The last two models introduce a possible effect of cell killing, as discussed in the previous section. In the mastitis study, model C was an improvement over model A (Land *et al.*, 1980), whereas in a separate analysis of the Canadian fluoroscopy study model A fitted well in the high-dose range (Miller *et al.*, 1987). The difference in the shape of the dose-response curve between these two studies in the high dose range (400–1000 rads) might be attributed to the higher dose rate, i.e., lower degree of fractionation, in the mastitis study. Apart from high doses in the mastitis series, model A gave an adequate fit to the different series of data, and the main findings of the different analyses can be summarized as follows:

(i) The dose-response appears linear throughout the range of dose observed (see Figure 6.10). A suggestion of a downturn at high dose levels, which might be predicted on the basis of models incorporating cell killing, is seen in the mastitis series, but not in the atomic bomb survivors nor in the Canadian fluoroscopy series.

Fig. 6.10   Increase in relative risk for breast cancer as radiation dose increases in the Canadian fluoroscopy (○) and atomic bomb (◆) studies

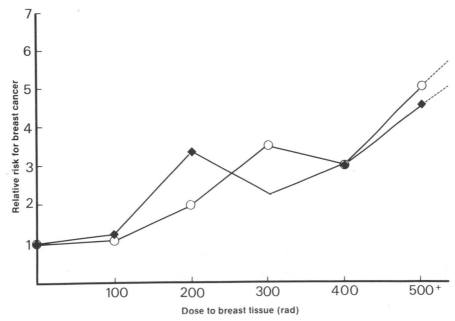

(ii) The excess relative risk appears some ten years after exposure, and continues thereafter at a roughly constant level. Even after 40 years, there is no indication of a diminution (see Figure 6.11). The absolute excess risk increases with time since exposure.

(iii) The excess relative risk is greater at younger ages at exposure, with little excess seen among women over 40 years of age when irradiated (Howe, 1982). Recent results from the atomic bomb survivors and from children irradiated for an enlarged thymus suggest that the excess relative risk is even higher among those exposed when aged 0–9 than among those aged 10–19 at exposure.

(iv) The absolute excess per unit dose in young Japanese women was similar to that seen in white American women, the excess relative risk being correspondingly larger. This finding is in contrast to the constancy of relative risk throughout the period of follow-up noted in point (ii) above, indicating that hypotheses of constant relative or constant absolute excess risks are both simplistic, and neither forms a sound basis for extrapolating results from one population to another.

(f) Radiation and bone tumours

This example contrasts the effect seen in two different studies of the different isotopes of radium, which after ingestion have been incorporated into the bone tissue. The first study is of radium dial painters (Rowland & Lucas, 1984), who by habitually

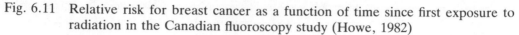

Fig. 6.11   Relative risk for breast cancer as a function of time since first exposure to radiation in the Canadian fluoroscopy study (Howe, 1982)

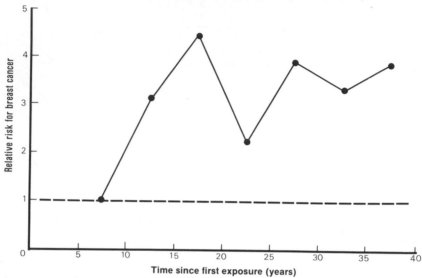

licking their paint brushes absorbed quantities of ^{226}Ra. The half life of ^{226}Ra is long (1600 years), so that exposure to the decay products continued virtually at constant levels after absorption of the radium. The effect on subsequent risk is shown in Figure 6.12A, with little indication of a decline in the number of cases even after 40 years. It is thought that most of the intake of ^{226}Ra occurred in the first ten years after entry, since brush-licking apparently stopped in 1926. The dose-response has also received close attention in this study, a function of the form

$$(\alpha + \beta \, \text{dose}^2) \exp(-\lambda \, \text{dose})$$

giving the best fit. As for the leukaemia dose-response, a cell sterilization term improves the fit.

The second study investigated ankylosing spondylitis patients in the Federal Republic of Germany who were given ^{224}Ra as treatment (Mays & Spiess, 1984). ^{224}Ra has a half-life of several days, so that exposure to the decay products effectively ceases a few days after treatment stops. The subsequent risk of bone tumours is shown in Figure 6.12B, in which a wave pattern to the excess risk is discernible, similar to that seen for leukaemia. The comparative behaviour of bone tumours and leukaemias in this study is given in Figure 6.13. Indications of a similar wavelike pattern to the excess risk of bone tumours are seen after short-term exposure to external gamma rays (Day & Boice, 1983; Kaldor *et al.*, 1987).

These two examples illustrate the care that is required in defining time since exposure; the relationship between tissue dose and external exposure requires close attention.

Fig. 6.12   (A) Bone sarcoma appearance times after exposure to ^{226}Ra (half-life, 1600 years). (B) Bone sarcoma appearance times after exposure to ^{224}Ra (half-life, 3.6 days). From Mays and Spiess (1984)

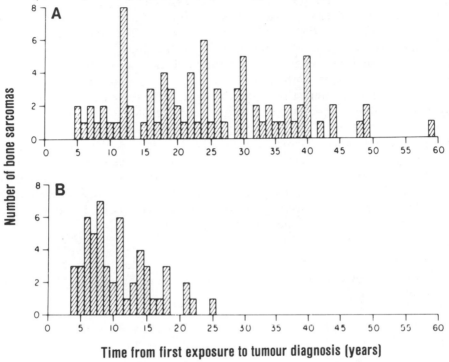

Time from first exposure to tumour diagnosis (years)

Fig 6.13   Appearance times of bone sarcomas in patients exposed to a short half-life radium isotope (●) and of leukaemias in the atomic bomb survivors (△). From Mays and Spiess (1984)

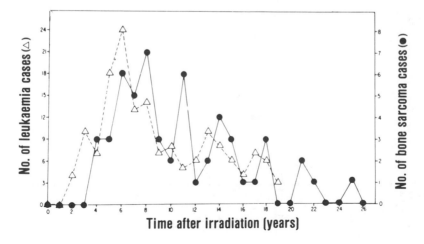

Time after irradiation (years)

(g) Bladder cancer and exposure to benzidine

The purpose of this example (Zavon *et al.*, 1973) is to illustrate the point that, even with a very small cohort and no clear measure of exposure (environmental measures of exposures related to different job categories varied by a factor of 10^4 in this study), an illuminating description of the excess risk can be given. The study relates to a small group of men employed in the manufacture of benzidine. Other exposures were recorded, but none represented a hazard for bladder cancer comparable to that of benzidine. Of the 28 men employed, 15 developed bladder cancer – a remarkable excess. Of even greater interest is to plot the cumulative increase in risk with years of employment for those who remained continuously employed, deriving Nelson plots (see Figure 6.14 and equation 5.16) such as are commonly used in the analysis of skin-painting experiments of carcinogenicity (IARC, 1982b). The cumulative risk of bladder cancer is 50% at 15 years, rising to 100% after 25 years. In this situation, such a presentation of the data essentially contains all the information in the results pertaining to bladder carcinogenesis. It is certainly much more informative than a statement that 15 bladder cancers were observed in a cohort of 28 workers, with an expected number (not given in the paper) of the order of 0.1.

Fig. 6.14   Cumulative absolute risk of developing a bladder tumour as a function of duration of continuous exposure to benzidine (from data of Zavon *et al.*, 1973). From IARC (1982b)

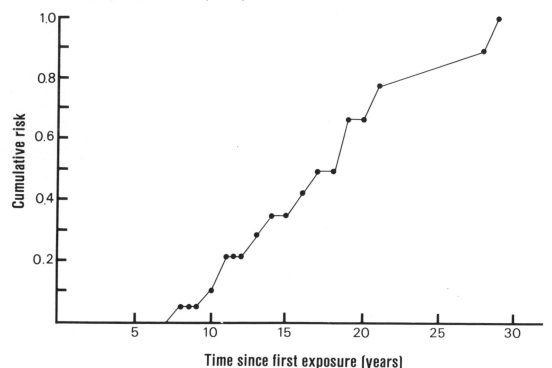

(h) Lung cancer among US uranium miners

The excess lung cancer risk seen among US uranium miners has been the subject of a number of reports (Waxweiler *et al.*, 1981), the most recent of which takes the follow-up to the end of 1977. Whittemore and McMillan (1983) focused their analysis on the joint effects of radiation (mainly alpha particles emitted during the radioactive decay of radon and its daughter products) and cigarette smoking. A case-control approach was adopted in which, for each lung cancer death, four control subjects were randomly selected from among those born within eight months of the case and known to survive him. The joint effects of radiation and smoking were modelled in a number of ways. First, radiation exposure was expressed as cumulative exposure in terms of working level months (WLM), based on extensive environmental measures of radon daughter levels, and cigarette smoke exposure was expressed in terms of total packs of cigarettes ever smoked (PKS). Both cumulative exposures were truncated ten years before the death of the lung cancer cases, and, for controls, ten years before the death of the matched case, as an approximate way of incorporating latency.

Since a case-control design was used, the relative risk was taken as the effect measure. A number of models were fitted, to investigate the following questions:

(1) Is the combined effect of radiation and smoking better described in additive or multiplicative terms?

(2) What is the shape of the dose-response curve?

(3) Does total amount smoked or average amount smoked per day provide a simpler description of tobacco-associated excess risk?

To investigate the first two issues, cumulative exposure to both factors was categorized. Writing the excess relative risk in the ith radiation category as $\beta_{i,R}$ and in the jth smoking category as $\beta_{j,S}$, alternative models representing multiplicative and additive joint action were fitted

$$RR_{ij} = (1 + \beta_{i,R})(1 + \beta_{j,S}) \quad \text{Multiplicative}$$
$$RR_{ij} = 1 + \beta_{i,R} + \beta_{j,S} \qquad \text{Additive}$$

and the two models compared with one describing general joint action

$$RR_{ij} = 1 + \beta_{ij},$$

where RR_{ij} is the risk for individuals in category i for radiation and category j for smoking, relative to those in the baseline category for both exposures.

The multiplicative model was not significantly worse than the general model, whereas the additive model fared badly. Thus, although the additive and multiplicative models were not compared directly, the latter certainly appeared to be preferable. This finding is in contrast to the interactive effect on lung cancer of smoking and radiation seen in the atomic bomb survivors study, which appeared to be additive or even subadditive (Prentice *et al.*, 1983). In the one case, there was continuous exposure to alpha particles, and in the other there was instantaneous exposure to gamma rays; whether this difference reflects different measurement errors or more basic differences in mode of joint action is unclear.

To investigate the shape of the dose-response curve, cumulative radiation exposure and cigarette smoking were introduced as quantitative variables. A number of models were considered, including

$$RR = (1 + \beta_1 WLM)(1 + \beta_2 PKS)$$
$$RR = 1 + \beta_1 WLM + \beta_2 PKS$$
$$RR = \exp(\beta_1 WLM + \beta_2 PKS)$$
$$RR = (WLM + BGR)^{\beta_1}(PKS + BGS)^{\beta_2},$$

(6.6)

where BGR and BGS are background rates for radiation and smoking exposures, respectively.

The first of these four models fit as well as the previous multiplicative model using categorized exposure variables, whereas the maximum achieved by the likelihood function under the other models was markedly less. Adding quadratic terms to give models such as

$$RR = \{1 + \beta_1 WLM + \beta_2 (WLM)^2\}(1 + \beta_3 PKS)$$

did not improve the fit appreciably.

The relative risk can thus be taken from these data to rise linearly with increasing cumulative exposure to each variable, the effect of the two variables combining multiplicatively.

Models using average number of cigarettes smoked per day were also investigated, but performed less well than the models given above using cumulative pack-years of cigarettes.

No effect on the relative risk of lung cancer was seen for age at start of underground mining after controlling for age at lung cancer death, year of birth and cumulative exposure to radiation and smoking.

It is interesting to note that total number of packs of cigarettes smoked is the most useful single measure of smoking, in contrast to the British doctors study where risk was modelled in terms of the number of cigarettes smoked per day. In that study, however, absolute rates were modelled, whereas relative rates were modelled in the miners study. If, among continuing smokers, absolute risk is proportional to:

$$(\text{Cigarettes per day})(\text{Duration of smoking})^4$$

and the baseline rates are proportional to the fourth power of age, then simple calculations show that the relative risks in different age groups are approximately equal among people who have smoked the same total number of cigarettes (up to ten years before death). Assuming that smoking started at 20 years of age gives Table 6.5, in which column 3 gives rates at different ages for smokers who smoke the same number of cigarettes per day, and column 5 gives rates at different ages for smokers who have smoked the same total number of cigarettes, excluding the last ten years.

The relative risks in the last column, which relates to total amount smoked truncated ten years before death, are almost constant, whereas in column 4 the risks vary fourfold (see Table 2.6 of Volume 1). The range of ages covers the great majority of deaths seen in the miners study so that a one-parameter model using total dose

Table 6.5 Comparison of the relative risk of lung cancer at different ages for continuing smokers classified either by number of cigarettes smoked per day (columns 3 and 4) or by total number of cigarettes smoked (columns 5 and 6)

Age at death (years)	Rate among non-smokers	Rate among smokers (constant no. of cigs/day)	Relative risk (col. 3/col. 2)	Rate among smokers (constant total no. of cigs)	Relative risk (col. 5/col. 2)
(1)	(2)	(3)	(4)	(5)	(6)
40	$\alpha_1 4^4$	$\alpha_2 2^4$	$\dfrac{k}{16}$	$4\alpha_2 \cdot 2^4$	$\dfrac{k}{4}$
50	$\alpha_1 5^4$	$\alpha_2 3^4$	$\dfrac{k}{7.7}$	$2\alpha_2 \cdot 3^4$	$\dfrac{k}{3.9}$
60	$\alpha_1 6^4$	$\alpha_2 4^4$	$\dfrac{k}{5.1}$	$\dfrac{4}{3}\alpha_2 \cdot 4^4$	$\dfrac{k}{3.8}$
70	$\alpha_1 7^4$	$\alpha_2 5^4$	$\dfrac{k}{3.8}$	$\alpha_2 5^4$	$\dfrac{k}{3.8}$
80	$\alpha_1 8^4$	$\alpha_2 6^4$	$\dfrac{k}{3.2}$	$\dfrac{4}{5}\alpha_2 \cdot 6^4$	$\dfrac{k}{3.9}$

Where $k = \alpha_2/\alpha_1$

is sufficient to describe smoking-associated variation in relative risk for the entire cohort.

This example indicates that the metameter of dose to use to achieve the simplest explanation may differ depending on whether absolute or relative risks are being investigated.

The preceding examples have demonstrated the important role in determining risk that may be played by time since first exposure, age at first exposure, and duration of exposure. In terms of defining metameters of dose, both dose rate and cumulative dose can offer advantages, depending in part on whether absolute or relative risks are being described. The use of duration of exposure can be considered a surrogate measure of cumulative dose in studies in which dose levels are inadequately measured.

In these examples we have not emphasized time since exposure stopped as an independent time variable, and it can obviously be derived from time since first exposure and duration of exposure. There may, however, be occasions on which it is the variable of major interest as an indicator of the effect to be expected from intervention measures. At times, also, risk may be more appropriately modelled in terms of duration of exposure and time since stopping exposure, so that time since first exposure would enter into the model only as their sum. Thus, for example, if relative risks are being modelled, then the lung cancer–cigarette smoking relationship for ex-smokers might be more simply modelled in terms of time since quitting and cumulative amount smoked (see Table 6.1), rather than in terms of a model incorporating time since smoking started.

6.3 Multistage models of carcinogenesis

A conceptual framework that facilitates understanding of the relationship between the different variables discussed in the previous section is provided by multistage models of carcinogenesis. A number of different models have been proposed at one time or another; we concentrate mainly on one of the simplest – the Armitage-Doll model (Armitage & Doll, 1961). Some of the details of the model may be uninterpretable biologically, but the broad features have gained increasing biological and experimental support in the past decade. It is these features that have value as an interpretive tool in epidemiology. It is not our purpose here to review in detail the role of multistage models, or the experimental evidence supporting the nature of the different stages (see, for example, Börzsönyi et al., 1984). The aim of this section is simply to indicate the aid to interpretation that these models can bring.

The Armitage–Doll model supposes that a cancer arises from a single, originally normal cell, which undergoes a series of transitions, after the last of which it is capable of uncontrolled malignant replication. The number of cells at risk at the start is assumed to be large and the probability of a transition assumed to be small for any individual cell. Cells are assumed to be in the initial, i.e., normal, stage at time zero, and k transitions are assumed to be required for malignancy.

Suppose the probability of a transition from stage i to stage $i + 1$ in time interval t, $t + \delta t$ is given by $\lambda_{i+1}(t)\delta t$, and that all transitions are independent of each other. Then, denoting by $N_i(t)$ the number of cells in stage i at time t, we can write down an expression for the rate of change of $N_i(t)$ with time, namely

$$\frac{dN_i(t)}{dt} = \lambda_i(t)N_{i-1}(t) - \lambda_{i+1}(t)N_i(t)$$

for $i = t, \ldots, k$.

We assume that transitions are rare, and that at time $t = 0$

$$N_i(0) = 0 \qquad i \geqslant 1$$
$$N_0(0) = N.$$

Putting $N_i(0)$ greater than zero for $i > 0$ would be a way of modelling genetic predisposition to cancer, as proposed by Knudson (1971). Since transitions are assumed to be rare, good approximate solutions to this set of differential equations are given by the simpler set of equations

$$\frac{dN_i(t)}{dt} = \lambda_i(t)N_{i-1}(t) \tag{6.7}$$

for $i = t, \ldots, k$.

The degree of approximation involved in (6.7) has been discussed by Moolgavkar (1978). For many tissues, when exposure consists largely of the background common to most individuals in a particular society, the transition rates may vary little with time. We then have $\lambda_i(t) = \lambda_i$ and

$$N_i(t) \propto t^i$$

for $i = 1, \ldots, k$.

The probability that a cancer occurs is the probability of a transition from stage $k - 1$ to stage k. If the transition rates are constant, this probability is simply proportional to the number of cells in stage $k - 1$, so that the incidence rate at time t, $I(t)$ say, is proportional to $N_{k-1}(t)$, given by

$$I(t) \propto t^{k-1}. \tag{6.8}$$

As is well known, plotting the logarithm of incidence against the logarithm of age results for many tumours in a straight line with a slope of between 4 and 5 (see Volume 1, Chapter 2, page 61; and Cook *et al.*, 1969), indicating that (6.8) is a good description of the background age-specific rates for many tumours in a variety of different populations, with k equal to 5 or 6.

This simple multistage model gives a reasonable description of the epidemiology of many nonhormonally-dependent cancers of epithelial origin, and can be modified straightforwardly to incorporate age-dependent hormonal changes. More general models have been developed which take account of time-varying cell kinetics and which fit the epidemiological behaviour of a wider range of malignancies, described, for example, by Moolgavkar and his coworkers (e.g., Moolgavkar *et al.*, 1980), to which the reader is referred for further details. A review by Knudson (1985) gives a good description of the biological background.

We now turn our attention to the effect on cancer incidence of exposure additional to the background, to examine how the types of behaviour described in the previous section can be predicted by multistage considerations.

(a) *Implication for the effect on tumour incidence of exposures of limited duration*

The effect of changing exposures is to change the transition rates given in expression (6.7). Thus, suppose that, during an interval extending from time t_0 to time t_1, the transition rates increase from λ_i to $\lambda_i + \mu_i$, for $i = 1, \ldots, k$. The extent to which the transition rates are modified, given by the μ_i, can be taken to represent the mode of action of the exposure in augmenting risk for a cancer. For example, when studying the induction of tumours on mouse skin by initiation-promotion experiments, initiating agents would be associated with large values of μ_1, whereas promoting agents would be associated with relatively large values of μ_{k-1} or μ_k.

The cancer incidence rates in times after t_0 would then be proportional to $N_{k-1}(t)$, given by:

$$N_{k-1}(t) = N \int_0^t \lambda_{k-1}^*(u_{k-1}) \int_0^{u_{k-1}} \lambda_{k-2}^*(u_{k-2}) \cdots \int_0^{u_1} \lambda_1^*(u_1) \, du_1 \, du_2, \ldots, du_{k-1}, \tag{6.9}$$

where

$$\lambda_i^*(t) = \lambda_i + \mu_i \quad \text{for} \quad t_0 < t < t_1$$
$$= \lambda_i \text{ otherwise.}$$

This expression is a polynomial of degree $k - 1$ in t. Attempts have been made to fit explicitly these expressions both to experimental (Lee, unpublished data, as quoted by Whittemore & Keller, 1978) and to epidemiological data (Thomas, D.C., 1982). Since no specific meaning can be given to the individual parameters, and epidemiological data will hardly ever be extensive or detailed enough to permit much precision in joint inferences for the full set of μ_i, this approach has not been widely adopted. It has been more common to use expression (6.9) in a heuristic way, to examine the behaviour predicted by the Armitage–Doll model in a few simple situations with plausible biological interpretation and to assess qualitatively the concordance between the observed epidemiological behaviour and the various paradigms (Day & Brown, 1980). Examination of these simple situations also provides insight into which variables to use to describe the effect of time on risk.

In the experimental situation, the separate effects of initiation and promotion have been demonstrated in the development of tumours at many sites (Börzsönyi et al., 1984). Although these terms have specific meanings, which it would be hazardous to apply outside a well-defined experimental situation, one might interpret them as indicating in a more general sense the possibility of action at early or at late stages in the carcinogenic process. We therefore examine the effect on incidence rates that this multistage model would predict for agents which act predominantly at early stages and for agents which act predominantly at late stages. An interesting discussion of the relationship between the terms 'early-stage' and 'late-stage', as used by epidemiologists, and 'initiation' and 'promotion', as used by experimentalists, is given by J. Peto (1984).

We consider an early-stage agent to be one that affects only the first transition rate, i.e., only μ_1 is nonzero, and a late-stage agent as one for which only μ_{k-1} is nonzero. It should be noted that a late-stage agent is taken to affect not the last but the penultimate transition. An agent that alters the rate of transition into the cancerous state would have an immediate effect on cancer rates, which is rarely observed. An effect on the penultimate transition appears to correspond to more frequently observed behaviour. We take k equal to 5, as suggested by Cook et al. (1969), to examine arithmetically the predicted behaviour.

For an early-stage carcinogen, acting between times t_0 and t_1, we have, from expression (6.9),

(i) before exposure $(t < t_0)$,

$I(t) \propto t^4$. There is clearly no excess risk and the expression is the same as (6.8).

(ii) during exposure $(t_0 < t < t_1)$,

$I(t) \propto t^4 + \beta(t - t_0)^4$. The excess absolute risk is proportional to a power of *duration of exposure* (or, equivalently, time since first exposure); the excess relative risk is given by $\beta(1 - t_0/t)^4$, which rises slowly to its asymptotic value of β. (The quantity β represents the potency of the extra agent, relative to the background, and is given by the ratio μ_1/λ_1.)

(iii) after exposure $(t > t_1)$,

$I(t) \propto t^4 + \beta\{(t - t_0)^4 - (t - t_1)^4\}$. The excess absolute risk is dominated by the term $(t - t_0)^4$, proportional to a *power of time since first exposure*. The excess relative risk is dominated by the term $\beta(1 - t_0/t)^4$, as if exposure had continued. The effect of the term $(t - t_1)^4$ in reducing the excess relative risk comes into play only slowly.

For a late-stage carcinogen acting between times t_0 and t_1, we have

(i) before exposure $(t > t_0)$,

$I(t) \propto t^4$ when $t > t_0$, as before.

(ii) during exposure $(t_0 < t < t_1)$,

$I(t) \propto t^4 + \gamma(t^4 - t_0^4)$, where $\gamma = \mu_4/\lambda_4$ is the potency of the extra late-stage agent, relative to the background. The excess relative risk is given by $\gamma\{1 - (t_0/t)^4\}$, which rises rapidly to a plateau at the value γ.

(iii) after exposure $(t > t_1)$,

$I(t) \propto t^4 + \gamma(t_1^4 - t_0^4)$. The excess absolute risk remains indefinitely at a *constant value*. The excess relative risk falls proportionately to a power of t, after exposure stops at t_1. The greater the age at which exposure stops, the more gradual is this fall.

The different effects on subsequent incidence rates thus described are shown schematically in Figures 6.15A and 6.15B. In Figure 6.15A, the effect of starting a continuous exposure at age 30 years is shown for an early-stage and a late-stage agent. In Figure 6.15B, the effect is shown of stopping at age 40 an exposure that has been operating throughout life, contrasting the effects of early- and late-stage agents. Risk rises more slowly after exposure starts, and falls more slowly after exposure ceases. As might be expected, the effect of changing exposure to early-stage agents is greatly delayed compared to the effect of changing exposure to late-stage agents. Thus, intervening to reduce exposure to late-stage agents will have a relatively rapid effect, whereas permitting even short-term exposure to early-stage agents will have long-term consequences.

There are also differences between early- and late-stage agents in the effect of the age at which exposure starts, as can be seen by the expressions given above. For an early-stage agent, the absolute excess risk depends only on time since first exposure (for continuing exposures) and is unaffected by age at first exposure. Since the background rates are rising with age, relative risks decrease with age at first exposure. By contrast, for continuous exposure to late-stage agents, the absolute excess risk increases with a power of age, and the excess relative risk, proportional to $1 - (t_0/t)^4$ is roughly independent of age at first exposure once t is appreciably greater than t_0.

For an agent that affects both early- and late-stage transitions, acting between times t_0 and t_1, the behaviour is a mixture of the two simpler models, given as follows:

$$\text{before exposure } I(t) \propto t^4, \quad t < t_0,$$

$$\text{during exposure } I(t) \propto t^4 + \beta(t - t_0)^4 + \gamma(t^4 - t_0^4)$$
$$+ \beta\gamma(t - t_0)^4 \quad \text{for} \quad t_0 < t < t_1$$

$$\text{and after exposure } I(t) \propto t^4 + \beta\{(t - t_0)^4 - (t - t_1)^4\} + \gamma(t_1^4 - t_0^4)$$
$$+ \beta\gamma(t_1 - t_0)^4 \quad \text{for} \quad t_1 < t.$$

The last two expressions have terms for the early-stage effect, the late-stage effect and both effects acting together. Which term predominates depends on the relative magnitudes of the early-stage effect, β, and the late-stage effect, γ; but if both effects

Fig. 6.15 (A) Age-specific cancer incidence for a cohort continuously exposed to a carcinogen from 20 years of age. (B) Effect of stopping exposure at 20 years of age when carcinogenic exposure started at birth: age-specific incidence. From Day and Brown (1980)

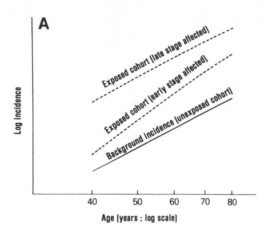

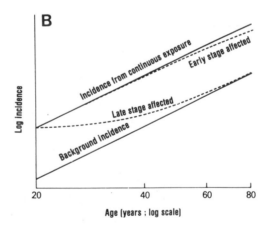

are appreciable then the combined effect, the term with $\beta\gamma$, would tend to dominate. In this case, while exposure lasts, the behaviour of the excess risk is dominated by the term $\beta\gamma(t-t_0)^4$, so that it resembles an early-stage agent. After exposure stops, the excess risk is dominated by the term $\beta\gamma(t_1-t_0)^4$, and so resembles a late-stage agent.

The distinguishing features of early- and late-stage agents, and those that affect both stages, are summarized in Table 6.6.

Table 6.6 Summary of the qualitative features of evolving risk following exposure to early-stage and late-stage carcinogens

	Early-stage	Late-stage	Both stages affected (about equally)
Evolution of risk during exposure	Time since first exposure of prime importance. Relative risk rises slowly to reach a plateau. Age at first exposure does not modify absolute excess risk. Relative risks decline with increasing age at first exposure, for given duration of exposure.	Age of primary importance. Relative risk rises rapidly to reach a plateau. Absolute excess risk increases with increasing age at first exposure. Relative risks nearly independent of age at first exposure, for given duration of exposure.	Behaviour may be more like an early-stage agent with main effect related to time since start of exposure (i.e., duration of exposure); absolute excess risk not related to age at start of exposure.
Evolution of risk after exposure stops	Absolute excess risk increases for many years as if exposure were continuous. Relative risk increases after exposure stops, then remains at a plateau.	Absolute excess risk remains constant at level attained when exposure stops. Relative risk declines rapidly.	Behaviour may be more like a late-stage agent with absolute excess risk remaining at level attained when exposure stopped, i.e., related to duration of exposure. Relative risk declines rapidly.

6.4 Interpretation of epidemiological data in terms of multistage models

One can now review some of the epidemiological behaviour described earlier in the chapter in the light of the multistage models of the preceding section. One should stress that the aim is not to classify the agent itself, but, more modestly, to indicate how the agent acts on a particular organ, in conjunction with whatever other carcinogenic factors may be present. Classification of carcinogens by their mode of action is still considered to be premature (IARC, 1983).

(a) Mesothelioma and asbestos

The induction of mesothelioma by asbestos corresponds closely to that expected from early-stage effects. The absolute excess risk is independent of the age at which exposure starts, and can be adequately described solely in terms of a power of time since first exposure (Peto, J. *et al.*, 1982).

(b) Lung cancer and smoking

The rates of lung cancer among smokers and ex-smokers are those to be expected if cigarette smoke affects both early and late stages. The absolute excess risk is well described in terms of a power of duration of exposure, both for those continuing to smoke and for those who have stopped smoking (Doll, 1971, 1978). A large case-control study has also shown that the greater the age at which smoking stopped, the smaller the fall in relative risk after quitting smoking (Lubin *et al.*, 1984).

(c) Lung cancer and asbestos

Asbestos behaves as a late-stage agent in the induction of lung cancer, the absolute excess risk rising rapidly with increasing age at first exposure and the relative risk remaining roughly constant. The risk increases much sooner after the start of exposure than does the risk for mesothelioma. The fact that the excess relative risk remains at roughly constant levels for several decades after external exposure stops is not consistent with a late-stage effect, but, as mentioned earlier, cessation of external exposure is not synonymous with stopping tissue exposure, since the asbestos fibres remain in the body.

(d) Radiation and breast cancer

The multistage models considered so far in this chapter have assumed homogeneity of the transition rates over age, implying that there is no age-related change in the susceptibility of the target tissue. This assumption must be relaxed for hormonally-dependent organs such as the breast. Modification of the assumption to incorporate the hormonal dependence of breast tissue leads to a model for breast cancer, which fits the epidemiological behaviour well (Moolgavkar *et al.*, 1980; Pike *et al.*, 1983). These modifications include decreasing susceptibility to early-stage effects with increasing parity, and hence in general with increasing age, and the existence of endogenous late-stage agents that are related to ovarian activity and so decrease at the menopause. The effect of short-term exposure to ionizing radiation is mainly that of an early stage agent, since susceptibility to early-stage events decreases with age. Thus the excess relative risk decreases with increasing age at exposure and, after exposure of short duration, rises to a plateau where it remains for at least 40 years. The excess risk induced by radiation increases more slowly with time the lower the age at exposure, and radiation-induced breast cancers occur only at ages when breast cancer arises spontaneously. Thus, for girls exposed when under ten years of age, the increase in incidence may take 30 years to become apparent, whereas for women over 30 years of age at exposure, an excess risk becomes appreciable within ten to 15 years. This effect of age may reflect the age-related changes in the strong endogenous late-stage factors.

6.5 Implications for the effect of dose on cancer incidence

(a) Form of the dose-response relationship

In the straightforward formulation of a multistage model given earlier, the incidence rate at age t is proportional to the product of the transition rates:

$$t^{k-1} \prod_{i=1}^{k} \lambda_i.$$

If the transition rates are increased by an additional exposure operating throughout life (λ_i increasing to $\lambda_i + \mu_i$), then the incidence rates will be proportional to

$$t^{k-1} \prod_{i=1}^{k} (\lambda_i + \mu_i). \tag{6.10}$$

It is often assumed that the transition rates are linearly related to dose rate, d, say, expressed, for example, in units of mg per kg per day; that is, one can express each μ_i as $\mu_i = \beta_i d$. This assumption has been the basis of much work on low dose extrapolation in the USA (Crump & Howe, 1984). The excess relative risk can then be expressed as a polynomial in dose rate of degree k or less with positive coefficients, at all ages. The excess absolute risk will, of course, increase steadily with a power of age.

Although fitting of low-order polynomials of dose rate is common practice, their uncritical use without prior examination of the general shape of the dose-response curve requires caution, for several reasons. First, most of the exposures in which we are interested are not continuous throughout life. They are often of limited duration, starting perhaps in early adult life, and, as seen in previous sections, the effect on excess risk may be more complex. Although for a given period of exposure the form of (6.9) indicates that the effect of dose is still through a low-order polynomial, the excess risk is dominated by the duration of the period of exposure and the age at which it occurred. Second, dose is seldom measured with great accuracy, and errors of measurement modify the observed dose-response relationship. More importantly perhaps, the observed exposure rates may be related only indirectly to tissue exposure rates. Thus, the dose-response of oesophageal cancer (see Volume 1, Chapter 6), and perhaps also bladder cancer, with cigarette smoking expressed in terms of cigarettes per day, appears to be sublinear, represented better by a square root transformation than by a low-order polynomial.

Third, the mechanism of action of the agent may be different from that assumed in this derivation of expression (6.10), and a dose-response curve of quite different shape may be appropriate. Two examples suffice to illustrate the point. The relative risk for oesophageal cancer rises exponentially with daily alcohol consumption (see Volume 1, Chapter 6). The mechanism of action of alcohol is at present unclear – apparently, it is not mutagenic and the oesophagus would probably not be exposed to its mutagenic metabolites, but it is difficult to see how an exponential dose-response would be generated by the mechanism described above. In the experimental field, the dose-response in CF1 mice (Tomatis *et al.*, 1972) relating hepatoma induction to DDT intake cannot be described in terms of a low-order polynomial with positive coefficients (see Fig. 6.16). Again, the mechanism of action of DDT as a carcinogen is not known; it may operate through modulations of enzyme systems. In order to determine whether unexpected behaviour of this type is occurring, plots of the risk against categorized levels of the exposure should be performed, to visualize the general shape of the dose-response curve, as stressed in Chapter 4.

(b) Metameters of dose suggested by multistage models when dose levels vary

For an exposure additional to background, which varies throughout life with intensity $f(t)$, the additional contribution to the incidence rate at time T depends on

Fig. 6.16   Prevalence of liver neoplasms among male CF1 mice fed differing doses of DDT. From Day (1985)

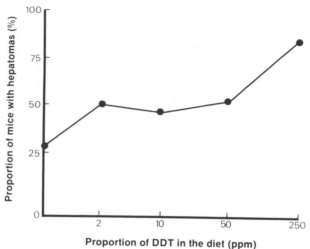

the mode of action. In terms of the Armitage–Doll model, if it affects only the first stage, it is given by

$$\int_0^T (T-t)^{k-2}f(t)\,\mathrm{d}t;\tag{6.11}$$

and if it affects only a late (penultimate) stage, it is given by

$$\int_0^T t^{k-2}f(t)\,\mathrm{d}t.\tag{6.12}$$

These two expressions clearly have different implications if one requires a simple summary measure of the excess exposure. In the first case, early exposure receives the heaviest weight, in the second case late exposure. The first expression (6.11) is in fact similar to (5.1), with a latency function $w(t-u)$ taken as a power of degree $k-2$. Peto, J. (1978) has proposed a weight function of this type for mesothelioma induction after asbestos exposure, with $k=4$ to give a quadratic. As we noted above, the epidemiology of mesothelioma induction fits well the description of early-stage action.

Functions other than a quadratic have been suggested to relate the incremental exposure to future incidence. The log-normal is one, with the rationale that cancers may have a 'latency period' which is log-normally distributed (Armenian & Lilienfeld, 1974; Thomas, D.C., 1982). The choice of a log-normal distribution appears to be based on an analogy with latent periods for infectious disease rather than a consideration of the process of carcinogenesis.

For late-stage agents, expression (6.12) above does not correspond to (5.1). Weight is given to recent exposure, since the late-stage agent acts on transitions that have already occurred. The concept of latency needs modification and cannot be simply expressed as a function such as (5.1).

For many agents, one might expect a mixture of early- and late-stage action (as seen for cigarette smoking). The appropriate weighting through the period of exposure would then be represented by a mixture of the two expressions above. In the absence of precise knowledge of the differential effects of the exposure on early and late stages, a rough approximation could be taken as constant weighting throughout the period, i.e., average dose rate, perhaps truncated some years before disease onset as in the analysis described earlier of the cohort of uranium miners.

(c) Effects of measurement error

The preceding discussion has assumed that exposure levels are measured without error. In many epidemiological situations, however, measurement error can be large. In cohort studies, one may be able to assume that the error distributions for cases and controls are the same, so that the unfortunate effects of differential misclassification are avoided. The effect of such errors on a single estimate of relative risk is to bias the estimate towards unity. The effect on dose-response curves, with categorized exposure data, is to decrease each point in the curve, so that the overall slope is lower. In addition, the curvature of the dose-response may be modified. The usual effect is to make the curve more concave downwards, or less convex upwards; for example, if a power of dose were to be fitted, the observed power would be less than the real power. Such an effect may be at the origin of the concave dose-response curves seen with regard to smoking for cancer of the bladder and of the oesophagus (see Fig. 6.17). Not only are smoking histories themselves in error, but it is also unclear how the effective dose should be measured. The correlation may not be high between the number of cigarettes smoked per day and the effective tissue exposure. Families of dose-response curves that allow for concavity of this type, such as

$$\text{Relative risk} = (1 + \beta \, \text{dose})^k \tag{6.13}$$

may therefore be appropriate.

It should be noted that the effect of misclassification is not always to induce greater concavity in the dose-response curve; the effect depends on the distribution of the exposure variable in the population. If the distribution is positively skewed, the curvature may increase; for example, a linear dose-response curve may appear convex upwards, or the estimate of k in the expression (6.13) may be biased upwards. Some examples are given in Table 1.10.

With the uncertainties surrounding the parametric form of dose-response curve that might be used, attempts have been made to develop nonparametric approaches to the estimation of a dose-response relationship. One method has been to assume nothing except that the relationship is monotone nondecreasing, and maximum likelihood can be used to estimate the best fitting nondecreasing curve. This approach has some appeal, its drawbacks being that monotonicity may not be a valid assumption, as in the leukaemia–radiation association, and that it does not provide a concise description of the data. This latter point will be particularly apposite when dose and time variables

Fig. 6.17   Relative risk for oesophageal cancer as a function of tobacco consumption.
            From Volume 1, p. 221

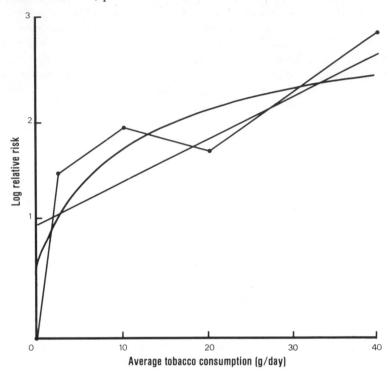

have to be considered jointly. A further advantage of the parametric approach is that
comparison between studies is facilitated.

(d) Implications for the joint effect of several exposures

With two agents, acting continuously, both of which affect some of the transition
rates, one can make a simple extension of expression (6.10). If the ith transition is
increased by μ_{1i} and μ_{2i} by the first and second agents respectively, then the incidence
at time t will be proportional to

$$t^{k-1} \prod_{i=1}^{k} (\lambda_i + \mu_{1i} + \mu_{2i}) \tag{6.14}$$

If the effect of both agents is confined to the same single transition, and if their
effects on this transition are independent, then the excess incidence at time t is simply
proportional to

$$(\mu_{1i} + \mu_{2i})t^{k-1},$$

the sum of the two separate effects. The joint action is additive.

If, on the contrary, the two agents affect different transitions, so that μ_{2i} is zero if μ_{1i} is non-zero, and *vice versa*, then the excess incidence will be proportional to the product of a term involving the μ_{1i} and a term involving the μ_{2i}, of the form

$$t^{k-1} \prod_{\substack{i \text{ for which} \\ \mu_{1i} \neq 0}} (\lambda_i + \mu_{1i}) \prod_{\substack{i \text{ for which} \\ \mu_{2i} \neq 0}} (\lambda_i + \mu_{2i}).$$

The joint effect is then multiplicative.

In all situations other than these two extremes, the joint effect will lie between the additive and multiplicative, provided that the transition rates are affected independently. On many occasions, of course, the assumption of independence would be questionable: a particular genotype might respond only to a specific exposure, one exposure might modify the enzyme systems mediating the effect of the second exposure, and so on. The issues are discussed by Siemiatycki and Thomas (1981). In simple terms, however, multistage models do suggest that both additive and multiplicative joint action are plausible models to investigate, at least initially.

6.6   Application to the analysis of the South Wales nickel refinery data

A number of papers have appeared in the past few years in which an epidemiological study is analysed to provide an interpretation in terms of multistage models (Brown & Chu, 1983a; Decarli *et al.*, 1985). We present here further analyses of the South Wales nickel workers study, extending those of Chapters 4 and 5. Interpretation of the results in terms of a multistage process derives principally from the variation of risk with a number of time variables, including time since first exposure, age at first exposure, duration of exposure and time since last exposure. Lack of information on exposure levels makes it difficult to ascertain when exposure started or stopped. We shall take time of first employment as an approximation to time of first exposure. From Table 4.24, it appears that little exposure to the agent of importance took place after 1925, which we shall take as the date at which exposure stopped. (This change corresponds to some of the process changes in the factory. In 1922, arsenical impurities were removed and respirator pads introduced, and in 1924 the calciners were altered to reduce dust emission. After 1932, the amount of copper in the raw material was reduced by about 90%, and the sulphur almost completely removed.) By the definition of the cohort, no one could have retired before 1925. All individuals thus have the same date of stopping exposure, and calendar time and time since last exposure are completely confounded. For this reason, the latter variable has not been considered as a separate risk-determining factor.

As described in Chapter 4, a case-control approach within a cohort was adopted to identify high-risk areas within the factory. The results are shown in Table 6.7 (Kaldor *et al.*, 1986), and the job categories classified as high risk are indicated. An exposure index based on years of employment in these job categories was constructed, as described in Chapter 4, and used as one of the four variables chosen for closer study, the other three being age at first employment, year of first employment, and time since first employment.

Table 6.7   Regression coefficients and standard errors (in parentheses) for duration in each job category, considering all categories simultaneously[a]

Category	Lung cancer	Nasal sinus cancer	Lung and nasal sinus cancer combined
Calcining I (general and furnace)	0.17[b] (0.052)	0.063 (0.075)	0.14[b] (0.042)
Calcining II (crushing)	0.27[b] (0.11)	0.081 (0.18)	0.21[b] (0.092)
Copper sulphate	0.094[b] (0.041)	0.070 (0.051)	0.087[b] (0.032)
Reduction	0.077[b] (0.043)	−0.030 (0.061)	0.039 (0.034)
Nickel sulphate	0.094 (0.059)	0.076 (0.070)	0.088[b] (0.046)
Furnaces	0.16[b] (0.058)	0.16[b] (0.071)	0.16[b] (0.046)
Concentrates	0.12[b] (0.067)	−0.054 (0.13)	0.067 (0.060)
Gas, steam and power production	0.024 (0.047)	−0.47 (0.19)	−0.047 (0.043)
General engineering	0.043 (0.048)	−0.021 (0.065)	0.021 (0.038)
General trades	−0.057 (0.049)	−0.10 (0.075)	−0.033 (0.040)

[a] From Kaldor et al. (1986)
[b] Ratio of the parameter to its standard error exceeds 1.645, indicating significance at the 0.05 level (one-sided test).

Two approaches were taken to describing the excess risk. One modelled the relative excess, giving parameters equivalent to SMRs, in terms of the expression

$$\lambda_k = E_k \cdot SMR_0 \exp(\boldsymbol{\beta}^T \mathbf{Z}_k), \tag{6.15}$$

where λ_k is the expected number of deaths in cell k, E_k is the expected number of deaths in cell k based on population rates, SMR_0 is the risk for the baseline category relative to the population rates (in this example given by the first level for each variable in Table 6.8), $\mathbf{Z}_k$ is a vector of indicator variables giving the value of each of the four exposure-related variables, and $\boldsymbol{\beta}$ is the vector of unknown parameters to be estimated. The elements of $\boldsymbol{\beta}$ correspond to the relative risks, or SMRs, associated with different levels of the exposure variables.

The second approach modelled the excess number of cases in each cell in terms of the number of person-years in that cell (P_k), the baseline rate (R_0) for the cell chosen as the reference and terms describing the relative effect on the absolute excess of the different levels of the exposure variables. Algebraically,

$$\lambda_k = E_k + P_k \cdot R_0 \exp(\boldsymbol{\beta}^T \mathbf{Z}_k). \tag{6.16}$$

In model 1, expression (6.15), the components of $\boldsymbol{\beta}$, when exponentiated, describe the relative effects of different exposure levels on the overall SMR for the cohort; in model 2, expression (6.16), the exponentiated components of $\boldsymbol{\beta}$ describe the relative effects of different exposure levels on the overall absolute excess mortality rate for the cohort, the EMR. Table 6.8 gives the results of fitting these two models for both lung and nasal sinus cancer, giving the estimated EMRs and SMRs associated with all four variables. For both cancers, there is a steady increase in risk with increasing exposure index, the increase being sharper for nasal sinus cancer. The effect of year of first employment,

Table 6.8   Estimated adjusted SMRs and EMRs for lung and nasal sinus cancer mortality[a]

Variable	Level	Lung cancer		Nasal sinus cancer	
		SMR[b]	EMR[b]	SMR[b]	EMR[b]
Age at first	<20	1.0	1.0	1.0	1.0
employment (years)	20–27.5	1.4	2.8[b]	3.3	5.1[c]
	27.5–35	1.3	2.9[b]	5.0[c]	10.9[d]
	35+	0.93	2.6	10.6[d]	36.6[d]
Year of first	<1910	1.0	1.0	1.0	1.0
employment	1910–1914	1.1	1.5	2.4[c]	2.4[c]
	1915–1919	0.57	0.95	2.9[c]	2.9[c]
	1920–1924	0.65	1.4	0.91	0.87
Exposure index	0	1.0	1.0	1.0	1.0
	1–4	1.9[d]	2.7[d]	4.7[d]	4.5[d]
	5–9	3.1[d]	4.4[d]	4.0[c]	3.9[d]
	10–14	2.6[d]	3.7[d]	12.7[d]	13.3[d]
	15+	4.2[d]	6.5[d]	20.5[d]	21.2[d]
Time since first	<20	1.0	1.0	1.0	1.0
employment (years)	20–29	0.74	2.8[c]	2.8	4.9
	30–39	0.47	4.9[d]	2.4	6.6[c]
	40–49	0.22[d]	4.8[d]	3.1	13.9[d]
	50+	0.11[d]	2.4	3.4	24.7[d]

[a] From Kaldor *et al.* (1986). Due to editing in progress, these analyses are based on a slightly modified version of the data given in Appendices VII and VIII. There are therefore some minor differences between this table and Table 4.25.
[b] Relative to the rate in the baseline category, which is arbitrarily fixed as 1.0
[c] Significantly different from the baseline at the 0.05 level of significance (two-tailed)
[d] Significantly different from the baseline at the 0.01 level of significance (two-tailed)

given the exposure index, is slight for both cancers. For age at first employment and time since first employment, however, the estimates are strikingly different for the two cancers.

The SMR for lung cancer varies little with age at first employment but decreases sharply with time since first employment – variables that can be considered as surrogates for age at first exposure and time since last exposure. The EMR, as a function of time since first employment, rises to a plateau then remains roughly constant. This behaviour of the SMR and the EMR corresponds well to that of a late-stage agent, as described in Table 6.6. There is some inconsistency with the behaviour of the EMR with age at first employment, which does not show the steady rise with age expected of a late-stage agent. The explanation may lie in changing underlying rates for lung cancer, since the relevant period is one in which the rate for lung cancer was increasingly rapidly. Those older at first employment would tend to have lower baseline rates.

For nasal sinus cancer, the EMR rises rapidly with time since first employment; the SMR rises initially and then plateaus. This behaviour corresponds to that of an early-stage agent. Both the EMR and SMR, however, rise steadily, the former more rapidly, with age at first employment, behaviour directly contrary to that predicted for an early-stage agent. This inconsistency may have arisen because age at first employment is still confounded with degree of exposure, even though an exposure index has been fitted in the model. In epidemiological data of this type, in which no concurrent measure of exposure is available, the retrospective construction of exposure indices may introduce problems of its own, and certainly cannot be guaranteed to summarize fully different exposures among individuals.

This example demonstrates that one cannot expect epidemiological observation to conform closely to the constraints of simple models, due, for example, to the effect of other variables for which there is no information, or to the inadequacy of exposure information for the variable of interest. The purpose of introducing multistage concepts is not to describe completely the complexities actually observed, but to explain, in terms of a fairly simple model of the carcinogenic process, major differences in behaviour.

7. DESIGN CONSIDERATIONS

CHAPTER 7

DESIGN CONSIDERATIONS

7.1 Introduction

In Chapter 1, we considered a range of questions concerned with the implementation of a cohort study. In this chapter, we concentrate on the more formal aspects of study design, in particular power, efficiency and study size. The design issues considered initially in this chapter are based, in large part, on the analytical methods of Chapters 2 and 3, comprising simple comparisons of a group with an external standard, internal comparisons within a cohort, and tests for trend using the approach of §3.6. Power considerations based on the modelling approach of Chapters 4 and 5 are only touched on.

The design of case-control studies is considered at some length. The motivation comes principally from the concept of risk-set sampling introduced in Chapter 5, but the results apply to general case-control studies. Topics discussed include the choice of matching criteria, the number of controls to select, and the effects that control of confounding or an interest in interaction will have on study size requirements. Attention is focused on the simple situation of one, or a small number, of dichotomous variables.

Two approaches are taken to the evaluation of different study designs; the first is based on calculation of the power function, the second is based on the expected standard errors of the relevant parameters. The power considerations are based on one-sided tests of significance unless specifically stated to the contrary, since in most studies the direction of the main effect of interest is an inherent part of the specification of the problem under study. The discussion of the design of cohort studies assumes that external rates are known, even though the analysis may be based on internal comparison and does not use external rates. The reason is evident – that evaluation of the potential performance of a study before it is carried out must be based on information exterior to the study. Since in this chapter all expected numbers are based on external rates, we have dispensed with the notation used in earlier chapters, where expected numbers based on external rates are starred.

It needs stressing strongly that power calculations are essentially approximate. The size, age composition and survival of the cohort will usually not be known with any great accuracy before the study is performed. In addition, calculations are generally based assuming a Poisson distribution for the observed events, since they derive from the statistical methods of Chapters 2 and 3. Many data may be affected by extra

Poisson variation, which will augment the imprecision in probability statements. Furthermore, the level of excess risk that one decides that it is important to detect is to some extent arbitrary.

7.2 Sample size for cohort studies – comparison with an external standard

This section considers the design of studies in which the total cohort experience is to be compared to an external standard. It is assumed that analyses are in terms of the SMR, with tests of significance and construction of confidence intervals following the methods of Chapter 2.

The number of deaths, D, of the disease of interest (or number of cases if cancer registry material is available) is to be determined in the cohort, and compared with the number expected, E, based on rates for some external population, whether national or local. The relative risk is measured by the ratio D/E, the SMR. Tests of significance for departures of the SMR from its null value of unity and the construction of confidence intervals were discussed in §2.3. The capacity of a given study design to provide satisfactory inferences on the SMR can be judged in two ways: first, in terms of the capacity of the design to demonstrate that the SMR differs significantly from unity, when in fact it does, and, second, in terms of the width of the resulting confidence intervals, and the adequacy of the expected precision of estimation.

The first approach proceeds as follows. For an observed number of deaths, D, to be significantly greater than the expected number, E, using a one-sided test at the $100\alpha\%$ level, it has to be greater than or equal to the α point of the Poisson distribution with mean E, a point that we shall denote by $C(E, \alpha)$. (For a two-sided test, α is replaced by $\alpha/2$.) Since the Poisson is a discrete distribution, the exact α point does not usually exist, and we take $C(E, \alpha)$ to be the smallest integer such that the probability of an observation greater than or equal to $C(E, \alpha)$ is less than or equal to α. Table 7.1 gives the value of $C(E, \alpha)$ for $\alpha = 0.05$ and 0.01, and a range of values of E. If, however, the true value of the SMR is equal to R, then the observed number of deaths will follow a Poisson distribution with mean RE. The probability of a significant result is then the probability that D, following a Poisson distribution with mean RE, is greater than or equal to $C(E, \alpha)$. For given values of E and α, this probability depends only on R. It is simple if somewhat laborious to calculate and is known as the power function of the study. Common practice is to choose a value of R that one feels is the minimum that should not pass undetected, and to calculate the power for this value. Table 7.2 gives the power for a range of values of E and R, for α equal to 0.05 and 0.01, respectively. The values in the column $R = 1$ are, of course, simply the probabilities of rejecting the null hypothesis when in fact it is true, and so give the real significance of the test, rather than the nominal 5% or 1%; one can see in Table 7.2a that they are all less than 5%, and in Table 7.2b all less than 1%.

Example 7.1

Suppose that with a given study cohort and the applicable mortality rates, there is an expected number of 20 deaths. Then, all observed values greater than or equal to 29 will be significant at the 5% level, and all values greater than or equal to 32 will be significant at the 1% level (Table 7.1). These are the values $C(20, 0.05)$ and $C(20, 0.01)$, respectively. If the true value of the relative risk is 1.5, then the true expected

Table 7.1   5% and 1% points of the Poisson distribution for different values of the mean. The numbers tabulated are the smallest integers for which the probability of being equalled or exceeded is less than 5% and 1% (designated $C(E, 0.05)$ and $C(E, 0.01)$), respectively.

Mean of Poisson distribution, E	$C(E, 0.05)$	$C(E, 0.01)$	Mean (E)	$C(E, 0.05)$	$C(E, 0.01)$
1	4	5	20	29	32
2	6	7	25	34	38
3	7	9	30	40	44
4	9	10	35	46	50
5	10	12	40	52	56
6	11	13	45	57	62
7	13	15	50	63	68
8	14	16	60	74	80
9	15	18	70	85	91
10	16	19	80	96	103
11	18	20	90	107	114
12	19	22	100	118	125
13	20	23			
14	21	24			
15	23	26			

Table 7.2   Comparison with an external standard

(a) Probability (%) of obtaining a result significant at the 0.05 level (one-sided) for varying values of the expected value E assuming no excess risk, and of the true relative risk R

Expected number of cases assuming no excess risk $(R = 1)$	True relative risk (R)									
	1.0	1.5	2.0	3.0	4.0	5.0	7.5	10.0	15.0	20.0
1.0	1.90	7	14	35	57	74	94	99	100	100
2.0	1.66	8	21	55	81	93	100			
3.0	3.35	17	39	79	95	99				
4.0	2.14	15	41	84	98	100				
5.0	3.18	22	54	93	100					
6.0	4.26	29	65	97	100					
7.0	2.70	26	64	98	100					
8.0	3.42	32	73	99	100					
9.0	4.15	38	79	100						
10.0	4.87	43	84	100						
11.0	3.22	39	83	100						
12.0	3.74	44	87	100						
13.0	4.27	48	90	100						
14.0	4.79	53	93	100						
15.0	3.27	49	92	100						
20.0	3.43	60	97	100						

Table 7.2   (*contd*)

Expected number of cases assuming no excess risk (R = 1)	True relative risk (R)									
	1.0	1.1	1.2	1.3	1.4	1.5	1.6	1.7	1.8	1.9
20.0	3.43	9	18	30	45	60	73	83	90	94
25.0	4.98	13	26	42	59	74	85	92	96	98
30.0	4.63	13	27	46	64	79	89	95	98	99
35.0	4.25	13	29	49	69	83	92	97	99	100
40.0	3.87	13	30	52	72	86	94	98	99	100
45.0	4.73	16	36	60	79	91	97	99	100	
50.0	4.24	16	37	61	81	93	98	99	100	
60.0	4.42	18	42	69	88	96	99	100		
70.0	4.48	19	47	75	92	98	100			
80.0	4.46	21	51	80	94	99	100			
90.0	4.39	22	55	83	96	99	100			
100.0	4.28	23	58	86	97	100				

(b) Probability (%) of obtaining a result significant at the 0.01 level (one-sided) for varying values of the expected value *E* assuming no excess risk, and of the true relative risk *R*

Expected number of cases assuming no excess risk (R = 1)	True relative risk (R)									
	1.0	1.5	2.0	3.0	4.0	5.0	7.5	10.0	15.0	20.0
1.0	0.37	2	5	18	37	56	87	97	100	100
2.0	0.45	3	11	39	69	87	99	100		
3.0	0.38	4	15	54	84	96	100			
4.0	0.81	8	28	76	96	99	100			
5.0	0.55	8	30	82	98	100				
6.0	0.88	12	42	91	99	100				
7.0	0.57	11	43	93	100					
8.0	0.82	16	53	97	100					
9.0	0.53	14	53	97	100					
10.0	0.72	18	62	99	100					
11.0	0.93	22	69	99	100					
12.0	0.61	20	69	100						
13.0	0.76	24	75	100						
14.0	0.93	28	80	100						
15.0	0.62	26	79	100						
20.0	0.81	38	91	100						

Table 7.2   (contd)

Expected number of cases assuming no excess risk (R = 1)	True relative risk (R)									
	1.0	1.1	1.2	1.3	1.4	1.5	1.6	1.7	1.8	1.9
20.0	0.81	3	7	14	25	38	52	66	77	86
25.0	0.92	3	9	19	33	49	65	78	87	93
30.0	0.97	4	11	23	40	58	74	85	93	97
35.0	0.98	4	12	27	46	65	81	91	96	98
40.0	0.97	5	14	31	52	71	86	94	98	100
45.0	0.93	5	15	34	57	76	89	96	99	100
50.0	0.89	5	17	37	61	81	92	97	99	100
60.0	0.78	5	19	43	68	87	96	99	100	
70.0	0.91	6	24	51	77	92	98	100		
80.0	0.76	6	25	55	81	95	99	100		
90.0	0.83	7	29	62	87	97	100			
100.0	0.88	9	34	68	91	98	100			

value will be $20 \times 1.5 = 30$. The probability that an observation from a Poisson distribution with mean 30 is greater than or equal to 29 is 60% (Table 7.2) and that it is greater than or equal to 32 is 38% (Table 7.2). There is thus 60% power of obtaining a result significant at the 5% level, and 38% power of obtaining a result significant at the 1% level, if the true relative risk is 1.5.

An alternative way of expressing the power of a study is to give the relative risk for which the power is equal to a certain quantity, such as 80% or 95%. Table 7.3 gives the relative risks for a range of values of E and of the power, for 0.05 and 0.01 levels of significance, respectively.

Example 7.1 (contd)

To continue the previous example, with E equal to 20, using a 5% significance test, 50% power is obtained if the relative risk is 1.43, 80% power if R is 1.67 and 95% power if R is 1.92. The corresponding figures for 1% significance are relative risks of 1.58, 1.83 and 2.09.

The values given in Tables 7.2 and 7.3 are based on exact Poisson probabilities. To calculate power values for other values of E and R, one can use one of the approximations to the Poisson distribution suggested in Chapter 2. For example, one can use expression (2.12), the square root transformation, from which the quantity

$$\chi = 2(D^{1/2} - E^{1/2})$$

is approximately a standard normal deviate. If Z_α is the α point of the normal distribution, then for D to be significant at the 5% level (one-sided as before) we must have

$$2(D^{1/2} - E^{1/2}) \geqslant Z_\alpha$$

or

$$D \geqslant \{E^{1/2} + (Z_\alpha)/2\}^2.$$

This value corresponds to the value $C(E, \alpha)$ of the discussion in the previous pages.

Table 7.3 Comparison with an external standard

(a) True value of the relative risk required to have given power of achieving a result significant at the 5% level (one-sided), for varying values of the expected value E assuming no excess risk (R = 1)

Expected cases (R = 1)	Probability of declaring significant ($p \leqslant 0.05$) difference				
	0.50	0.80	0.90	0.95	0.99
1.0	3.67	5.52	6.68	7.75	10.05
2.0	2.84	3.95	4.64	5.26	6.55
3.0	2.22	3.03	3.51	3.95	4.86
4.0	2.17	2.84	3.25	3.61	4.35
5.0	1.93	2.50	2.84	3.14	3.76
6.0	1.78	2.28	2.57	2.83	3.36
7.0	1.81	2.27	2.54	2.78	3.26
8.0	1.71	2.13	2.37	2.58	3.02
9.0	1.63	2.01	2.24	2.43	2.83
10.0	1.57	1.92	2.13	2.31	2.67
11.0	1.61	1.95	2.15	2.32	2.66
12.0	1.56	1.88	2.06	2.22	2.55
13.0	1.51	1.82	1.99	2.14	2.45
14.0	1.48	1.77	1.93	2.08	2.36
15.0	1.51	1.79	1.95	2.09	2.37
20.0	1.43	1.67	1.80	1.92	2.15
25.0	1.35	1.55	1.67	1.77	1.96
30.0	1.32	1.51	1.61	1.70	1.87
35.0	1.30	1.47	1.57	1.65	1.81
40.0	1.29	1.45	1.54	1.61	1.76
45.0	1.26	1.41	1.49	1.55	1.69
50.0	1.25	1.39	1.47	1.53	1.66
60.0	1.23	1.35	1.42	1.48	1.59
70.0	1.21	1.32	1.39	1.44	1.54
80.0	1.20	1.30	1.36	1.41	1.50
90.0	1.19	1.28	1.34	1.38	1.47
100.0	1.18	1.27	1.32	1.36	1.45

(b) True value of the relative risk required to have given power of achieving a result significant at the 1% level (one-sided), for varying values of the expected value E assuming no excess risk (R = 1)

Expected cases (R = 1)	Probability of declaring significant ($p \leqslant 0.01$) difference				
	0.50	0.80	0.90	0.95	0.99
1.0	4.67	6.72	7.99	9.15	11.60
2.0	3.33	4.54	5.27	5.92	7.29
3.0	2.89	3.79	4.33	4.81	5.80
4.0	2.42	3.13	3.55	3.93	4.70
5.0	2.33	2.96	3.32	3.64	4.30
6.0	2.11	2.65	2.96	3.24	3.80

Table 7.3 (*contd*)

Expected cases (R = 1)	Probability of declaring significant ($p \leqslant 0.01$) difference				
	0.50	0.80	0.90	0.95	0.99
7.0	2.10	2.59	2.88	3.13	3.64
8.0	1.96	2.40	2.66	2.89	3.34
9.0	1.96	2.38	2.62	2.83	3.26
10.0	1.87	2.25	2.48	2.67	3.06
11.0	1.79	2.15	2.35	2.53	2.90
12.0	1.81	2.15	2.35	2.52	2.86
13.0	1.74	2.07	2.26	2.42	2.74
14.0	1.69	2.00	2.18	2.33	2.63
15.0	1.71	2.01	2.18	2.33	2.62
20.0	1.58	1.83	1.97	2.09	2.33
25.0	1.51	1.72	1.84	1.95	2.15
30.0	1.46	1.65	1.76	1.85	2.03
35.0	1.42	1.60	1.69	1.78	1.94
40.0	1.39	1.55	1.64	1.72	1.87
45.0	1.37	1.52	1.61	1.68	1.82
50.0	1.35	1.50	1.58	1.64	1.77
60.0	1.33	1.46	1.53	1.59	1.70
70.0	1.30	1.41	1.48	1.53	1.64
80.0	1.28	1.39	1.45	1.50	1.60
90.0	1.26	1.37	1.42	1.47	1.56
100.0	1.25	1.34	1.40	1.44	1.52

When rounded up to the next integer value, one obtains exactly the same result as in Table 7.1 on almost every occasion.

If the true value of the relative risk is R, then the observation D will have a distribution such that

$$2\{D^{1/2} - (RE)^{1/2}\}$$

is a standard normal distribution. To achieve significance at the α level, we must have

$$D \geqslant \{E^{1/2} + (Z_\alpha)/2\}^2,$$

which will occur with probability β when

$$(RE)^{1/2} - (E)^{1/2} = (Z_\alpha + Z_{1-\beta})/2,$$

where $Z_{1-\beta}$ is the $(1 - \beta)$ point of the standard normal distribution. In other words, to have probability β of obtaining a result significant at the α level when the true relative risk is R, one needs a value of E equal to or greater than

$$(Z_\alpha + Z_{1-\beta})^2/4(R^{1/2} - 1)^2. \tag{7.1}$$

As can be simply verified, use of this expression gives values close to those shown in Tables 7.2 and 7.3. For example, with $\alpha = 1 - \beta = 0.05$, for which $Z_\alpha = Z_{1-\beta} = 1.645$, a value of R equal to 2.31 requires a value of E equal to 10.01 from expression (7.1), and a value of 10.0 from Table 7.3. Use of expression (2.11) based on the cube root transformation will give slightly improved accuracy for small values of E – say, less than 10 – whereas use of expression (2.10), the usual χ^2 statistic, will give somewhat less accurate results. Only for very small studies in which large relative risks are expected would the accuracy of the simple expression (7.1) be inadequate.

The other approach to assessing the capacity of a given study design to respond to the questions for which answers are sought is in terms of the expected widths of the resulting confidence intervals. These widths are given, in proportional terms, in Table 2.11. Given an expected number E based on external rates and a postulated value R for the relative risk, one can read off, from Table 2.11, the lower and upper multipliers one would expect to apply to the observed SMR to construct a confidence interval.

Thus, for $E = 20$ and for different values of R, we have the following 95% confidence intervals for R if D takes its expected value of RE:

	Lower bound	Upper bound
$R = 1.5$	1.01	2.09
$R = 2.0$	1.43	2.67
$R = 3.0$	2.29	3.81

The investigator would have to decide whether confidence intervals of this expected width satisfy the objectives of the study, or whether attempts would be needed to augment the size of the study.

For values of E and R not covered in Table 2.11, we can use as before the square root transformation (see expression 2.15). For a given value of E and R, the square root of the observed number of deaths, $D^{1/2}$, will be approximately normally distributed, with mean $(ER)^{1/2}$ and variance 1/4. The resulting $100(1 - \alpha)\%$ confidence intervals if D took its expected value would thus be given by

$$\{(ER)^{1/2} \pm Z_{\alpha/2}/2\}^2/E$$

or

$$R \pm Z_{\alpha/2}\left(\frac{R}{E}\right)^{1/2} + Z_{\alpha/2}^2/4E.$$

The upper limit is improved by incorporating the modification of (2.15), replacing R by $R(D + 1)/D$.

7.3 Sample size for cohort studies – comparison with an internal control group

In this section, we outline power and sample size determination when it is envisaged that the main comparisons of interest will be among subgroups of the study cohort, using the analytical methods of Chapter 3. We start by considering the simplest situation, in which the comparison of interest is between two subgroups of the study cohort, one considered to be exposed, the other nonexposed. Rates for the disease of interest are to be compared between the two groups. The situation corresponds to that of §3.4, with two dose levels. As argued in the preceding chapters, use of an internal control group is often important in order to reduce bias. Suppose that the two groups are of equal size and age structure, and that we observe O_1 events in one group (the exposed) and O_2 in the other. Since the age structures are the same, age is not a confounder, and no stratification is necessary. Following §3.4, inferences on the relative risk R are based on the binomial parameter of a trial in which O_1 successes have occurred from $O_1 + O_2$ observations, the binomial parameter, π say, and R being related by

$$R = \pi/(1 - \pi) \quad \text{or} \quad \pi = \frac{R}{(R + 1)}$$

as in expression (3.6).

Now if R is equal to unity, π is equal to $1/2$, and the test of significance can be based on the tail probabilities of the exact binomial distribution given by

$$\sum_{x=O_2}^{O_+} \binom{O_+}{x} 2^{-O_+},$$

where $O_+ = O_1 + O_2$. For a fixed value of O_+, the power of the study can be evaluated for different values of R, using the binomial distribution with parameter $R/(R + 1)$. O_+, however, is not fixed, but a random variable following a Poisson distribution with mean $E(1 + R)$, where E is the expected number of events in the nonexposed group. The power for each possible value of O_+ needs to be calculated, and the weighted sum computed, using as weights the corresponding Poisson probabilities. This weighted sum gives the unconditional power.

When the groups are of unequal size, but have the same age structure, a similar approach can be adopted. Suppose that E_1 events are expected in the exposed group under the null hypothesis, and that E_2 events are expected in the control group. Then, under the null hypothesis, the number of events in the exposed group, given O_+ the total number of events, will follow a binomial distribution with probability parameter $E_1/(E_1 + E_2)$. Under the alternative hypothesis with relative risk R, the binomial distribution will have parameter $RE_1/(RE_1 + E_2)$. The power can be evaluated for each value of O_+, and the weighted sum computed using as weights the probabilities of the Poisson distribution with mean $RE_1 + E_2$. Gail (1974) has published power calculations when E_1 equals E_2, and Brown and Green (1982) the corresponding values when E_1 is not equal to E_2. Table 7.4 gives the expected number of events in the control group, E_2, for power of 80% and 90% and significance (one-sided) of 5% and 1% for various values of R and of the ratio E_2/E_1 (written as k).

On many occasions, particularly when O_1 and O_2 are large, the formal statistical test is unlikely to be based on the binomial probabilities, but on a normal approximation using either a corrected or uncorrected χ^2 test.

In the case of equal-sized exposed and control cohorts, the observed proportion $p = O_1/(O_1 + O_2)$ is compared with the proportion under the null hypothesis, namely $1/2$, using as variance that under the null. The uncorrected χ^2 test statistic is equivalent to comparing

$$2\sqrt{O_+}(p - \tfrac{1}{2})$$

with a standard normal distribution.

Table 7.4 Comparison with an internal control group

(a) Expected number of cases in the control group required to detect a
difference with 5% significance and given power, for given relative risk,
when the control group is k times the size of the exposed group (using
exact Poisson distribution)

k^a	Relative risk[b]							
	2	3	4	5	6	8	10	20
1/10	11.3	3.86	2.16	1.47	1.10	0.712	0.528	0.212
	15.0	5.00	2.75	1.84	1.36	0.881	0.639	0.262
1/5	12.3	4.23	2.37	1.60	1.18	0.770	0.566	0.236
	16.2	5.45	3.03	2.03	1.50	0.958	0.696	0.283
1/2	15.1	5.18	2.85	1.93	1.45	0.954	0.706	0.299
	20.2	6.80	3.74	2.48	1.83	1.19	0.873	0.363
1	20.0	6.70	3.71	2.52	1.89	1.25	0.923	0.392
	27.0	8.89	4.90	3.27	2.43	1.58	1.17	0.485
2	29.6	9.91	5.40	3.58	2.59	1.63	1.19	0.498
	40.3	13.5	7.26	4.82	3.54	2.22	1.59	0.642
5	58.6	19.5	10.8	7.21	5.21	3.33	2.44	1.00
	80.1	26.3	14.5	9.76	7.19	4.50	3.25	1.33
10	107	35.0	19.5	13.0	9.52	6.00	4.29	1.67
	146	48.2	26.5	17.7	13.0	8.27	5.93	2.31

(b) Expected number of cases in the control group required to
detect a difference with 1% significance and given power, for
given relative risk, when the control group is k times the size of the
exposed group (using exact Poisson distribution)

k^a	Relative risk[b]							
	2	3	4	5	6	8	10	20
1/10	17.9	6.06	3.38	2.26	1.69	1.10	0.805	0.336
	22.5	7.51	4.12	2.76	2.03	1.30	0.952	0.387
1/5	19.4	6.55	3.63	2.44	1.82	1.19	0.864	0.275
	24.5	8.15	4.47	2.97	2.20	1.42	1.03	0.416
1/2	23.9	8.03	4.46	2.96	2.19	1.41	1.03	0.431
	30.3	10.0	5.57	3.69	2.70	1.73	1.25	0.508
1	31.2	10.5	5.73	3.82	2.85	1.87	1.38	0.567
	39.8	13.2	7.27	4.79	3.52	2.28	1.68	0.689
2	46.1	15.1	8.33	5.42	3.91	2.49	1.82	0.775
	59.2	19.4	10.6	7.02	5.08	3.17	2.29	0.946
5	90.5	29.2	15.9	10.6	7.76	4.80	3.41	1.38
	116	37.9	20.5	13.6	10.0	6.32	4.47	1.75
10	164	52.8	28.5	18.6	13.5	8.50	6.07	2.41
	213	69.0	37.3	24.3	17.7	11.2	7.98	3.15

[a] Ratio of E_2/E_1, where E_2 is the number of events expected in the control group and E_1
the number expected in the exposed group under the null hypothesis
[b] The top number corresponds to a power of 80% and the bottom to a power of 90%

Under the alternative of a relative increase in risk of R, p has mean $R/(R+1)$ and variance $R/\{O_+(R+1)^2\}$. The required sample size is then given by

$$O_+ = \frac{\left(\frac{1}{2}Z_\alpha + Z_{1-\beta}\sqrt{\dfrac{R}{(R+1)^2}}\right)^2}{\left(\dfrac{R}{R+1} - \dfrac{1}{2}\right)^2} = \frac{\{(R+1)Z_\alpha + 2Z_{1-\beta}\sqrt{R}\}^2}{(R-1)^2}. \tag{7.2}$$

When R is close to unity, approximate solutions are given by approximating $R/(R+1)^2$ by $1/4$ and rewriting the equation

$$O_+ = E_2(1+R) = (Z_\alpha + Z_{1-\beta})^2\left(\frac{R+1}{R-1}\right)^2.$$

When the two groups are of unequal size, n_1 and n_2, say, but the same age distribution, then we have

$$O_+ = \frac{\left(\sqrt{\dfrac{n_1 n_2}{(n_1+n_2)^2}}\, Z_\alpha + \sqrt{\dfrac{Rn_1 n_2}{(Rn_1+n_2)^2}}\, Z_{1-\beta}\right)^2}{\left(\dfrac{Rn_1}{Rn_1+n_2} - \dfrac{n_1}{n_1+n_2}\right)^2}. \tag{7.3}$$

Following Casagrande et al. (1978b) and Ury and Fleiss (1980), more accurate values are given by incorporating Yates' correction in the χ^2 significance test, which for groups of equal size results in multiplying the right-hand side of (7.3) by the term

$$\tfrac{1}{4}[1 + \sqrt{1 + 4(p_1 - p_2)/A}]^2,$$

where

$$A = \left(\tfrac{1}{2}Z_\alpha + \frac{\sqrt{R}}{(R+1)}Z_{1-\beta}\right)^2, \qquad p_1 = \frac{R}{R+1}, \qquad p_2 = \tfrac{1}{2}.$$

When the groups are of unequal size, n_1 and n_2, respectively, the corresponding correction factor is given by

$$\tfrac{1}{4}[1 + \sqrt{1 + A'}]^2,$$

where

$$A' = 2\left(\frac{Rn_1}{Rn_1+n_2} - \frac{n_1}{n_1+n_2}\right)\bigg/\left(Z_\alpha\sqrt{\frac{n_1 n_2}{(n_1+n_2)^2}} + Z_{1-\beta}\sqrt{\frac{Rn_1 n_2}{(Rn_1+n_2)^2}}\right)^2. \tag{7.4}$$

Table 7.5 gives the number of cases that would need to be expected in the nonexposed group for a range of values of the relative risk R, of the relative sizes of the exposed and unexposed group, and of α and β. The numbers are based on expression (7.3), modified by incorporating Yates' correction. The values in Table 7.5 are very close to the corresponding values based on exact binomial probabilities given in Table 1 of Brown and Green (1982). They are slightly smaller than the values in Table 7.4 for the more extreme values of R and of the ratio of the sizes of the two groups; the values in Table 7.4 took account of the Poisson variability of O_+.

Table 7.5 Sample size requirements in cohort studies when the exposed group is to be compared with a control group of k times the size. The numbers in the table are those expected in the control group (using χ^2 approximation)

	k	Relative risk				
		1.5	2.0	2.5	5.0	10.0
Significance, 5%	1.00	30.9	10.0	5.5	1.5	0.6
Power, 50%	2.00	43.7	13.7	7.3	1.9	0.7
	4.00	69.2	20.9	10.9	2.6	0.9
	10.00	145.6	42.8	21.7	4.9	1.7
	100.00	1292.6	370.1	184.4	38.9	12.3
	0.50	24.6	8.2	4.6	1.3	0.5
	0.25	21.4	7.3	4.1	1.2	0.5
	0.10	19.5	6.7	3.8	1.1	0.5
Significance, 5%	1.00	64.9	19.8	10.3	2.4	0.8
Power, 80%	2.00	95.4	28.7	14.8	3.3	1.1
	4.00	156.5	46.6	23.8	5.2	1.7
	10.00	340.0	100.5	51.1	11.2	3.5
	100.00	3094.3	911.3	463.0	102.0	33.0
	0.50	49.7	15.4	8.1	2.0	0.7
	0.25	42.2	13.2	7.0	1.7	0.6
	0.10	37.6	11.9	6.3	1.6	0.6
Significance, 5%	1.00	88.1	26.4	13.5	3.0	1.0
Power, 90%	2.00	131.1	39.0	19.9	4.3	1.4
	4.00	217.5	64.6	32.9	7.1	2.2
	10.00	477.1	142.0	72.4	15.8	4.9
	100.00	4374.8	1305.8	669.8	151.3	49.7
	0.50	66.7	20.1	10.4	2.4	0.8
	0.25	56.0	17.0	8.9	2.1	0.7
	0.10	49.7	15.2	8.0	1.9	0.7
Significance, 5%	1.00	110.0	32.6	16.6	3.6	1.1
Power, 95%	2.00	165.1	48.9	24.8	5.3	1.6
	4.00	275.8	82.0	41.7	8.9	2.6
	10.00	608.7	182.0	93.2	20.3	6.2
	100.00	5607.8	1689.6	872.6	200.7	66.7
	0.50	82.6	24.6	12.5	2.8	0.9
	0.25	69.0	20.6	10.6	2.4	0.8
	0.10	60.9	18.3	9.4	2.2	0.7
Significance, 1%	1.00	58.0	18.2	9.7	2.5	0.9
Power, 50%	2.00	81.7	24.6	12.7	3.1	1.1
	4.00	128.9	37.3	18.8	4.2	1.4
	10.00	270.5	75.5	37.0	7.6	2.4
	100.00	2394.9	649.1	310.2	58.0	16.7
	0.50	46.2	15.0	8.2	2.2	0.9
	0.25	40.3	13.4	7.4	2.1	0.8
	0.10	36.8	12.4	7.0	2.0	0.8

Table 7.5   (contd)

	k	Relative risk				
		1.5	2.0	2.5	5.0	10.0
Significance, 1%	1.00	103.2	31.2	16.1	3.8	1.3
Power, 80%	2.00	150.2	44.4	22.6	5.0	1.6
	4.00	244.2	71.0	35.7	7.6	2.4
	10.00	526.4	150.9	75.1	15.5	4.7
	100.00	4761.5	1352.1	688.4	136.4	41.4
	0.50	79.8	24.6	12.9	3.1	1.1
	0.25	68.1	21.3	11.3	2.8	1.0
	0.10	61.1	19.4	10.4	2.6	1.0
Significance, 1%	1.00	132.3	39.5	20.2	4.5	1.5
Power, 90%	2.00	194.7	57.3	29.0	6.3	2.0
	4.00	319.8	93.3	46.9	9.8	3.0
	10.00	695.8	201.7	101.0	21.0	6.3
	100.00	6338.3	1831.8	917.5	194.0	60.4
	0.50	101.2	30.6	15.9	3.7	1.3
	0.25	85.7	26.2	13.7	3.3	1.1
	0.10	76.4	23.6	12.4	3.0	1.1
Significance, 1%	1.00	159.1	47.1	23.9	5.0	1.7
Power, 95%	2.00	235.9	69.3	34.9	7.4	2.3
	4.00	390.2	114.1	57.4	12.0	3.6
	10.00	854.0	249.4	125.6	26.3	7.8
	100.00	7816.1	2286.2	1155.3	250.3	79.3
	0.50	120.8	36.1	18.5	4.2	1.4
	0.25	101.7	30.7	15.9	3.7	1.2
	0.10	90.3	27.5	14.3	3.4	1.2

Comparison of Table 7.5 with Table 7.2 indicates that, for given α, β and R, roughly twice as many cases must be expected in the nonexposed control group when an internal comparison group of equal size is used. Since there are two groups, this implies that roughly four times as many individuals must be followed. This increase represents the price to be paid for using internal rather than external comparisons.

Since power calculations are essentially approximate, an alternative and simple approach is obtained by using the variance stabilizing arcsin transformation, given by

$$\arcsin[\{O_1/(O_1 + O_2)\}^{1/2}].$$

This transformed variable is approximately normally distributed with variance equal to $1/\{4(O_1 + O_2)\}$. The mean if the two groups are of equal size is given by $\arcsin\{R/(R + 1)\}^{1/2}$.

Under the null hypothesis, R equals unity, so that a result significant at the α level is obtained if

$$\arcsin\{O_1/(O_1 + O_2)\}^{1/2} \geqslant \arcsin(\tfrac{1}{2})^{1/2} + 0.5Z_\alpha(O_1 + O_2)^{-1/2}.$$

If the relative risk among the exposed is equal to R, then this inequality will hold with probability at least β if

$$(O_1 + O_2) \geq (Z_\alpha + Z_{1-\beta})^2/4 \left\{ \arcsin\left(\frac{1}{R+1}\right)^{1/2} - \arcsin(\tfrac{1}{2})^{1/2} \right\}^2, \qquad (7.5)$$

whre $Z_{1-\beta}$ is the $(1 - \beta)$ point of the normal distribution.

This expression gives the total number of events expected in the two groups combined that are required to have probability β of achieving a result significant at the α level if the true relative risk is R. An approximation closer to the equivalent χ^2 test with the continuity correction is given if one adds a correction term to the arcsin transformation, replacing, for a binomial with proportion p and denominator n, $\arcsin(p)^{1/2}$ by $\arcsin(p - \tfrac{1}{2}n)^{1/2}$. In the present context n is given by $O_1 + O_2$, so that (7.5) would no longer give an explicit expression for E, but would require an iterative solution. Usually one iteration would suffice.

If the exposed and nonexposed groups are not of equal size, but the age distributions are the same, then a minor modification can be made to the above inequality. The binomial parameter, previously $R/(R + 1)$, now becomes $Rn_1/(Rn_1 + n_2)$, where n_1 and n_2 are the numbers of individuals in the two groups. Expression (7.2) then becomes

$$(O_1 + O_2) \geq (Z_\alpha + Z_{1-\beta})^2/4 \left\{ \arcsin\left(\frac{Rn_1}{Rn_1 + n_2}\right)^{1/2} - \arcsin\left(\frac{n_1}{n_1 + n_2}\right)^{1/2} \right\}^2.$$

When the age structures of the two groups are dissimilar, one could use the approach of §3.4 or §3.5, and replace n_1 and n_2 in expressions (7.3), (7.4) and (7.5) by E_1 and E_2, the expected number of cases in the two groups based on an external standard or on the pooled rates for the two groups. If the confounding due to age is at all severe, however, this procedure will suffer from appreciable bias, and one should use the preferred methods of §3.6, basing power considerations on the variance of the Mantel–Haenszel estimate of relative risk (expression 3.17) (Muñoz, 1985). The effect of confounding on sample size requirements is discussed in more detail in §7.7.

If more emphasis is to be put on the precision of estimates of relative risk, rather than on detection of an effect, then the width of expected confidence intervals is of more relevance. The equations given by (3.19) can be solved to give upper and lower limits, or alternatively one can use the simpler expression (3.18).

7.4 Tests for trend

The results of a cohort study will be more persuasive of a genuine effect of exposure on risk if one can demonstrate, in addition to a difference between an exposed and an unexposed group, a smoothly changing risk with changing exposure. It is thus important that the study be designed with this aim in view. Under favourable circumstances, one will have not just two groups – one exposed and one nonexposed – but a number of groups, each with different exposures. In the analysis of the results of such a study, the single most powerful test for an effect of exposure on risk will normally be a trend test. It will therefore be useful, when assessing the value of a given study design, to examine the power of a trend test. For the sake of simplicity, we consider the situation in which we have K exposure groups but no further stratification by age or other confounding variables. Using the notation of Chapter 3, we shall investigate the power of the test statistic (3.12), given by

$$\chi^2 = \{\sum x_k(O_k - \bar{E}_k)\}^2 / \{\sum x_k^2 \bar{E}_k - (\sum x_k \bar{E}_k)^2 / \sum \bar{E}_k\},$$

where the $\bar{E}_k$ are expectations based on external rates, but normalized so that

$$\sum \bar{E}_k = \sum O_k; \quad \text{i.e.,} \quad \bar{E}_k = E_k \frac{\sum O_j}{\sum E_j}.$$

For a one-sided test of size α for positive slope, and writing the denominator in the above expression as V, we need

$$\sum x_k(O_k - \bar{E}_k) \geq \sqrt{V} \cdot Z_\alpha \qquad (7.6)$$

to achieve significance.

V is given by

$$\{\sum x_k^2 E_k - (\sum x_k E_k)^2 / \sum E_k\} \frac{\sum O_k}{\sum E_k}$$

and so, being a multiple of $\sum O_k$, will have a Poisson distribution, multiplied by a scale factor involving the x_k and E_k. $V^{1/2}$ will then be approximately normal, with standard deviation given by 1/2 times the scale factor

If E_k are the expectations based on external rates, then the left-hand side of expression (7.6) can be written as

$$\sum_k O_k \left\{ x_k - \left(\sum_j x_j E_j / \sum_j E_j \right) \right\}.$$

In order to assess the probability that the inequality (7.6) will hold, we have to specify a range of distributions for the O_k alternative to the null distribution that $E(O_k) = E_k$ for all k.

A simple family of alternatives representing a linear trend in risk is given by

$$E(O_k) = (1 + \delta x_k)E_k,$$

from which we have

$$\text{Expectation } (\bar{E}_k) = E_k \left(1 + \frac{\delta \sum x_j E_j}{\sum E_j} \right).$$

The power is then given by the probability that the following inequality holds:

$$\sum O_k \{x_k - (\sum x_j E_j / \sum E_j)\} - Z_\alpha . \sqrt{V} \geq 0.$$

Writing

$$V = W \sum O_k,$$

where W is a function of the x_k and E_k, then under the family of alternative distributions given above, the left-hand side will have mean m approximated by

$$m = \sum \delta x_k E_k \{x_k - (\sum x_j E_j / \sum E_j)\} - Z_\alpha W^{1/2} \{\sum (E_k + \delta x_k E_k)\}^{1/2}$$

and variance s^2 by

$$s^2 = \sum (1 + \delta x_k) E_k \{x_k - (\sum x_j E_j / \sum E_j)\}^2$$

$$- Z_\alpha W^{1/2} \sum \delta x_k E_k \{x_k - (\sum x_j E_j / \sum E_j)\} (\sum E_k)^{-1/2} + z_\alpha^2 W / 4.$$

The power is then approximately the probability corresponding to the normal deviate $Z_{1-\beta}$ given by $m = s \cdot Z_{1-\beta}$.

An alternative approach to the power of tests for linear trend was given by Chapman and Nam (1968) based on the noncentral χ^2 distribution.

Example 7.2

We consider a hypothetical example, comparing power considerations based on a trend test with those based on two alternative dichotomizations of the data. Let us suppose that we have four exposure levels, 0, 1, 2, 3, and that the groups at each level are of the same size and age structure. Under the null hypothesis, they therefore have the same expected numbers of events, E, say, in each group.

We consider a family of alternative hypotheses in which the relative risk is given as above by

$$1 + \delta x_k,$$

where x_k takes the values 0, 1, 2, 3. Substituting into the expression for m and s^2 gives

$$5\delta\sqrt{E} = Z_\alpha\sqrt{(5 + 7.5\delta)} + Z_{1-\beta}\{(5 + 7.5\delta) - 5\delta E^{-1/2} Z_\alpha (5/16)^{1/2} + 5Z_\alpha^2/16E\}^{1/2},$$

an equation that can be solved for β given δ and E or, conversely, solved for E given δ and β.

It is interesting to compare the results of power calculations for the trend test to the results one would obtain by dichotomizing the data, grouping, for example, the two highest and the two lowest exposed groups. We would then have a relative risk between the two groups of

$$(2 + 5\delta)/(2 + \delta),$$

and each of the two groups would be twice the size of the original four groups.

Substituting these values in expression (7.5) gives

$$2E\left(1 + \frac{2 + 5\delta}{2 + \delta}\right) = (Z_\alpha + Z_{1-\beta})^2/4\left\{\arcsin\left(\frac{2 + 5\delta}{4 + 6\delta}\right)^{1/2} - \arcsin(\tfrac{1}{2})^{1/2}\right\}^2$$

(the 2 at the start of the left-hand side arises since we have the sum of two groups each of size E), again an equation that can be solved for either E or for β.

Alternatively, one could base power calculations on a comparison between the two groups with highest and lowest exposure, respectively, the risk of the former relative to the latter being $1 + 3\delta$.

The three approaches give the following result for the expected number E required in each group, using a test with $\alpha = 0.05$ and $\beta = 0.95$:

δ	Trend test	Dichotomy into two equal groups	Highest against lowest
0.25	46.8	66.2	51.6
0.5	14.6	22.9	16.4
1.0	5.0	9.5	6.0
2.0	1.8	4.9	2.4

The trend test is considerably more powerful in this example than the test obtained by dichotomizing the study cohort, and marginally more powerful than the simple test of highest against lowest.

7.5   Restriction of power considerations to the follow-up period of interest

The discussion so far has treated observed and expected deaths as if all periods of follow-up were of equal interest. Usually, however, one would expect any excess risk to be concentrated in particular periods of follow-up, as outlined in Chapter 6. The carcinogenic effect of many exposures is not seen for ten years or more since the start of exposure. One is clearly going to overestimate the power of a study if one groups together all person-years of follow-up. An example comes from a study of the later cancer experience among women diagnosed with cancer of the cervix (Day & Boice, 1983). The purpose of the study was to investigate the occurrence of second cancers induced by radiotherapy given for the cervical cancer. For this purpose, three cohorts were assembled: women with invasive cancer of the cervix treated by radiotherapy, women with invasive cancer of the cervix not treated by radiotherapy, and women with in-situ carcinoma of the cervix not treated by radiotherapy. Table 7.6 gives the woman-years in different follow-up periods for the three groups, and the expected numbers of cancers in the first group, excluding the first year, and excluding the first ten years of follow-up. One can see that in the in-situ group 90% of the person-years of follow-up occurred in the first ten years, with a corresponding figure of over 70% for the women with invasive cancer. This example is extreme in the sense that cohort membership for the invasive cases is defined in terms of a life-shortening condition,

Table 7.6a   Woman–years at risk by time since entry into the cohort (i.e., diagnosis of cervical cancer)

Time since diagnosis (years)	Invasive cancer		In-situ cancer
	Treated by radiotherapy	Not treated by radiotherapy	
0–9	445 990 (71%)	89 719 (74%)	485 026 (90%)
10–19	149 772	27 945	53 621
20+	29 676	3 961	2 265
Total	625 438	121 625	540 912

Table 7.6b   Expected number of second cancers at selected
sites among the radiation-treated group

	Excluding the first year of follow-up	Excluding the first ten years of follow-up
Stomach	210.4	86.1
Rectum	157.4	68.6
Breast	804.4	304.6
Multiple myeloma	33.9	14.8

and large-scale identification of in-situ cases by mass screening did not occur until the mid-1960s or later in many of the participating areas. For most of the cancers of interest, excesses were not seen until at least ten years after entry, so that power considerations based on the full follow-up period would seriously overestimate the potential of the study, especially in assessing the value of the in-situ cohort as a comparison group.

7.6   Case-control sampling within a cohort

(a) *Basic considerations of case-control design*: *dichotomous exposure – unmatched design*

Before discussing the specific issues of concern when sampling from a risk set in the context of §5.4, we review more generally design aspects of case-control studies. We begin with the simplest situation, of a single dichotomous exposure variable. The problem is that of comparing two independent binomial distributions, one corresponding to the cases, one to the control population, with binomial probabilities, respectively, of p_1 and p_2, say.

The approach to the comparison of two proportions that we have taken in these two volumes has been based on the exact conditional distribution of a 2×2 table, expressed in terms of the odds ratio. Tests of the null hypothesis were derived either from this exact distribution, or from the approximation to it given by the χ^2 test with continuity correction. Since sample size and power calculations should refer to the statistical test that is going to be used, most of the subsequent discussions of power refer to the exact test, or approximations to it.

When the samples of cases and controls are of the same size, n, say, then for a χ^2 test without the continuity correction the power and sample sizes are related by the equation

$$n = (Z_\alpha \sqrt{2\bar{p}\bar{q}} + Z_{1-\beta} \sqrt{p_1 q_1 + p_2 q_2})^2/(p_1 - p_2)^2, \qquad (7.7)$$

where α is the size of the test, β the power, p_1 the proportion exposed among the cases and p_2 the proportion exposed among the controls (and with $q_i = 1 - p_i$, $i = 1$, 2 and $\bar{p} = 1 - \bar{q} = (p_1 + p_2)/2$.)

Incorporating the continuity correction into the χ^2 test, to make it approach the exact test more closely, results in multiplying the right-hand side of (7.7) by the factor

(Casagrande *et al.*, 1978b)

$$\tfrac{1}{4}\{1 + \sqrt{1 + 4(p_1 - p_2)/A}\}^2,$$

where

$$A = (Z_\alpha \sqrt{2\bar{p}\bar{q}} + Z_{1-\beta} \sqrt{p_1 q_1 + p_2 q_2})^2.$$

From this expression, one can either calculate the power β from a given sample size, or the sample size n required to achieve a given power.

This result has been extended by Fleiss *et al.* (1980) to the situation of unequal sample sizes. If we have a sample of size n from the population of cases (with parameter p_1) and size nk from the controls ($0 < k < \infty$), then to have probability β of achieving significance at the α level, we need

$$n = A \cdot W / k(p_1 - p_2)^2,$$

where

$$A = \left(Z_\alpha \sqrt{(k+1)\bar{p}\bar{q}} + Z_{1-\beta} \sqrt{kp_1 q_1 + p_2 q_2} \right)^2,$$

$$W = \frac{1}{4}\left(1 + \sqrt{1 + \frac{2(k+1)(p_1 - p_2)}{A}} \right)^2,$$

and

$$\bar{p} = 1 - \bar{q} = (p_1 + kp_2)/(1 + k).$$

In any particular study, sample size considerations would normally be based on an estimate of p_2, the prevalence of the exposure in the general population, and a value R for the relative risk that the investigator feels it would be important not to miss. In terms of the previous discussion, we would then have

$$\frac{p_1(1 - p_2)}{p_2(1 - p_1)} = R$$

or $p_1 = Rp_2/(1 - p_2 + Rp_2)$.

Table 7.7 gives the required number of cases for a range of values of R, p_2, α, β and k, the ratio of the number of controls to the number of cases, for the χ^2 test with continuity correction. The values are close to those obtained using the exact conditional test (Casagrande *et al.*, 1978a).

An alternative, simple approximation is obtained using the variance stabilizing arcsin transformation, with which the sample size needed from each of the two populations to achieve one-sided significance at the α level with probability β is given by

$$n = (Z_\alpha + Z_{1-\beta})^2 / 2(\arcsin p_1^{1/2} - \arcsin p_2^{1/2})^2.$$

If there are nk controls and n cases, this expression becomes

$$n = (k + 1)(Z_\alpha + Z_{1-\beta})^2 / 4k(\arcsin p_1^{1/2} - \arcsin p_2^{1/2})^2. \tag{7.8}$$

Consideration has recently been given to exact unconditional tests for equality of two proportions (Suissa & Shuster, 1985), approximations to which would be given by the

Table 7.7 Unmatched case-control studies. Number of cases required in an unmatched case-control study for different values of the relative risk, proportion of exposed among controls, significance level, power and number of controls per case. The three numbers in each cell refer to case-control ratios of 1:1, 1:2 and 1:4.

(a) *Significance = 0.05; power = 0.80*

Relative risk	Proportion exposed in control group											
	0.01	0.05	0.10	0.15	0.20	0.25	0.30	0.40	0.50	0.60	0.70	0.80
1.5	6672	1415	763	550	448	390	356	325	325	352	419	571
	4901	1041	563	407	332	290	265	243	244	265	317	434
	4009	854	462	335	274	240	219	202	203	222	266	365
2.0	2087	449	246	181	150	133	123	115	119	133	162	226
	1512	327	180	133	110	98	91	86	89	100	123	173
	1220	264	146	108	90	81	75	72	75	84	104	146
2.5	1114	243	135	101	84	76	71	69	72	82	102	146
	799	175	98	74	62	56	53	51	54	62	78	112
	638	140	79	60	51	46	43	42	45	52	66	95
3.0	732	161	91	69	58	53	50	49	53	61	78	112
	521	116	66	50	43	39	37	37	40	47	59	86
	412	92	53	40	35	32	31	31	33	39	50	73
4.0	420	94	55	42	37	34	33	33	37	43	56	82
	296	67	39	31	27	25	24	25	28	33	43	64
	231	53	31	25	22	20	20	21	23	28	36	54
5.0	290	66	39	31	27	26	25	26	29	35	46	69
	203	47	28	22	20	19	19	20	22	27	36	54
	157	37	22	18	16	15	15	16	19	23	30	46
7.5	161	39	24	20	18	17	17	19	22	27	36	55
	112	27	17	14	13	13	13	14	17	21	28	43
	85	21	13	11	10	10	10	12	14	17	24	36
10.0	111	28	18	15	14	14	14	16	19	24	32	50
	77	20	13	11	10	10	11	12	14	18	25	39
	58	15	10					10	12	15	21	33
15.0	69	19	13	11	11	11	12	13	16	21	29	45
	48	13						10	12	16	22	35
	36	10							10	13	19	29
20.0	51	15	10	10		10	10	12	15	19	27	42
	35	10							11	15	21	33
	26									12	17	28

(b) *Significance = 0.05; power = 0.95*

Relative risk	Proportion exposed in control group											
	0.01	0.05	0.10	0.15	0.20	0.25	0.30	0.40	0.50	0.60	0.70	0.80
1.5	11381	2413	1301	938	763	665	606	553	553	600	713	974
	8527	1808	975	703	572	498	454	414	414	449	534	730
	7089	1503	811	585	476	415	378	345	345	374	445	607
2.0	3505	753	413	302	250	221	205	193	199	221	271	379
	2622	564	309	226	187	166	154	144	149	166	203	284
	2171	467	256	188	155	138	128	120	123	138	168	235

Table 7.7　(contd)

(b) Significance = 0.05; power = 0.95

Relative risk	Proportion exposed in control group											
	0.01	0.05	0.10	0.15	0.20	0.25	0.30	0.40	0.50	0.60	0.70	0.80
2.5	1852	403	224	166	139	125	117	113	119	135	169	241
	1383	301	167	124	104	93	88	84	89	101	126	180
	1140	248	138	103	86	77	73	70	74	84	104	149
3.0	1208	265	149	112	95	86	82	80	86	100	127	184
	900	198	111	84	71	64	61	60	64	75	94	137
	739	163	92	69	59	53	50	50	53	62	78	113
4.0	685	153	88	68	58	54	52	53	58	70	90	133
	509	114	66	50	44	40	39	39	44	52	67	99
	416	93	54	41	36	33	32	32	36	42	55	81
5.0	469	107	63	49	43	40	39	41	46	56	74	111
	348	79	47	36	32	30	29	31	34	42	55	82
	283	65	38	30	26	25	24	25	28	34	45	67
7.5	258	61	37	30	27	26	27	29	34	42	57	88
	191	45	28	22	20	20	20	21	25	31	42	65
	154	37	22	18	17	16	16	17	20	25	34	52
10.0	177	43	27	23	21	21	21	24	29	37	50	78
	131	32	20	17	16	15	16	18	21	27	37	57
	105	26	16	14	13	12	13	14	17	22	30	46
15.0	109	28	19	17	16	16	17	20	24	32	44	70
	81	21	14	12	12	12	12	14	18	23	32	51
	64	17	11	10		10	10	11	14	18	26	40
20.0	80	22	15	14	14	14	15	18	22	30	42	66
	59	16	11	10	10	10	11	13	16	21	30	48
	47	13						10	13	17	24	38

(c) Significance = 0.01; power = 0.80

Risk ratio	Proportion exposed in control group											
	0.01	0.05	0.10	0.15	0.20	0.25	0.30	0.40	0.50	0.60	0.70	0.80
1.5	10583	2245	1211	873	711	620	565	515	515	559	664	906
	7698	1638	887	642	524	458	419	385	387	422	505	693
	6247	1332	724	525	430	377	346	319	323	354	425	585
2.0	3266	703	386	283	234	207	192	181	186	207	253	354
	2328	504	278	206	171	153	142	135	140	158	194	274
	1851	403	224	166	139	125	117	112	117	133	165	234
2.5	1728	377	210	156	131	118	110	106	112	128	159	226
	1214	267	150	113	95	86	82	80	85	98	123	177
	950	210	119	90	77	70	67	66	71	82	104	151
3.0	1128	249	140	106	90	82	78	76	82	95	119	173
	784	175	100	76	65	60	57	57	62	73	93	136
	606	136	79	61	52	48	47	47	52	61	79	116
4.0	641	144	84	64	56	52	50	51	56	66	85	126
	439	100	59	46	40	38	37	38	43	51	67	100
	333	77	46	36	32	31	30	31	36	43	57	86

Table 7.7 (contd)

(c) Significance = 0.01; power = 0.80

Risk ratio	Proportion exposed in control group											
	0.01	0.05	0.10	0.15	0.20	0.25	0.30	0.40	0.50	0.60	0.70	0.80
5.0	440	101	60	47	41	39	38	40	45	54	70	105
	298	70	42	33	30	28	28	30	34	42	56	84
	223	53	32	26	24	23	23	25	29	35	47	72
7.5	243	58	36	29	27	26	26	28	33	41	55	83
	162	40	25	21	19	19	19	21	25	32	44	67
	119	30	19	16	15	15	16	18	21	27	37	58
10.0	167	42	27	23	21	21	21	24	28	36	48	74
	111	28	19	16	15	15	16	18	22	28	39	60
	80	21	14	13	12	12	13	15	18	24	33	52
15.0	104	28	19	17	16	16	17	20	24	31	43	67
	68	19	13	12	12	12	13	15	19	25	34	54
	49	14	10			10	10	12	16	21	29	47
20.0	76	22	16	14	14	14	15	18	22	29	40	63
	50	15	11	10	10	11	12	14	17	23	32	51
	35	11						11	14	19	28	44

(d) Significance = 0.01; power = 0.95

Risk ratio	Proportion exposed in control group											
	0.01	0.05	0.10	0.15	0.20	0.25	0.30	0.40	0.50	0.60	0.70	0.80
1.5	16402	3478	1875	1352	1100	959	874	797	797	865	1028	1404
	12155	2580	1393	1006	820	715	653	597	598	650	775	1060
	10016	2128	1151	832	679	593	542	496	498	542	647	886
2.0	5018	1078	591	433	359	317	294	276	285	317	388	543
	3686	794	437	321	266	236	219	207	214	239	293	412
	3007	649	358	264	219	195	181	172	178	199	245	345
2.5	2639	574	319	237	199	178	167	161	170	193	241	344
	1926	420	235	175	147	132	125	121	128	146	183	261
	1557	341	191	143	121	109	103	100	106	122	152	219
3.0	1715	377	212	160	135	123	116	114	123	142	180	261
	1245	275	156	118	100	91	87	86	92	107	137	199
	1000	222	126	96	82	75	71	71	77	89	114	166
4.0	968	217	125	96	83	77	74	75	83	99	128	189
	698	157	91	70	61	57	55	56	62	74	97	144
	554	126	73	57	50	46	45	46	52	62	81	120
5.0	662	151	88	69	61	57	56	58	66	80	105	157
	474	109	64	51	45	42	41	43	49	60	79	120
	373	86	51	41	36	34	34	36	41	50	66	99
7.5	362	86	52	43	39	37	38	41	48	60	81	123
	258	62	38	31	28	28	28	30	36	45	61	94
	200	48	30	25	23	22	23	25	29	37	50	78
10.0	248	61	38	32	30	30	30	34	41	52	71	110
	176	44	28	24	22	22	22	25	30	39	54	84
	136	34	22	19	18	18	18	20	25	32	44	69
15.0	153	40	27	23	22	23	24	28	34	45	62	98
	108	29	19	17	17	17	18	21	26	34	47	74
	82	22	15	13	13	13	14	17	21	27	38	61
20.0	111	31	21	19	19	20	21	25	32	41	58	92
	79	22	16	14	14	15	16	19	23	31	44	70
	60	17	12	11	11	12	12	15	19	25	36	57

χ^2 test without continuity correction. Sample sizes for the latter can be calculated directly from expression (7.7).

A comparison of the sample size requirements, for 80% power and a test at the 0.05 level, is given in Table 7.8, for the exact conditional test, the exact unconditional test, the χ^2 test with and without correction, and for the arcsin approximation. It is noteworthy that in each case the exact unconditional test is more powerful than the exact conditional test. At present, however, the advantages of working within a unified structure of inference based on Cox regression methods and conditional likelihood, of which the conditional exact test is an example, more than outweigh this slight loss of power.

(b) Basic considerations of case-control design: dichotomous exposure – matched design

In matched designs, two problems have to be faced: how many controls to choose per case, and how many case-control sets to include, given the number of controls per case. We consider the second question first.

For the sake of simplicity, we shall assume that each case is matched to the same number of controls, k, say. The method of analysis is described in Chapter 5 of Volume 1. When $k = 1$, a matched-pairs design, the analysis concentrates on the discordant pairs. Suppose we have T discordant pairs, among O_1 of which the case is exposed. If risk for disease is unaffected by exposure, then O_1 is binomially distributed with proportion $1/2$. If exposure increases the relative risk by R, then O_1 is binomially distributed with proportion $R/(R + 1)$. The situation is discussed in §7.3, and similar power considerations apply.

Expression (7.2), with the continuity correction factor and with $n_1 = n_2$, gives the number of discordant case-control pairs that will be required to detect a relative risk of R with probability β at significance level α. Table 7.5, based on expression (7.2) and in the context of a cohort study, gives the expected number of cases required in the nonexposed group. To obtain the expected number of discordant case-control pairs required in a 1:1 matched case-control study, which corresponds to the total number of cases in the exposed and nonexposed groups combined in the context of Table 7.5, the quantities in the part of Table 7.5 referring to equal numbers in the exposed and nonexposed groups must be multiplied by $(1 + R)$.

The total number of case-control pairs that is required must be evaluated. If, as in the previous section, the probability of exposure is p_1 among the cases and p_2 among the controls, then the probability of a pair being discordant is simply

$$p_1(1 - p_2) + p_2(1 - p_1).$$

In a situation in which a matched design is thought appropriate, the probability of exposure would vary among pairs. The above expression then, strictly speaking, requires integration over the distribution of exposure probabilities. For the approximate purposes of sample size determination, however, it would usually be sufficient to use the average exposure probabilities, $\bar{p}_1$ and $\bar{p}_2$. The number of matched pairs, M,

Table 7.8 Comparison of minimum sample sizes to have 80% power of achieving 5% significance for comparing two independent binomial proportions[a], for five different test procedures[b]

p_2	p_1	n_e	n_r	n_p	n_{as}	n^*
0.05	0.15	126	130	111	105	107
	0.20	67	72	59	55	56
	0.25	45	48	39	35	38
	0.30	34	36	28	25	28
	0.35	25	28	21	19	22
	0.40	20	22	17	15	18
	0.45	17	19	14	12	13
0.10	0.25	89	92	79	76	79
	0.30	56	58	49	47	49
	0.35	39	42	34	32	35
	0.40	30	31	25	24	26
	0.45	24	25	20	19	21
	0.50	19	20	16	15	17
	0.55	16	17	13	12	13
	0.60	13	14	11	10	10
0.15	0.30	106	108	95	94	96
	0.35	65	67	57	56	59
	0.40	46	46	39	38	40
	0.45	34	35	28	28	29
	0.50	26	27	22	21	23
	0.55	22	22	17	17	18
	0.60	17	18	14	13	14
	0.65	15	15	11	11	13
0.20	0.35	121	122	109	108	111
	0.40	73	74	64	64	68
	0.45	49	50	43	42	45
	0.50	36	37	31	30	32
	0.55	27	28	23	23	26
	0.60	23	23	18	18	20
	0.65	17	18	14	14	15
	0.70	15	15	12	12	13
0.25	0.40	132	133	120	119	123
	0.45	78	79	70	69	71
	0.50	54	53	46	46	48
	0.55	37	39	32	32	33
	0.60	30	30	24	24	26
	0.65	23	23	19	19	20
	0.70	18	19	15	15	17
	0.75	15	15	12	12	13

[a] From Suisa and Shuster (1985)
[b] n_e = Fisher's exact test; n_r = corrected chi-squared approximation; n_p = uncorrected chi-squared approximation; n_{as} = arcsin formula; n^* = unconditional exact test; p_2 = proportion exposed in control group; p_1 = proportion exposed among cases

Table 7.8   (contd)

p_2	p_1	n_e	n_r	n_p	n_{as}	n^*
0.30	0.45	142	141	128	128	132
	0.50	84	83	74	73	77
	0.55	55	55	48	48	50
	0.60	41	40	33	33	37
	0.65	31	30	25	25	27
	0.70	23	23	19	19	20
0.35	0.50	143	147	134	134	136
	0.55	85	86	76	76	79
	0.60	56	56	49	49	51
	0.65	41	40	34	34	37
0.40	0.55	144	149	136	136	144
	0.60	85	86	77	77	79

required is then given by

$$T/\{\bar{p}_1(1-\bar{p}_2)+\bar{p}_2(1-\bar{p}_1)\},$$

where T is the number of discordant pairs. Table 7.9 with $M = 1$ indicates the number of matched pairs required for different values of R, p_2, α and β.

For studies involving $1:M$ matching, the approach is similar, if more complicated. We use the data layout and notation of §5.14, Volume 1, as below:

		Number of controls positive			
		0	1	...	M
Cases	Positive	$n_{1,0}$	$n_{1,1}$	$n_{1,2}$	$n_{1,M}$
	Negative	$n_{0,0}$	$n_{0,1}$	$n_{0,2}$	$n_{0,M}$

and we write $T_i = n_{1,i-1} + n_{0,i}$.

The usual test of the null hypothesis without the continuity correction is

$$\chi = \frac{\left\{\sum_{m=1}^{M}\left(n_{1,m-1} - \frac{mT_m}{(M+1)}\right)\right\}}{\left\{\frac{1}{(M+1)^2}\sum_{m=1}^{M} T_m m(M-m+1)\right\}^{1/2}}, \qquad (7.9)$$

which, for significance at level α, we can write in the form

$$\sum_{m=1}^{M} n_{1,m-1} - E_{R=1}\left(\sum_{m=1}^{M} n_{1,m-1}\right) \geq Z_\alpha\left\{\text{Var}_{R=1}\left(\sum_{m=1}^{M} n_{1,m-1}\right)\right\}^{1/2}.$$

Under the alternative hypothesis of a non-null relative risk R, we have (see §5.3, Volume 1)

$$E_R(n_{1,m-1}) = \frac{T_m mR}{mR + M - m + 1}$$

Table 7.9 Matched case-control studies. Number of case-control sets in a matched case-control study required to achieve given power at the given level of significance, for different values of the relative risk and different matching ratios

M^a	Relative risk								
	1.5	2.0	2.5	3.0	3.5	4.0	4.5	5.0	10.0
Proportion exposed = 0.1; significance = 5%; power = 80%									
1	757	241	131	87	65	52	43	37	17
2	559	176	95	63	46	37	30	26	11
4	460	144	77	51	37	29	24	21	9
10	400	124	66	43	32	25	21	17	7
20	380	118	63	41	30	24	19	16	7
Proportion exposed = 0.1; significance = 5%; power = 95%									
1	1283	398	211	138	101	79	65	55	23
2	963	299	158	103	76	59	48	41	17
4	804	250	133	87	63	49	40	34	14
10	708	221	118	77	56	44	36	31	12
20	677	211	113	74	54	42	35	29	12
Proportion exposed = 0.1; significance = 1%; power = 80%									
1	1204	380	206	137	102	81	67	58	27
2	881	274	146	96	71	56	46	40	18
4	720	221	117	76	56	44	36	31	13
10	623	189	99	64	47	36	30	25	10
20	591	178	93	60	44	34	28	23	10
Proportion exposed = 0.1; significance = 1%; power = 95%									
1	1855	575	305	200	147	115	95	81	35
2	1380	425	224	147	107	84	69	58	24
4	1142	351	185	120	88	68	56	47	19
10	1000	306	161	105	76	59	49	41	16
20	953	292	153	100	72	56	46	39	16
Proportion exposed = 0.3; significance = 5%; power = 80%									
1	355	122	71	50	39	32	28	25	14
2	264	90	52	37	29	24	20	18	10
4	219	74	43	30	23	19	17	15	8
10	191	65	37	26	20	17	14	13	7
20	182	62	35	24	19	16	13	12	6
Proportion exposed = 0.3; significance = 5%; power = 95%									
1	602	201	114	79	60	49	42	37	19
2	452	152	86	59	46	37	32	28	14
4	377	126	72	49	38	31	26	23	12
10	331	111	63	43	33	27	23	20	10
20	316	106	60	41	32	26	22	19	10

[a] M = number of controls per case

Table 7.9 (*contd*)

M	Relative risk								
	1.5	2.0	2.5	3.0	3.5	4.0	4.5	5.0	10.0
Proportion exposed = 0.3; significance = 1%; power = 80%									
1	565	192	111	78	61	51	44	39	22
2	419	142	81	57	44	37	32	28	16
4	346	116	66	46	36	30	25	22	12
10	301	101	57	40	31	25	22	19	10
20	287	95	54	37	29	24	20	18	10
Proportion exposed = 0.3; significance = 1%; power = 95%									
1	870	291	165	114	88	72	62	54	29
2	651	217	123	85	65	54	46	40	21
4	540	180	102	70	54	44	38	33	17
10	474	157	89	61	47	38	32	28	15
20	452	150	84	58	44	36	31	27	14
Proportion exposed = 0.5; significance = 5%; power = 80%									
1	324	118	72	52	42	36	31	28	18
2	243	89	54	39	32	27	24	21	13
4	203	74	45	33	26	22	20	18	11
10	178	65	39	29	23	20	17	16	10
20	170	62	37	27	22	19	16	15	9
Proportion exposed = 0.5; significance = 5%; power = 95%									
1	550	195	115	83	65	55	48	42	24
2	413	147	87	63	50	42	36	32	18
4	344	123	73	52	41	35	30	27	15
10	302	108	64	46	36	30	26	23	13
20	289	102	61	43	34	29	25	22	13
Proportion exposed = 0.5; significance = 1%; power = 80%									
1	516	187	112	82	66	56	49	45	28
2	387	140	85	62	50	42	37	34	21
4	323	117	70	51	41	35	31	28	17
10	284	103	62	45	36	31	27	24	15
20	271	98	59	43	34	29	26	23	14
Proportion exposed = 0.5; significance = 1%; power = 95%									
1	795	282	167	120	95	80	69	62	36
2	597	212	126	91	72	61	53	47	28
4	498	177	105	76	60	50	44	39	23
10	437	155	92	66	52	44	38	34	20
20	417	148	88	63	50	42	36	33	19

Table 7.9   (*contd*)

M	Relative risk								
	1.5	2.0	2.5	3.0	3.5	4.0	4.5	5.0	10.0

Proportion exposed = 0.7; significance = 5%; power = 80%

M	1.5	2.0	2.5	3.0	3.5	4.0	4.5	5.0	10.0
1	417	160	100	75	61	53	47	43	28
2	316	122	77	58	47	41	37	34	22
4	265	102	65	49	40	35	31	29	19
10	234	91	57	43	36	31	28	26	17
20	224	87	55	42	34	30	27	25	16

Proportion exposed = 0.7; significance = 5%; power = 95%

M	1.5	2.0	2.5	3.0	3.5	4.0	4.5	5.0	10.0
1	707	263	161	118	95	81	71	64	39
2	531	199	122	90	73	62	55	49	30
4	443	166	102	75	61	52	46	41	25
10	390	146	90	66	54	46	40	37	23
20	372	139	86	63	51	44	39	35	22

Proportion exposed = 0.7; significance = 1%; power = 80%

M	1.5	2.0	2.5	3.0	3.5	4.0	4.5	5.0	10.0
1	663	252	157	117	96	83	74	67	44
2	504	193	121	91	75	65	58	53	35
4	424	163	103	78	64	56	50	46	31
10	376	146	92	70	57	50	45	41	28
20	360	140	88	67	55	48	43	40	27

Proportion exposed = 0.7; significance = 1%; power = 95%

M	1.5	2.0	2.5	3.0	3.5	4.0	4.5	5.0	10.0
1	1022	381	233	172	138	118	104	94	58
2	771	289	178	132	107	91	81	73	46
4	645	242	150	111	90	77	68	62	39
10	569	214	132	98	80	69	61	55	35
20	544	205	127	94	76	66	58	53	34

Proportion exposed = 0.9; significance = 5%; power = 80%

M	1.5	2.0	2.5	3.0	3.5	4.0	4.5	5.0	10.0
1	1045	417	268	205	170	148	134	123	83
2	798	322	209	161	134	118	107	98	68
4	674	275	179	139	116	103	93	86	60
10	599	246	162	125	106	93	85	79	56
20	575	237	156	121	102	90	82	76	54

Proportion exposed = 0.9; significance = 5%; power = 95%

M	1.5	2.0	2.5	3.0	3.5	4.0	4.5	5.0	10.0
1	1772	688	432	323	264	226	201	182	113
2	1331	519	327	246	202	174	155	141	90
4	1111	434	275	207	170	147	132	120	78
10	979	384	244	184	152	132	118	108	71
20	936	367	233	177	146	127	113	104	68

Table 7.9   (contd)

M	Relative risk								
	1.5	2.0	2.5	3.0	3.5	4.0	4.5	5.0	10.0

Proportion exposed = 0.9; significance = 1%; power = 80%

1	1663	657	421	320	266	232	208	191	129
2	1278	514	333	256	214	188	170	157	109
4	1086	442	289	224	188	166	150	139	99
10	970	399	262	204	172	152	139	129	92
20	932	384	254	198	167	148	135	125	90

Proportion exposed = 0.9; significance = 1%; power = 95%

1	2562	993	624	468	383	329	293	266	168
2	1942	760	481	363	299	259	231	211	137
4	1631	643	409	311	257	223	200	183	122
10	1445	573	367	279	232	202	181	167	112
20	1384	549	352	269	233	195	175	161	109

and

$$\mathrm{Var}_R(n_{1,m-1}) = T_m \frac{mR(M-m+1)}{(mR+M-m+1)^2}.$$

Sample size requirements are therefore determined from the equation

$$\sum_{m=1}^{M} \{E_R(n_{1,m-1}) - E_{R=1}(n_{1,m-1})\}$$

$$= Z_\alpha \left\{ \sum_{m=1}^{M} \mathrm{Var}_{R=1}(n_{1,m-1}) \right\}^{1/2} + Z_{1-\beta} \left\{ \sum_{m=1}^{M} \mathrm{Var}_R(n_{1,m-1}) \right\}^{1/2}. \quad (7.10)$$

This equation involves the quantities $T_1, \ldots, T_M$. The probability P_m that an individual matched set contributes to a specific T_m is given in terms of p_1 and p_2 by

$$P_m = Pr(\text{matched set contributes to } T_m)$$

$$= \binom{M}{m}(1-p_1)p_2^m(1-p_2)^{M-m} + \binom{M}{m-1}p_1 p_2^{m-1}(1-p_2)^{M-m+1}. \quad (7.11)$$

As in the case of matched pairs, for approximate sample size calculations we can use the mean values of p_1 and p_2 over all matched sets in this expression, rather than integrating it over the distribution of the p's over the matched sets. The quantities T_m in expression (7.10) are then replaced by NP_m, where N is the total number of matched sets and P_m is evaluated for the mean values of p_1 and p_2. Expression (7.10) can then be solved for N given α, β, p_1, p_2 and M.

More complex situations in which the number of controls per case varies can clearly be handled in the same way (Walter, 1980), with the numerator and denominator of (7.9) summed over all relevant sets. There is usually little point, however, in introducing fine detail into what are essentially rather crude calculations.

A continuity correction can be incorporated into the test given by expression (7.9) by subtracting one half from the absolute value of the numerator. The resulting sample sizes differ from those obtained by omitting the continuity correction by a factor A, given by

$$A = \tfrac{1}{4}\{1 + \sqrt{1 + 2(E_R - E_{R=1})/(Z_\alpha V_{R=1}^{1/2} + Z_{1-\beta} V_R^{1/2})^2}\}^2, \tag{7.12}$$

where

$$E_R = \sum_{m=1}^{M} E_R(n_{1,m-1})$$

and

$$V_R = \sum_{m=1}^{M} \mathrm{Var}_R(n_{1,m-1}).$$

Sample size calculations incorporating the continuity correction into the statistical test are comparable to the sample sizes given in Table 7.7 for unmatched studies.

Table 7.9 gives the number of matched sets required for a range of values of M, R, p_2, α and β using the continuity correction. The values can be compared with those in Table 7.7 for the number of cases required in unmatched analyses, to indicate the effect of matching on the sample size. As a case of special interest, we have included in Table 7.9 a large value of M. This corresponds to the situation in which one uses all available individuals as controls, of interest in the context of §5.4, where the entire risk set is potentially available.

We now turn to the question of how many controls should be selected for each case. There are several contexts in which this issue can be discussed, as outlined in Chapter 1. We may be in a situation, as in §5.4, in which all data are available and sampling from the risk sets is done solely for convenience and ease of computing. We should then want the information in the case-control series to correspond closely to the information in the full cohort, and we should select sufficient controls per case for the information loss to be acceptably small. Thus, in Table 7.9, we compare the power achieved by a given value of M with the value obtained when M is infinite, or, more generally, use expression (7.11) to evaluate the power (i.e., $Z_{1-\beta}$) for a range of values of M and R.

In other situations, the cohort may be well defined and the cases identified but information on the exposures of interest not readily available and the cost of obtaining it a serious consideration. One should then assess the marginal gain in power associated with choosing more controls.

On other occasions, as would arise in many conventional case-control studies, the investigator may be able to decide on both the number of case-control sets and the number of controls per case. The question would then be to decide on the optimal combination of controls per case and number of cases.

Several authors have considered optimal designs in terms of the costs of inclusion in the study of cases and controls (Schlesselman, 1982). On occasion, the separate costs of cases and controls may be available, and a formal economic calculation can then be made. The more usual situation, however, is one in which one wants to know the cost in terms of the number of individuals required in the study, for different case-control ratios. For example, the rate at which cases are registered may be a limiting factor, and one would like to assess the cost, in terms of the number of extra controls required, of reducing the duration of the study by half, i.e., halving the number of cases, keeping the power constant.

The values in Table 7.9 can be used to provide answers to all three of these questions.

7.7   Efficiency calculations for matched designs

As an alternative to the criterion of power to compare different designs, one can use the efficiency of estimation of the parameter of interest, given by the expectation of the inverse of the variance of the estimate. The parameter of interest is often taken as the logarithm of the relative risk. As a comparative measure, the efficiency has attractions, since interest is usually centred more on parameter estimation than on hypothesis testing. For parameter values close to the null, power and efficiency considerations give, of course, very similar results. For parameter values distant from the null, however, the two approaches may diverge considerably. Efficiency considerations have the additional advantage that, at least in large samples, they can be derived directly from the second derivative of the likelihood function evaluated at just one point in the parameter space (see §7.11).

(a) Relative size of the case and control series in unmatched studies

In the simplest situation, of a single dichotomous variable, the results of a case-control study can be expressed as

	Exposure		Total
	$+$	$-$	
Case	a	b	n_1
Control	c	d	n_2

If p_1 is the probability of exposure for a case, and p_2 the corresponding probability for a control, then

$$E(a) = n_1 p_1 \qquad E(c) = n_2 p_2,$$

and in large samples the variance of the estimate of $\log R$ is given by

$$\frac{1}{n_1 p_1} + \frac{1}{n_1(1 - p_1)} + \frac{1}{n_2 p_2} + \frac{1}{n_2(1 - p_2)}. \tag{7.13}$$

When n_2 is large compared to n_1, as it typically would be in a cohort study, the variance is dominated by the first two terms. If we write $n_2 = k n_1$, so that k is the number of controls per case, then we can clearly evaluate (7.13) for different values of

p_2, R and k. When the relative risk is close to unity, then the efficiency relative to using the entire cohort for different values of k is well approximated by $(1 + 1/k)^{-1}$. The relative efficiency with $k = 1$ is thus 50%, and with $k = 4$ is 80%. Clearly, the marginal increase in relative efficiency as k increases beyond 4 becomes slight, hence, the conventional dictum that it is not worth choosing more than four controls per case. This is true, however, only when the expected relative risk is close to unity. As the relative risk diverges from one, considerably more than four controls per case may be necessary to achieve results close to those given by the entire cohort. Figure 7.1A

Fig. 7.1 Efficiency of case-control designs for differing values of the relative risk for a single dichotomous exposure E

The efficiency of a design, defined as v_k/v_∞, where v_k represents the asymptotic variance of the estimated log relative risk when using k controls per case, depends on both the relative risk and the control exposure probability p_2. Efficiencies for unmatched designs were computed from the unconditional likelihood (A). From Whittemore and McMillan (1982). Efficiencies for matched designs were computed from the conditional likelihood, assuming control exposure probabilities p_2 are constant across matching strata (B). From Breslow *et al.* (1983)

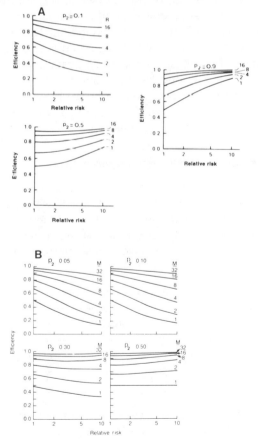

shows the change in efficiency for changing k, relative to using the entire cohort, for a number of values of p_2 and R.

(b) Number of controls per case in a matched study

With M controls per case and the layout of §7.6(b), the maximum likelihood equation for R is given by

$$\sum_{m=1}^{M} n_{1,m-1} = \sum_{m=1}^{M} \frac{T_m mR}{mR + M - m + 1}$$

(see §5.17 in Volume 1), from which the expectation of the inverse of the variance of $\log R$ is given by

$$[\text{Var} \log R]^{-1} = \sum_{m=1}^{M} \frac{T_m mR(M - m + 1)}{(mR + M - m + 1)^2}. \tag{7.14}$$

Using approximate values for T_m given by (7.11), we can evaluate this expression for given values of R, M and p_2. As in the previous paragraph, large values of M correspond to the inclusion of the entire risk set (see §5.4), and the relative values one obtains for small M give the relative efficiency of choosing a small number of controls per risk set. Results are given in Figure 7.1B, taken from Breslow et al. (1983), which can be compared with Figure 7.1A. From both figures it is clear that as the relative risk increases, for small values of p_2, a substantial loss is sustained by selecting only a small number of controls. When $R = 1$, one has the same result as in the previous section, that the efficiency relative to a large number of controls is given by $M/(M + 1)$. This result is a convenient rule of thumb when R is close to 1; but, as R increases, for many values of p_2 it becomes increasingly misleading.

7.8 Effect of confounding on sample size requirements

We now consider the effect on the required sample size if account must be taken of a confounding factor. We consider the situation in which we have a single polytomous confounding variable, C, which can take K different values. We assume that the situation is given by the following layout for each stratum, and for simplicity treat the case of equal numbers of cases and controls. We assume further that there is no interaction.

Exposure	Total control population	Stratum i (C takes value i)	
		Number of controls	Relative risk of disease
$E+$	nP	nPp_{1i}	$R_E R_{C_i}$
$E-$	$n(1 - P)$	$n(1 - P)p_{2i}$	R_{C_i}

where n is the total number of controls. Thus, R_E is the exposure-related relative risk for disease given C, R_{C_i} is the relative risk of the ith level of the confounder given E,

p_{1i} is the proportion of those exposed to E also exposed to C_i, p_{2i} is the proportion of those not exposed to E who are exposed to C_i, and P is the proportion exposed to E in the control population. We have taken $R_{C_1} = 1$.

When C is not a confounder, inferences on R_E can be based on the pooled table given by

	Case	Control
Exposed	nPR_E/Σ	nP
Not exposed	$n(1-P)/\Sigma$	$n(1-P)$

where $\Sigma = (PR_E + 1 - P)$.

For a given value of R_E, power β and significance α, the required number of cases is obtained by solving the equation

$$\log R_E = Z_\alpha \sqrt{V_N} + Z_{1-\beta} \sqrt{V_A}, \tag{7.15}$$

where V_N is the variance of the estimate of $\log R_E$ under the null hypothesis that $R_E = 1$, and V_A the equivalent variance with the given value of R_E. They are given when inferences are based on the pooled table by

$$nV_N = 4\Sigma[1/\{P(R_E + \Sigma)\} + 1/(1-P)(1+\Sigma)]$$

and

$$nV_A = \left(\frac{1}{P} + \frac{1}{1-P} + \frac{\Sigma}{PR_E} + \frac{\Sigma}{1-P}\right).$$

When C is a confounder, then stratification is required to give unbiased estimates of R_E. The variances in equation (7.15) now have to be replaced by the variances of the stratified estimate of R_E. An approximation to the variance of the Wolff estimate of the logarithm of R_E (see expression 3.16) which has often been used in the past (Gail, 1973; Thompson, W.D. et al., 1982, Smith & Day, 1984) is given by

$$V_W = \left(\Sigma \frac{1}{V_i}\right)^{-1},$$

where V_i is the variance of the logarithm of the odds ratio derived from stratum i (given by the expression from stratum i corresponding to V_N and V_A of the previous paragraph). V_W can be calculated for the null case ($R_E = 1$), $V_{W,N}$, say, and for values of R_E of interest $V_{W,A}$, say. We then solve for

$$\log R_E = Z_\alpha \sqrt{V_{W,N}} + Z_{1-\beta} \sqrt{V_{W,A}}.$$

Writing

$$\Sigma' = PR_E \sum_{i=1}^{K} p_{1i} R_{C_{2i}} + (1-P) \sum_{i=1}^{K} p_{2i} R_{C_{1i}}$$

we have

$$nV_{i,A} = \frac{1}{Pp_{1i}} + \frac{1}{(1-P)p_{2i}} + \frac{\Sigma'}{Pp_{1i} R_{C_i} R_E} + \frac{\Sigma'}{(1-P)p_{2i} R_{C_i}}$$

and

$$nV_{i,N} = T_i^3/W_{1i}W_{2i}W_{3i}W_{4i},$$

where

$T_i = W_{1i} + W_{2i} = W_{3i} + W_{4i}$

$W_{1i} = Pp_{1i} + (1 - P)p_{2i}$ = proportion of controls in stratum i

$W_{2i} = (Pp_{1i}R_{C_i}R_E + (1 - P)p_{2i}R_{C_i})/\Sigma'$ = proportion of cases in stratum i

$W_{3i} = Pp_{1i}(1 + R_{C_i}R_E/\Sigma')$ = proportion exposed in stratum i

$W_{4i} = (1 - P)p_{2i}(1 + R_{C_i}/\Sigma')$ = proportion nonexposed in stratum i.

In the situation with only two strata, extensive tabulations have been published (Smith & Day, 1984) for a range of values of P, p_{1i}, p_{2i}, R_E and R_C. Some of the results are given in Table 7.10. The main conclusion to be drawn is that, unless C and E are strongly related, or C strongly related to disease (meaning by 'strongly related' an odds ratio of 10 or more), an increase of more than 10% in the sample size is unlikely to be needed. An alternative approach is through approximations to the variance of estimates obtained through the use of logistic regression, which has been used to investigate the joint effect of several confounding variables (Day et al., 1980). Results using this approach restricted to the case of two dichotomous variables are also given in Table 7.10; for values of R_C near to one, the approximation is close to the approach given above. For several confounding variables that are jointly independent, conditional on E, as a rough guide one could add the extra sample size requirements for each variable separately.

7.9   Change in sample size requirements effected by matching

If a matched design is adopted, then equal numbers of cases and controls are included in each stratum. Usually, the numbers in each stratum would be determined by the distribution of cases rather than of controls (i.e., one chooses controls to match the available cases), so that they would be given by n times the W_{2i} of the preceding section. The computation then proceeds along similar lines to that of the previous section, and the sample size is given by

$$\log R_E = Z_\alpha\sqrt{V^1_{W,N}} + Z_{1-\beta}\sqrt{V^1_{W,A}},$$

where $V^1_{W,N}$ and $V^1_{W,A}$ correspond to $V_{W,A}$ and $V_{W,N}$ but with the constraint of matching. Alternatively, one can compare the relative efficiencies of matched and unmatched designs, in terms of the variance of the estimates. Table 7.11, from Smith and Day (1981), compares the efficiency of the matched and unmatched designs. The main conclusion is that unless C is strongly related to disease (odds ratio greater than 5) there is little benefit from matching. A similar derivation is given by Gail (1973).

Table 7.10 Increase in sample size required to test for a main effect if the analysis must incorporate a confounding variable. The ratio ($\times 100$) of the sample sizes, n_C and n, required to have 95% power to detect an odds ratio associated with exposure, R_E, at the 5% level of significance (one-sided) where n_C = sample size required allowing for stratification on confounding variable C and n = sample size required if stratification on C is ignored

P	p_1	p_2	R_{CE}	[a]	$R_E = 2.0$ $R_C=$ 1.0	2.0	5.0	10.0	$R_E = 5.0$ $R_C=$ 1.0	2.0	5.0	10.0	$R_E = 10.0$ $R_C=$ 1.0	2.0	5.0	10.0
0.1	0.5	0.5	1.0	100	100	102	113	124	100	102	113	124	100	102	114	125
	0.6	0.4	2.3	102	101	100	105	112	102	103	111	119	103	106	116	126
	0.7	0.3	5.4	107	109	103	103	107	112	111	117	123	116	119	130	139
	0.8	0.2	16.0	120	126	115	112	113	138	135	140	146	148	153	167	177
	0.9	0.1	81.0	164	185	164	154	154	223	218	225	234	256	269	297	315
0.5	0.5	0.5	1.0	100	100	102	114	125	100	102	114	125	100	102	113	123
	0.6	0.4	2.3	104	104	109	124	138	103	112	131	146	103	113	133	150
	0.7	0.3	5.4	119	118	127	149	166	117	133	163	187	115	135	170	197
	0.8	0.2	16.0	156	155	171	204	230	151	180	232	270	145	182	245	290
	0.9	0.1	81.0	278	275	310	378	431	264	331	443	523	248	330	465	561
0.9	0.5	0.5	1.0	100	100	102	113	124	100	102	111	121	100	101	109	117
	0.6	0.4	2.3	102	101	110	132	151	100	111	131	149	100	111	131	148
	0.7	0.3	5.4	107	105	123	159	192	103	123	161	193	102	124	162	194
	0.8	0.2	16.0	120	115	145	207	265	110	143	211	271	107	143	214	275
	0.9	0.1	81.0	164	148	203	327	456	134	193	328	466	125	187	328	470

P	p_1	p_2	R_{CE}	[a]	$R_E = 0.5$ $R_C=$ 1.0	2.0	5.0	10.0	$R_E = 0.2$ $R_C=$ 1.0	2.0	5.0	10.0	$R_E = 0.1$ $R_C=$ 1.0	2.0	5.0	10.0
0.1	0.5	0.5	1.0	100	100	102	113	124	100	102	111	121	100	101	109	117
	0.6	0.4	2.3	102	101	97	100	106	100	96	97	101	100	94	93	96
	0.7	0.3	5.4	107	105	95	92	94	103	92	86	87	102	89	81	80
	0.8	0.2	16.0	120	115	98	89	87	110	91	80	77	107	86	73	69
	0.9	0.1	81.0	164	148	118	100	94	134	101	81	75	125	91	70	64
0.5	0.5	0.5	1.0	100	100	102	114	125	99	102	114	125	100	102	113	123
	0.6	0.4	2.3	104	104	104	113	123	103	101	107	114	103	99	102	108
	0.7	0.3	5.4	119	118	116	123	132	117	109	109	114	115	104	100	102
	0.8	0.2	16.0	156	155	149	153	162	151	134	127	128	145	122	109	107
	0.9	0.1	81.0	278	275	258	259	270	264	221	196	192	248	194	159	149
0.9	0.5	0.5	1.0	100	100	102	114	125	100	102	113	124	100	102	113	124
	0.6	0.4	2.3	102	101	109	128	145	102	107	123	138	103	106	119	133
	0.7	0.3	5.4	107	109	122	152	180	112	120	142	165	116	119	135	154
	0.8	0.2	16.0	120	126	148	197	245	138	150	184	221	148	151	173	201
	0.9	0.1	81.0	164	185	224	319	421	223	244	307	381	256	259	296	349

[a] Approximation to $(n_C/n) \times 100$ based on the normal approximation to logistic regression $= 1/(1 - q^2)$, where q = correlation coefficient between E and C, $q^2 = P(1 - P)(p_1 - p_2)^2/\{(Pp_1 + (1 - P)p_2)(1 - Pp_1 - (1 - P)p_2)\}$. See Smith and Day (1984).

P = proportion of controls exposed to E;
p_1 = proportion exposed to E who were also exposed to C;
p_2 = proportion not exposed to E who were exposed to C;
R_{CE} = odds ratio measure of association between E and C

Table 7.11 Relative efficiency of an unmatched to a matched design, in both cases with a stratified analysis, when the extra variable is a positive confounder. The body of table shows the values of $100 \times V_{MS}/V_S$[a] (where MS = 'matched stratified'; S = 'stratified')

P	p_1	p_2	R_{CE}	$R_E = 2.0$ $R_C =$ 1.0	2.0	5.0	10.0	$R_E = 5.0$ $R_C =$ 1.0	2.0	5.0	10.0	$R_E = 10.0$ $R_C =$ 1.0	2.0	5.0	10.0
0.1	0.5	0.5	1.0	100	97	87	79	100	98	88	79	100	98	89	80
	0.6	0.4	2.3	99	91	78	69	98	90	78	70	98	91	79	71
	0.4	0.2	2.7	99	90	73	60	98	90	74	62	98	90	76	64
	0.8	0.6	2.7	99	92	84	80	98	91	84	79	97	91	84	79
	0.7	0.3	5.4	98	84	69	60	93	82	68	61	92	82	71	63
	0.9	0.1	81.0	89	69	51	43	79	66	53	47	80	71	62	57
0.3	0.5	0.5	1.0	100	97	87	79	100	97	87	80	100	97	88	81
	0.6	0.4	2.3	100	95	84	77	101	97	88	80	102	100	91	84
	0.4	0.2	2.7	100	96	83	71	101	99	88	76	102	102	92	82
	0.8	0.6	2.7	100	96	89	85	100	97	91	87	102	100	94	90
	0.7	0.3	5.4	99	93	82	74	102	99	89	81	107	106	96	88
	0.9	0.1	81.0	96	88	76	69	108	105	94	85	130	129	115	102
0.5	0.5	0.5	1.0	100	97	88	80	100	97	89	83	100	98	91	87
	0.6	0.4	2.3	100	99	90	82	101	100	93	87	102	101	96	91
	0.4	0.2	2.7	101	100	90	79	101	102	94	84	102	102	97	89
	0.8	0.6	2.7	100	99	93	89	101	100	96	93	102	101	98	95
	0.7	0.3	5.4	101	100	92	84	105	106	99	92	107	108	102	96
	0.9	0.1	81.0	106	107	98	90	129	133	121	108	152	157	139	122
0.7	0.5	0.5	1.0	100	97	88	82	100	98	91	87	100	99	94	91
	0.6	0.4	2.3	101	101	93	87	101	101	96	91	101	101	97	94
	0.4	0.2	2.7	101	102	95	84	101	102	97	89	101	102	98	93
	0.8	0.6	2.7	101	101	96	93	101	101	98	96	101	101	99	97
	0.7	0.3	5.4	102	105	99	92	104	106	102	96	103	105	102	98
	0.9	0.1	81.0	112	122	117	107	131	141	133	120	138	146	137	124
0.9	0.5	0.5	1.0	100	97	89	83	100	98	93	89	100	99	96	94
	0.6	0.4	2.3	100	102	96	90	100	101	97	94	100	100	98	96
	0.4	0.2	2.7	100	103	98	88	100	101	97	92	100	101	98	95
	0.8	0.6	2.7	100	102	98	95	100	101	99	97	100	101	99	98
	0.7	0.3	5.4	101	106	103	97	101	104	101	98	101	102	101	99
	0.9	0.1	81.0	109	125	128	120	112	122	122	116	109	115	115	111

[a] From Smith and Day (1981)

7.10 Interaction and matching

Occasionally, the major aim of a study is not to investigate the main effect of some factor, but to examine the interaction between factors. One might, for example, want to test whether obesity is equally related to pre- and post-menopausal breast cancer, or whether the relative risk of lung cancer associated with asbestos exposure is the same among smokers and nonsmokers. The basic question of interest is whether two relative risks are equal, rather than if a single relative risk is equal to unity. For illustrative purposes, we consider the simplest situation of two 2×2 tables, with a layout as before but restricted to two strata and with an interaction term, R_I, added.

Exposure	Proportion of population	Confounder	Proportion of population	Relative risk of disease
$E+$	P	$C+$	Pp_1	$R_E R_C R_I$
		$C-$	$P(1-p_1)$	R_E
$E-$	$1-P$	$C+$	$(1-P)p_2$	R_C
		$C-$	$(1-P)(1-p_2)$	1

If $\hat{\psi}_1$ is the odds ratio associating E with disease in the stratum with $C+$, and $\hat{\psi}_2$ the corresponding estimate in the stratum with $C-$, then

$$\mathrm{Var}(\log R_I) = \mathrm{Var}\{\log(\hat{\psi}_1/\hat{\psi}_2)\} = \mathrm{Var}(\log \hat{\psi}_1) + \mathrm{Var}(\log \hat{\psi}_2),$$

and the required sample size is given by the solution of

$$(\log R_I)^2 = (Z_\alpha \sqrt{V_N} + Z_{1-\beta} \sqrt{V_A}),$$

where V_N is the expected value of $\mathrm{Var}(\log R_I)$ in the absence of interaction, and V_A is the expected value of $\mathrm{Var}(\log R_I)$ at the value R_I. Some results are shown in Figures 7.2, 7.3 and 7.4. The most striking results are perhaps those of Figure 7.4, in which the

Fig. 7.2 Sample size for interaction effects between dichotomous variables. Size of study required to have 95% power to detect, using a one-sided test at the 5% level, the difference between a two-fold increased risk among those exposed to E and C and no increased risk among those exposed to E but not to C ($R_E = 1$; $R_I = 2$). The variable C is taken to be not associated with exposure ($p_1 = p_2 = p$) and not associated with disease among those not exposed to E ($R_C = 1$). From Smith and Day (1984)

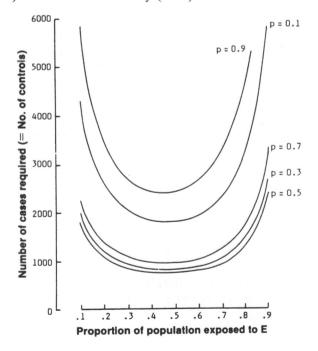

Fig. 7.3 Sample size for interaction effects between dichotomous variables. Size of study required to have 95% power to detect, using a one-sided test at the 5% level, the difference between no increased risk among those exposed to E but not to C ($R_E = 1$) and an R_I-fold increased risk among those exposed to both E and C. It has been assumed that 50% of the population are exposed to C ($p_1 = p_2 = 0.5$) and C is not associated with disease among those not exposed to E ($R_C = 1$). From Smith and Day (1984)

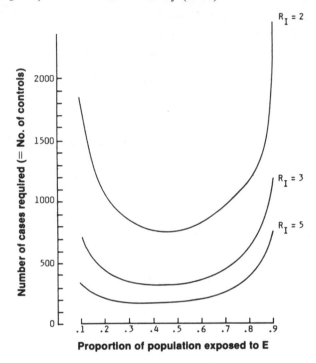

sample size required to detect an interaction of size R_I is compared to the sample size required to detect a main effect of the same size. The former is always at least four times the latter, and often the ratio is considerably larger. This difference can be seen intuitively, for, whereas

$$\text{Var}(\log R_I) = v_1 + v_2,$$

we have

$$\text{Var}(\log R_E) = v_1 v_2 / (v_1 + v_2), \quad \text{approximately,}$$

and the ratio $(v_1 + v_2)^2 / v_1 v_2$ is always greater than or equal to 4, increasing the greater the disparity between v_2 and v_1.

One might imagine that matching, by tending to balance the strata, would improve tests for interaction, but in general the effect is slight (Table 7.12). Matching can, on occasion, have an adverse effect.

Fig. 7.4 Ratio of sample sizes required to have 95% power to detect, using a one-sided test at the 5% level, (i) an interaction of strength R_I and (ii) a main effect of strength R_I (relative risk of R_E for exposure to E for both levels, assuming 50% of the population exposed to E, $p_1 = p_2 = p$ and C not associated with disease among those not exposed to E ($R_C = 1$)). From Smith and Day (1984)

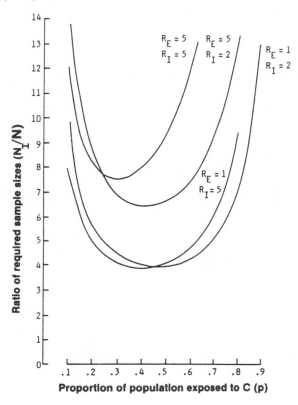

7.11 More general considerations

The previous sections have considered the simple case of dichotomous variables and power requirements for essentially univariate parameters. A more comprehensive approach can be taken in terms of generalized linear models. If interest centres on a p-dimensional parameter $\boldsymbol{\theta}$, then asymptotically the maximum likelihood estimate of $\boldsymbol{\theta}$, $\hat{\boldsymbol{\theta}}$, say, is normally distributed with mean $\boldsymbol{\theta}_0$, the true value, and variance covariance matrix given by the inverse of $I(\boldsymbol{\theta})$, the expected information matrix, the i,jth term of which is given by

$$-E\left[\frac{\partial^2 \ell(\boldsymbol{\theta})}{\partial \theta_i \, \delta \theta_j}\right], \qquad j = 1, \ldots, p,$$

Table 7.12 Effect of matching on testing for a non-null interaction. The ratio (×100) of the sample sizes, $n_I(MS)$ and $n_I(S)$ required to have 95% power to detect a difference at the 5% level of significance between an odds ratio associated with exposure E of R_E among those not exposed to C and an odds ratio for E of $R_E R_I$ among those exposed to C, where $n_I(MS)$ = sample size required in a matched stratified study and $n_I(S)$ = sample size required in an unmatched study[a]

P		$R_I = 2.0$						$R_I = 0.5$					
		$R_E = 1.0$			$R_E = 2.0$			$R_E = 1.0$			$R_E = 2.0$		
	$p_1(=p_2)$	$R_C = 1.0$	2.0	5.0	1.0	2.0	5.0	1.0	2.0	5.0	1.0	2.0	5.0
0.1	0.1	96	72	57	92	67	52	87	67	60	78	62	59
	0.3	98	93	107	96	93	112	96	102	135	96	109	158
	0.5	100	112	147	101	118	165	106	134	197	115	155	246
	0.7	102	129	176	106	141	207	116	164	244	133	200	315
	0.9	105	145	197	110	163	240	126	191	279	151	243	368
0.5	0.1	84	64	53	82	65	55	64	53	53	65	57	61
	0.3	93	92	107	93	93	109	92	101	126	95	106	125
	0.5	102	114	140	102	114	135	113	131	149	114	126	134
	0.7	109	130	158	110	128	148	128	144	154	124	130	131
	0.9	116	143	168	117	137	154	137	149	155	125	128	128
0.9	0.1	76	59	50	82	68	60	54	47	52	67	61	70
	0.3	90	91	107	94	95	107	91	103	120	99	110	121
	0.5	102	113	132	102	110	120	112	120	121	112	116	114
	0.7	111	126	144	108	116	123	117	118	115	112	111	107
	0.9	118	132	144	111	118	123	113	112	110	105	104	102

P		$R_I = 0.5$						$R_I = 0.2$					
		$R_E = 2.0$			$R_E = 4.0$			$R_E = 5.0$			$R_E = 10.0$		
	$p_1(=p_2)$	$R_C = 1.0$	2.0	5.0	1.0	2.0	5.0	1.0	2.0	5.0	1.0	2.0	5.0
0.1	0.1	105	73	48	110	72	46	126	77	43	151	89	46
	0.3	102	88	89	106	87	86	116	87	76	133	93	74
	0.5	100	102	123	101	101	125	106	97	111	115	98	106
	0.7	98	114	145	96	115	156	96	107	137	96	102	134
	0.9	96	124	158	92	127	178	87	115	152	78	106	156
0.5	0.1	116	88	62	117	93	67	137	115	80	125	115	90
	0.3	109	95	92	110	97	92	128	109	92	124	111	95
	0.5	102	101	116	102	100	112	113	101	103	114	103	100
	0.7	93	106	134	93	103	126	92	93	112	95	93	105
	0.9	84	111	147	82	106	137	64	84	119	65	81	109
0.9	0.1	118	98	74	111	99	81	113	111	98	105	106	99
	0.3	111	99	94	108	99	95	117	111	99	112	108	99
	0.5	102	100	112	102	100	106	112	103	100	112	104	100
	0.7	90	101	126	94	100	115	91	89	101	99	94	100
	0.9	76	102	138	82	100	123	54	71	103	67	79	100

[a] From Smith and Day (1984)

where $\ell(\boldsymbol{\theta})$ is the logarithm of the likelihood function. An overall test that $\boldsymbol{\theta} = \boldsymbol{\theta}_0$ is given by comparing

$$(\hat{\boldsymbol{\theta}} - \boldsymbol{\theta}_0)' I(\boldsymbol{\theta}_0)(\hat{\boldsymbol{\theta}} - \boldsymbol{\theta}_0) \tag{7.16}$$

with a χ^2 distribution on p degrees of freedom.

Power and sample size considerations are then approached through the distribution of the quadratic form (7.16) under alternative values for the true value of $\boldsymbol{\theta}$. In the general case, for an alternative $\boldsymbol{\theta}_1$, $\hat{\boldsymbol{\theta}}$ will have mean $\boldsymbol{\theta}_1$ and variance–covariance matrix $I^{-1}(\boldsymbol{\theta}_1)$, which will differ from $I^{-1}(\boldsymbol{\theta}_0)$. Power calculations will then require evaluation of the probability that a general quadratic form exceeds a certain value, necessitating direct numerical integration. Some special situations, however, give more tractable results. Whittemore (1981), for example, has given a sample size formula for the case of multiple logistic regression with rare outcomes. In the univariate case, expression (7.16) leads directly to the following relationship between sample size N and power β:

$$N = \{Z_\alpha I^{-1/2}(\theta_0) + Z_{1-\beta} I^{-1/2}(\theta_1)\}/(\theta_1 - \theta_0)^2,$$

where now I refers to the expected information in a single observation.

Table 7.13 Degree of approximation in sample size calculation assuming that the test statistic has the same variance under the alternative as under the null hypothesis – example of an unmatched case-control study with no continuity correction in the test statistic; equal number of cases and controls. Significance = 0.05; power = 0.80

(a) Sample sizes calculated using expression (7.7), without the continuity correction

Proportion exposed in control population	Relative risk				
	1.5	2.0	2.5	5.0	10.0
0.1	717	223	119	32	13.5
0.3	334	111	62	20	10.6
0.5	305	107	63	24	14.3
0.7	393	146	90	38	25
0.9	992	387	247	114	81

(b) Sample sizes calculated using expression (7.17)

Proportion exposed in control population	Relative risk				
	1.5	2.0	2.5	5.0	10.0
0.1	764	247	136	40	19.0
0.3	357	124	72	26	15.4
0.5	325	120	73	30	20.0
0.7	420	163	103	74	33
0.9	1056	430	282	140	103

More generally, in the multivariate situation, asymptotically only alternatives close to θ_0 are of interest, since power for distant alternatives will approach 100%. One can then take $I(\theta_1)$ to be approximately the same as $I(\theta_0)$. Under the alternative hypothesis, the statistic

$$(\hat{\theta} - \theta_0)'I(\theta_0)(\hat{\theta} - \theta_0)$$

will then follow a noncentral χ^2 distribution on p degrees of freedom, with noncentrality parameter

$$(\theta_1 - \theta_0)'I(\theta_0)(\theta_1 - \theta_0),$$

and the power will be given by the probability that this noncentral χ^2 distribution exceeds the α point of the central χ^2 distribution on p degrees of freedom. Greenland (1985) discusses this approach in a number of situations.

An example of the degree of approximation used in this approach is given in Table 7.13, for unmatched case-control studies without the continuity correction. The relationship between power and sample size provided by this approach is, using the notation of expression (7.7),

$$n = (Z_\alpha\sqrt{2\bar{p}\bar{q}} + Z_{1-\beta}\sqrt{2\bar{p}\bar{q}})/(p_1 - p_2)^2. \tag{7.17}$$

In Table 7.13, the results of using this expression in place of (7.7) are compared, no continuity correction being used in the latter. For moderate values of the relative risk, the difference is some 5% to 10%; for values of the relative risk of 5 or greater, the approximation can overestimate the required sample size by as much as 50%.

Since, on many occasions, the likelihood function and its derivatives take relatively simple values under the null hypothesis, this approach clearly has considerable utility when interest centres mainly on detecting weak or moderate excess risks.

REFERENCES

REFERENCES

Acheson, E.D. & Gardner, M.J. (1980) *Asbestos: scientific basis for environmental control of fibres*. In: Wagner, J.C., ed., *Biological Effects of Mineral Fibres* (*IARC Scientific Publications No. 30*), Lyon, International Agency for Research on Cancer, pp. 737–754

Adelhardt, M., Møller Jensen, O. & Sand Hansen, H. (1985) Cancer of the larynx, pharynx and oesophagus in relation to alcohol and tobacco consumption among Danish brewery workers. *Dan. med. Bull.*, **32**, 119–123

Andersen, P.K. & Gill, R.D. (1982) Cox's regression model for counting processes: a large sample study. *Ann. Statist.*, **10**, 1110–1120

Andersen, P.K. & Rasmussen, N.K. (1982) *Admissions to Psychiatric Hospitals among Women Giving Birth and Women Having Induced Abortion. A Statistical Analysis of a Counting Process Model.* Unpublished technical report from Statistical Research Unit, Copenhagen

Andersen, P.K., Borch–Johnsen, K., Deckert, T., Green, A., Hougaard, P., Keiding, N. & Kreiner, S. (1985) A Cox regression model for the relative mortality and its application to diabetes mellitus survival data. *Biometrics*, **41**, 921–932

Anderson, S., Auquier, A., Hauck, W.W., Oakes, D., Vandaele, W. & Weisberg, H.I. (1980) *Statistical Methods for Comparative Studies*, New York, Wiley

Aranda-Ordaz, F.J. (1983) An extension of the proportional hazards model for grouped data. *Biometrics*, **39**, 109–117

Armenian, K. & Lilienfeld, A.M. (1974) The distribution of incubation periods of neoplastic diseases. *Am. J. Epidemiol.*, **99**, 92–100

Armitage, P. (1955) Tests for linear trend in proportions and frequencies. *Biometrics*, **11**, 375–386

Armitage, P. (1966) The chi-square test for heterogeneity in proportions after adjustment for stratification. *J. R. stat. Soc. B*, **26**, 150–163

Armitage, P. (1971) *Statistical Methods in Medical Research*, Oxford, Blackwell

Armitage, P. & Doll, R. (1961) *Stochastic models for carcinogenesis*. In: *Proceedings of the 4th Berkeley Symposium on Mathematical Statistics and Probability: Biology and Problems of Health*, Berkeley, University of California Press, pp. 19–38

Baker, R. J. & Nelder, J.A. (1978) *The GLIM System: Release 3*, Oxford, Numerical Algorithms Group

Barlow, W.E. (1986) General relative risk models in stratified epidemiologic studies. *Appl. Stat.*, **34**, 246–257

Bartholomew, D.J. (1963) The sampling distribution of an estimate arising in life testing. *Technometrics, 5,* 361–374

Beasley, R.P., Hwang, L.Y., Lin, C.C. & Chien, C.S. (1981) Hepatocellular carcinoma and hepatitis B virus. A prospective study of 22,707 men in Taiwan. *Lancet,* **ii,** 1129–1133

Beebe, G.W., Ishida, M. & Jablon, S. (1962) Studies of the mortality of A-bomb survivors. I. Plan of study and mortality in the medical subsample (selection 1), 1950–1958. *Radiat. Res.,* **16,** 253–280

Beebe, G.W., Kato, H. & Land, C.E. (1977) *Mortality Experience of Atomic Bomb Survivors 1950–74, Life Span Study Report 8 (Technical Report RERF TR 1–77),* Hiroshima, Radiation Effects Research Foundation

Benjamin, B. (1968) *Health and Vital Statistics,* London, Allen & Unwin

Beral, V. (1974) Cancer of the cervix: a sexually transmitted infection? *Lancet,* **i,** 1037–1040

Beral, V., Fraser, P. & Chilvers, C. (1978) Does pregnancy protect against ovarian cancer? *Lancet,* **i,** 1083–1087

Bernstein, L., Anderson, J. & Pike, M.C. (1981) Estimation of the proportional hazard in two treatment clinical trials. *Biometrics,* **37,** 513–519

Berry, G. (1980) Dose-response in case-control studies. *J. Epidemiol. Community Health,* **34,** 217–222

Berry, G., Gilson, J.C., Holmes, S., Lewinsohn, H.A. & Roach, S.A. (1979) Asbestosis: a study of dose-response relationship in an asbestos textile factory. *Br. J. ind. Med.,* **36,** 98–112

Bithell, J. & Stewart, A. (1975) Pre-natal irradiation and childhood malignancy: a review of British data from the Oxford survey. *Br. J. Cancer,* **31,** 271–287

Bjarnason, O., Day, N.E., Snaedal, G. & Tulinius, H. (1974) The effect of year of birth on breast cancer incidence in Iceland. *Int. J. Cancer,* **13,** 689–696

Blot, W.J., Morris, L.E., Stroube, R., Tagnon, I. & Fraumeni, J.F. (1980) Lung and laryngeal cancers in relation to shipyard employment in coastal Virginia. *J. natl Cancer Inst.,* **65,** 571–575

Boice, J.D., Jr & Monson, R.R. (1977) Breast cancer in women after repeated fluoroscopic examinations of the chest. *J. natl Cancer Inst.,* **59,** 823–832

Boice, J.D. & Day, N.E.; Andersen, A., Brinton, L.A., Brown, R., Choi, N.W., Clarke, E.A., Coleman, M.P., Curtis, R.E., Flannery, J.T., Hakama, M., Hakulinen, T., Howe, G.R., Jensen, O.M., Kleinerman, R.A., Magnin, D., Magnus, K., Makela, K., Malker, B., Miller, A.B., Nelson, N., Patterson, C.C., Pettersson, F., Pompe-Kirn, V., Primic-Zakelj, M., Prior, P., Ravnihar, B., Skeet, R.G., Skjerven, J.E., Smith, P.G., Sok, M., Spengler, R.F., Storm, H.H., Stovall, M., Tomkins, G.W.O. & Wall, C. (1985) Second cancers following radiation treatment for cervical cancer. An international collaboration among cancer registries. *J. natl Cancer Inst.,* **74,** 955–975

Borgan, O. (1984) Maximum likelihood estimation in parametric counting process models, with applications to censored failure time data. *Scand. J. Stat.,* **11,** 1–16

Börzsönyi, M., Day, N.E., Lapis, K. & Yamasaki, H., eds (1984) *Models, Mechanisms and Etiology of Tumour Promotion* (*IARC Scientific Publications No. 56*), Lyon, International Agency for Research on Cancer

Breslow, N.E. (1974) Covariance analysis of censored survival data. *Biometrics*, **30**, 89–100

Breslow, N.E. (1975) Analysis of survival data under the proportional hazards model. *Int. stat. Rev.*, **43**, 55–68

Breslow, N.E. (1976) Regression analysis of the log odds ratio: a method for retrospective studies. *Biometrics*, **32**, 409–416

Breslow, N.E. (1979) Statistical methods for censored survival data. *Environ. Health Perspect.*, **32**, 181–192

Breslow, N.E. (1981) Odds ratio estimators when the data are sparse. *Biometrika*, **68**, 73–84

Breslow, N.E. (1984a) Extra-Poisson variation in log-linear models. *Appl. Stat.*, **33**, 38–44

Breslow, N.E. (1984b) Elementary methods of cohort analysis. *Int. J. Epidemiol.*, **13**, 112–115

Breslow, N.E. (1985a) Multivariate cohort analysis. *Natl Cancer Inst. Monogr*, **67**, 149–156

Breslow, N.E. (1985b) *Cohort analysis in epidemiology*. In: Atkinson, A.C. & Fienberg, S.E. eds, *A Celebration of Statistics*, New York, Springer, pp. 109–143

Breslow, N.E. & Crowley, J.C. (1974) A large sample study of the life table and product limit estimators under random censorship. *Ann. Stat.*, **2**, 437–453

Breslow, N.E. & Day, N.E. (1975) Indirect standardization and multiplicative models for rates, with reference to the age adjustment of cancer incidence and relative frequency data. *J. chron. Dis.*, **28**, 289–303

Breslow, N.E. & Day, N.E. (1980) *Statistical Methods in Cancer Research, Vol. I, The Analysis of Case-Control Studies* (*IARC Scientific Publications No. 32*), Lyon, International Agency for Research on Cancer

Breslow, N.E. & Day, N.E. (1985) *The standardized mortality ratio*. In: Sen, P.K., ed., *Biostatistics: Statistics in Biomedical, Public Health and Environmental Sciences*, New York, Elsevier, pp. 55–74

Breslow, N.E. & Langholz, B. (1987) Nonparametric estimation of relative mortality functions. *J. chron. Dis.* (in press)

Breslow, N.E. & Patton, J. (1979) *Case-control analysis of cohort studies*. In: Breslow, N.E. & Whittemore, A.S., eds, *Energy and Health*, Philadelphia, SIAM, pp. 226–242

Breslow, N.E. & Storer, B.E. (1985) General relative risk functions for case-control studies. *Am. J. Epidemiol.*, **122**, 149–162

Breslow, N.E., Lubin, J.H., Marek, P. & Langholz, B. (1983) Multiplicative models and cohort analysis. *J. Am. stat. Assoc.*, **78**, 1–12

Breslow, N.E., Edler, L. & Berger, J. (1984) A two-sample censored data rank test for acceleration. *Biometrics*, **40**, 1049–1062

Brown, C.C. (1977) The shape of the dose-response curve for radiation carcinogenesis: extrapolation to low doses. *Radiat. Res.*, **71**, 34–50

Brown, C.C. & Chu, K. (1987) Use of multistage models to infer stage affected by carcinogenic exposure: example of lung cancer and cigarette smoking. *J. chron. Dis.* (in press)

Brown, C.C. & Chu, K.C. (1983a) A new method for the analysis of cohort studies: implications of the multistage theory of carcinogenesis applied to occupational arsenic exposure. *Environ. Health Perspect.,* **150,** 293–308

Brown, C.C. & Chu, K.C. (1983b) Implications of the multi-stage theory of carcinogenesis applied to occupational arsenic exposure. *J. natl Cancer Inst.,* **70,** 455–463

Brown, C.C. & Green, S.B. (1982) Additional power computations for designing comparative Poisson trials. *Am. J. Epidemiol.,* **115,** 752–758

Buckley, J.D., Harris, R.W.C., Doll, R., Vessey, M.P. & Williams, P.T. (1981) Case-control study of the husbands of women with dysplasia or carcinoma of the cervix uteri. *Lancet,* **ii,** 1010–1015

Casagrande, J.T., Pike, M.C. & Smith, P.G. (1978a) The power function of the exact test for comparing two binomial distributions. *Appl. Stat.,* **27,** 1–35

Casagrande, J.T., Pike, M.C. & Smith, P.G. (1978b) An improved approximate formula for calculating sample sizes for comparing two binomial distributions. *Biometrics,* **34,** 483–486

Case, R.A.M. & Pearson, J.T. (1954) Tumours of the urinary bladder in workmen engaged in the manufacture and use of certain dyestuff intermediates in the British chemical industry. Part II. Further considerations of the role of aniline and of the manufacture of auramine and magenta (fuchsine) as possible causative agents. *Br. J. ind. Med.,* **11,** 213–216

Case, R.A.M. & Pearson, J.T. (1957) *Tables for comparative composite cohort analysis.* In: *Cancer Statistics for England and Wales, 1901–55,* London, Her Majesty's Stationery Office, pp. 37–99

Case, R.A.M., Hosker, M.E., McDonald, D.B. & Pearson, J.T. (1954) Tumours of the urinary bladder in workmen engaged in the manufacture and use of certain dyestuff intermediates in the British chemical industry. Part I. The role of aniline, benzidine, alpha-naphthylamine and beta-naphthylamine. *Br. J. ind. Med.,* **11,** 75–104

Chapman, D.G. & Nam, J.M. (1968) Asymptotic power of chi square tests for linear trends in proportions. *Biometrics,* **16,** 315–327

Chiang, C.L. (1961) *Standard Error of the Age-adjusted Death Rate (Vital Statistics – Special Report. Selected Studies No. 9),* Washington DC, US Department of Health, Education, and Welfare

Clayton, D.G. (1982) The analysis of prospective studies of disease aetiology. *Commun. Stat. Theory. Meth.,* **11,** 2129–2155

Clayton, D.G. (1985) Using test-retest reliability data to improve estimates of relative risk: an application of latent class analysis. *Stat. Med.,* **4,** 445–455

Clayton, D.G. & Kaldor, J.M. (1985) Heterogeneity models as an alternative to proportional hazards in cohort study data. *Bull. Int. stat. Inst.,* 3.2, 1–16

Clayton, D.G. & Kaldor, J.M. (1987) Diagnostic plots for departures from proportional hazards in cohort study data. *J. chron. Dis.* (in press)

Coleman, M., Douglas, A., Hermon, C. & Peto, J. (1986) Cohort study analysis with a FORTRAN computer program. *Int. J. Epidemiol.,* **15,** 134–137

Committee on the Biological Effects of Ionizing Radiation (1980) *The Effects on Populations of Exposure to Low Levels of Ionizing Radiation*, National Academy of Sciences – National Research Council, Washington DC, National Academy Press

Cook, P.J., Doll, R. & Fellingham, S.A. (1969) A mathematical model for the age distribution of cancer in man. *Int. J. Cancer*, **4**, 93–112

Cook, R.D. & Weisberg, S. (1982) *Residuals and Influence in Regression*, London, Chapman & Hall

Cornfield, J. (1951) A method of estimating comparative rates from clinical data. Application to cancer of the lung, breast and cervix. *J. natl Cancer Inst.*, **11**, 1269–1275

Cornfield, J. (1956) *A statistical problem arising from retrospective studies*. In: Neyman, J., ed, *Proceedings of the Third Berkeley Symposium*, Vol. IV, Berkeley, University of California Press, pp. 133–148

Court Brown, W.M. & Doll, R. (1957) Mortality from cancer and other causes after radiotherapy for ankylosing spondylitis. *Br. med. J.*, **ii**, 1327–1332

Cox, D.R. (1972) Regression models and life tables (with discussion). *J. R. stat. Soc. B*, **34**, 187–220

Cox, D.R. (1975) Partial likelihood. *Biometrika*, **62**, 269–276

Cox, D.R. & Hinkley, D.V. (1974) *Theoretical Statistics*, London, Chapman & Hall

Cox, D.R. & Oakes, D. (1984) *Analysis of Survival Data*, London, Chapman & Hall

Crump, K.S. & Howe, R.B. (1984) The multi-stage model with a time dependent dose pattern: application to carcinogenic risk assessment. *Risk Anal.*, **4**, 163–176

Darby, S.C. (1984) *Modelling age- and time-dependent changes in the rates of radiation-induced cancers*. In: Prentice, R.L. & Thompson, D.J., eds, *Atomic Bomb Survivor Data: Utilization and Analysis*, Philadelphia, SIAM, pp. 67–80

Darby, S.C., Nakashima, E. & Kato, H. (1985) A parallel analysis of cancer mortality among atomic bomb survivors and with ankylosing spondylitis given X-ray therapy. *J. natl Cancer Inst.*, **75**, 1–21

Day, N.E. (1976) *A new measure of age standardized incidence, the cumulative rate*. In: Waterhouse, J.A.H., Muir, C.S., Correa, P. & Powell, J., eds, *Cancer Incidence in Five Continents, Vol. III (IARC Scientific Publications No. 15)*, Lyon, International Agency for Research on Cancer, pp. 443–452

Day, N.E. (1985) *Epidemiological methods for the assessment of human cancer risk*. In: Krewski, D., Munro, I. & Clayson, D., eds, *Toxicological Risk Assessment*, New York, CRC Press, pp. 3–15

Day, N.E. & Boice, J.D., Jr, eds (1983) *Second Cancer in Relation to Radiation Treatment for Cervical Cancer. A Cancer Registry Collaboration (IARC Scientific Publications No. 52)*, Lyon, International Agency for Research on Cancer

Day, N.E. & Brown, C.C. (1980) Multistage models and the primary prevention of cancer. *J. natl Cancer Inst.*, **64**, 977–989

Day, N.E. & Byar, D.P. (1979) Testing hypotheses in case-control studies – equivalence of Mantel–Haenszel statistics and logit score tests. *Biometrics*, **35**, 623–630

Day, N.E., Byar, D.P. & Green, S.B. (1980) Overadjustment in case-control studies. *Am. J. Epidemiol.*, **112**, 696–706

Day, N.E., Boice, J.D., Jr, Andersen, A., Brinton, L.A., Brown, R., Choi, N.W., Clarke, E.A., Coleman, M.P., Curtis, R.E., Flannery, J.T., Hakama, M., Hakulinen, T., Howe, G.R., Jensen, O.M., Kleinerman, R.A., Magnin, D., Magnus, K., Makela, K., Malker, B., Miller, A.B., Nelson, N., Patterson, C.C., Pettersson, F., Pompe–Kirn, V., Primic-Zakelj, M., Prior, P., Ravnihar, B., Skeet, R.G., Skjerven, J.E., Smith, P.G., Sok, M., Spengler, R.F., Storm, H.H., Tomkins, G.W.O. & Wall, C. (1983) *Summary chapter.* In: Day, N.E. & Boice, J.R., Jr, eds, *Second Cancer in Relation to Radiation Treatment for Cervical Cancer. A Cancer Registry Collaboration (IARC Scientific Publications No. 52),* Lyon, International Agency for Research on Cancer, pp. 137–181

Decarli, A., Peto, J., Piolatto, G. & La Vecchia, C. (1985) Bladder cancer mortality of workers exposed to aromatic amines: analysis of models of carcinogenesis. *Br. J. Cancer,* **51,** 707–712

Decouflé, P., Thomas, T.L. & Pickle, L.W. (1980) Comparison of the proportionate mortality ratio and standardized mortality ratio risk measures. *Am. J. Epidemiol.,* **111,** 263–269

Doering, C.R. & Forbes, A.L. (1939) Adjusted death rates. *Proc. natl Acad. Sci. USA,* **25,** 461–467

Doll, R. (1971) The age distribution of cancer: implications for models of carcinogenesis. *J. R. stat. Soc. A,* **134,** 133–156

Doll, R. (1978) An epidemiological perspective of the biology of cancer. *Cancer Res.,* **38,** 3573–3583

Doll, R. & Cook, P.J. (1967) Summarizing indices for comparison of cancer incidence data. *Int. J. Cancer,* **2,** 269–279

Doll, R. & Hill, A.B. (1950) Smoking and carcinoma of the lung. Preliminary report. *Br. med. J.,* **iii,** 739–748

Doll, R. & Hill, A.B. (1952) A study of the aetiology of carcinoma of the lung. *Br. med. J.,* **iv,** 1271–1286

Doll, R. & Hill, A.B. (1954) The mortality of doctors in relation to their smoking habits. A preliminary report. *Br. med. J.,* **ii,** 1451–1455

Doll, R. & Hill, A.B. (1966) Mortality of British doctors in relation to smoking: observations on coronary thrombosis. *Natl Cancer Inst. Monogr.,* **19,** 205–268

Doll, R. & Peto, R. (1976) Mortality in relation to smoking: 20 years' observations on male British doctors. *Br. med. J.,* **ii,** 1525–1536

Doll, R. & Peto, R. (1978) Cigarette smoking and bronchial carcinoma: dose and time relationships among regular smokers and life-long non-smokers. *J. Epidemiol. Community Health,* **32,** 303–313

Doll, R., Fisher, R.E.W., Gammon, E.J., Gunn, W., Hughes, G.O., Tyrer, F.H. & Wilson, W. (1965) Mortality of gasworkers with special reference to cancers of the lung and bladder, chronic bronchitis, and pneumoconiosis. *Br. J. ind. Med.,* **22,** 1–12

Doll, R., Muir, C. & Waterhouse, J., eds (1970a) *Cancer Incidence in Five Continents, Vol. II,* Heidelberg, Springer-Verlag

Doll, R., Morgan, L.G. & Speizer, F. (1970b) Cancers of the lung and nasal sinuses in nickel workers. *Br. J. Cancer,* **24,** 623–632

Doll, R., Vessey, M.P., Beasley, R.W.R., Buckley, A.R., Fear, E.C., Fisher, R.E.W., Gammon, E.J., Gunn, W., Hughes, G.O., Lee, K., & Norman-Smith, B. (1972) Mortality of gasworkers – final report of a prospective study. *Br. J. ind. Med.*, **29**, 394–406

Doll, R., Gray, R., Hafner, B. & Peto, R. (1980) Mortality in relation to smoking: 22 years' observations on female British doctors. *Br. med. J.*, **ii**, 967–971

Duck, B.W. & Carter, J.T. (1976) Letter to the editor. *Lancet*, **ii**, 195

Duck, B.W., Carter, J.T. & Coombes, E.J. (1975) Mortality study of workers in a polyvinyl-chloride production plant. *Lancet*, **ii**, 1197–1199

Elveback, L.R. (1966) Discussion of 'Indices of mortality and tests of their statistical significance'. *Human Biol.*, **38**, 322–324

Enterline, P.E. (1975) Not uniformly true for each cause of death (letter). *J. occup. Med.*, **17**, 127–128

Enterline, P.E. (1976) Pitfalls in epidemiologic research: an examination of the asbestos literature. *J. occup. Med.*, **18**, 150–156

Epstein, B. (1954) Truncated life tests in the exponential case. *Ann. math. Stat.*, **23**, 555–564

Fienberg, S.E. (1980) *The Analysis of Cross-classified Categorical Data*, Cambridge, Mass., MIT Press

Fleiss, J.L. (1973) *Statistical Methods for Rates and Proportions*, New York, Wiley

Fleiss, J.L., Tytun, A. & Ury, H.K. (1980) A simple approximation for calculating sample sizes for comparing independent proportions. *Biometrics*, **36**, 343–346

Fox, A.J. & Goldblatt, P.O. (1982) *Longitudinal Study. Socio-demographic Mortality Differentials*, London, Her Majesty's Stationery Office

Freeman, D.H. & Holford, T.R. (1980) Summary rates. *Biometrics*, **36**, 195–203

Frome, E.L. (1983) The analysis of rates using Poisson regression models. *Biometrics*, **39**, 665–674

Frome, E.L. & Checkoway, H. (1985) Use of Poisson regression models in estimating incidence ratios and rates. *Am. J. Epidemiol.*, **121**, 309–323

Fujita, S. (1984) *Potential additional data sources for dosimetry and biological re-evaluation*. In: Prentice, R.L. & Thompson, D.J., eds, *Atomic Bomb Survivor Data: Utilization and Analysis*, Philadelphia, SIAM, pp. 183–193

Gail, M. (1973) The determination of sample sizes for trials involving several independent 2×2 tables. *J. chron. Dis.*, **226**, 669–673

Gail, M. (1974) Power computations for designing comparative Poisson trials. *Biometrics*, **30**, 231–237

Gail, M.H., Lubin, J.H. & Rubinstein, L.V. (1981) Likelihood calculations for matched case-control studies and survival studies with tied death times. *Biometrika*, **68**, 703–707

Gardner, M.J. & Munford, A.G. (1980) The combined effect of two factors on disease in a case-control study. *Appl. Stat.*, **29**, 276–281

Gart, J.J. (1971) The comparison of proportions: a review of significance tests, confidence intervals, and adjustments for stratification. *Int. stat. Rev.*, **39**, 148–169

Geser, A. & de-Thé, G.B. (1972) *Does the Epstein–Barr virus play an etiological role in Burkitt's lymphoma? The planning of a longitudinal seroepidemiological survey in the West Nile district, Uganda.* In: Biggs, P.M., de-Thé, G. & Payne, L.N., eds, *Oncogenesis and Herpesviruses* (*IARC Scientific Publications No. 2*), Lyon, International Agency for Research on Cancer, pp. 372–375

Gilbert, E.S. (1983) An evaluation of several methods for assessing the effects of occupational exposure to radiation. *Biometrics,* **39,** 161–171

Gilbert, E.S. (1984) *The effects of random dosimetry errors and the use of data on acute symptoms for dosimetry evaluation.* In: Prentice, R.L. & Thompson, D.J., eds, *Atomic Bomb Survivor Data*: *Utilization and Analysis,* Philadelphia, SIAM, pp. 170–182

Gilbert, E.S. & Buchanan, J.A. (1984) An alternative approach to analyzing occupational mortality data. *J. occup. Med.,* **11,** 822–828

Gilbert, E.S. & Marks, S. (1979) An analysis of the mortality of workers in a nuclear facility. *Radiat. Res.,* **79,** 122–148

Gillespie, M.J. & Fisher, L. (1979) Confidence bounds for the Kaplan-Meier survival curve estimate. *Ann. Stat.,* **7,** 920–924

Greenland, S. (1982) Interpretation and estimation of summary ratios under heterogeneity. *Stat. Med.,* **1,** 217–227

Greenland, S. (1985) Power, sample size and smallest detectable effect determination for multivariate studies. *Stat. Med.,* **4,** 117–127

Greenwood, M. (1926) *The Errors of Sampling of the Survivorship Tables* (*Reports on Public Health and Statistical Subjects No. 33*), London, His Majesty's Stationery Office, Appendix 1

Grove, R.D. & Hetzel, A.M. (1968) *Vital Statistics Rates in the United States, 1940–1960.* Washington DC, National Center for Vital Statistics

Haberman, S.J. (1974) *The Analysis of Frequency Data,* Chicago, University of Chicago Press

Haenszel, W. (1950) A standardized rate for mortality defined in units of lost years of life. *Am. J. public Health,* **40,** 17–26

Haenszel, W., Loveland, D. & Sirken, M.G. (1962) Lung cancer mortality as related to residence and smoking histories. *J. natl Cancer Inst.,* **28,** 947–1001

Hall, W.J. & Wellner, J.A. (1980) Confidence bands for a survival curve from censored data. *Biometrika,* **67,** 133–143

Hamilton, M.A. (1982) Detection of interactive effects in carcinogenesis. *Biometr. J.,* **24,** 483–491

Hammond, E.C. (1966) Smoking in relation to the death rates of one million men and women. *Natl Cancer Inst. Monogr.,* **19,** 127–204

Hammond, E.C., Selikoff, I.J. & Seidman, H. (1979) Asbestos exposure, cigarette smoking and death rates. *Ann. N.Y. Acad. Sci.,* **330,** 473–490

Hartge, P., Hoover, R.N., West, D.W. & Lyon, J.L. (1983) Coffee drinking and risk of bladder cancer. *J. natl Cancer Inst.,* **70,** 1021–1024

Hill, I.D. (1972) Computing man years at risk. *Br. J. prev. soc. Med.,* **26,** 132–134

Hirayama, T. (1975) *Smoking and cancer*: *a prospective study on cancer epidemiology based on a census population in Japan.* In: *Proceedings of the Third World Conference on Smoking and Health,* Vol. II, Washington DC, Department of Health, Education, and Welfare, pp. 65–72

Hoaglin, D.C. & Welsh, R.F. (1978) The hat matrix in regression and ANOVA. *Am. Stat.*, **32**, 17–22

Hobbs, M.S.T., Woodward, S., Murphy, B., Musk, A.W. & Elder, J.E. (1980) *The incidence of pneumoconiosis, mesothelioma and other respiratory cancer in men engaged in mining and milling crocidolite in Western Australia.* In: Wagner, J.C., ed., *Biological Effects of Mineral Fibres (IARC Scientific Publications No. 30)*, Lyon, International Agency for Research on Cancer, pp. 615–625

Hoem, J.M. (1984) Statistical analysis of a multiplicative model and its application to the standardization of vital rates. A review. *Int. stat. Rev.* (in press)

Holford, T.R. (1980) The analysis of rates and of survivorship using log-linear models. *Biometrics*, **36**, 229–306

Howe, G.R. (1982) *Epidemiology of radiogenic breast cancer.* In: Boice, J.D., Jr & Fraumeni, J.R., Jr, eds, *Radiation Carcinogenesis. Epidemiology and Biological Significance*, New York, Raven Press, pp. 119–129

Huber, P.J. (1983) *Robust Statistics*, New York, Wiley

Hutchinson, W.B., Thomas, D.B., Hamlin, W.B., Roth, G.J., Peterson, A.V. & Williams, B.J. (1980) Risk of breast cancer in women with benign breast disease. *J. natl Cancer Inst.*, **65**, 13–20

Hutchison, G.B. (1968) Leukemia in patients with cancer of the cervix uteri treated with radiation. A report covering the first 5 years of an international study. *J. natl Cancer Inst.*, **40**, 951–982

IARC (1982a) *IARC Monographs on the Evaluation of the Carcinogenic Risk of Chemicals to Humans*, Supplement 4, *Chemicals, Industrial Processes and Industries Associated with Cancer in Humans (IARC Monographs, Volumes 1 to 29)*, Lyon, International Agency for Research on Cancer

IARC (1982b) *IARC Monographs on the Evaluation of the Carcinogenic Risk of Chemicals to Humans*, Vol. 29, *Some Industrial Chemicals and Dyestuffs*, Lyon, International Agency for Research on Cancer, pp. 93–184

IARC (1983) *Approaches to Classifying Chemical Carcinogens According to Mechanism of Action (IARC Internal Technical Report No. 83/001)*, Lyon, International Agency for Research on Cancer

Infante, P.F., Rinsky, R.A., Wagoner, J.K. & Young, R.J. (1977) Leukaemia in benzene workers. *Lancet*, **ii**, 76–78

Ishimaru, T., Otake, M. & Ichimaru, M. (1979) Dose-response relationship of neutrons and γ rays to leukemia incidence among atomic-bomb survivors in Hiroshima and Nagasaki by type of leukemia, 1950–1971. *Radiat. Res.*, **77**, 377–394

Jensen, O.M. (1979) Cancer morbidity and causes of death among Danish brewery workers. *Int. J. Cancer*, **23**, 454–463

Johansen, S. (1981) Discussion of paper by D. Oakes. *Int. stat. Rev.*, **49**, 258–262

Kahn, H. (1966) The Dorn study of smoking and mortality among US veterans: report on eight and one-half years of observation. *Natl Cancer Inst. Monogr.*, **19**, 1–129

Kalbfleisch, J.D. & Prentice, R.L. (1980) *The Statistical Analysis of Failure Time Data*, New York, Wiley

Kaldor, J.M., Peto, J., Easton, D., Doll, Hermon, C. & Morgan, L. (1986a) Models for respiratory cancer in nickel refinery workers. *J. natl Cancer Inst.*, **77**, 841–848

Kaldor, J.M., Day, N.E., Bana, P., Choi, N.W., Clarke, E.A., Coleman, M.P., Hakama, M., Koch, M., Langmark, F., Neal, F.E., Pettersson, F., Pompe-Kim, V., Prior, P. & Storm, H.H. (1987) Second malignancies following testicular cancer, ovarian cancer and Hodgkin's disease: an international collaborative study among cancer registries. *Int. J. Cancer* (in press)

Kark, J.D., Smith, A.H., Switzer, B.R. & Hames, C.G. (1981) Serum vitamin A (retinol) and cancer incidence in Evans County, Georgia. *J. natl Cancer Inst.*, **66**, 7–16

Keiding, N. (1985a) Standardized mortality ratio and statistical analysis: historical perspective. *Biometrics*, **41**, 109–116

Keiding, N. (1985b) *The Method of the Expected Number of Deaths, 1786–1886–1986 (Research Report No. 85/6)*, University of Copenhagen, Statistical Research Unit

Keiding, N. (1987) The method of the expected number of deaths, 1786–1886–1986. *Int. Stat. Rev.*, **55**, 1–20

Kerridge, D. (1958) A new method of standardizing death rates. *Br. J. prev. soc. Med.*, **2**, 154–155

Keyfitz, N. (1966) Sampling variance of the standardized mortality rates. *Human. Biol.*, **38**, 309–317

Kilpatrick, S.J. (1962) Occupational mortality indices. *Pop. Stud.*, **16**, 175–183

Kilpatrick, S.J. (1963) Mortality comparisons in socio-economic groups. *Appl. Stat.*, **12**, 65–86

Kinlen, L.J. (1982) Meat and fat consumption and cancer mortality: a study of strict religious orders in Britain. *Lancet*, **i**, 946–949

Knox, E.G. (1973) Computer simulation of industrial hazards. *Br. J. ind. Med.*, **30**, 54–63

Knudson, A.G. (1971) Mutation and cancer: statistical study of retinoblastoma. *Proc. natl Acad. Sci. USA*, **68**, 820–823

Knudson, A.G. (1985) Hereditary cancer, oncogenes, and antioncogenes. *Cancer Res.*, **45**, 1437–1443

Koopman, J. (1982) Analysing different types of multiple causation (abstract). *Am. J. Epidemiol.*, **116**, 586

Kupper, L.L., McMichael, A.J., Symons, M.J. & Most, B.M. (1978) On the utility of proportional mortality analysis. *J. chron. Dis.*, **31**, 15–22

Land, C.E., Boice, J.D., Jr, Shore, R.E., Norman, J.E. & Tokunaga, M. (1980) Breast risk from low-dose exposures to ionizing radiation: results of parallel analysis of three exposed populations of women. *J. natl Cancer Inst.*, **65**, 353–376

Lee, A.M. & Fraumeni, J.F., Jr (1969) Arsenic and respiratory cancer in man: an occupational study. *J. natl Cancer Inst.*, **42**, 1045–1052

Lee, P.N. (1975) *A model of experimental carcinogenesis and experiments to test it.* In: *Tobacco Research Council Review of Activities, 1970–74*, London, Tobacco Research Council, pp. 28–32

Lee-Feldstein, A. (1983) Arsenic and respiratory cancer in humans: follow-up of copper smelter employees in Montana. *J. natl Cancer Inst.*, **70**, 601–610

Lehman, E.L. (1959) *Testing Statistical Hypotheses*, New York, Wiley

Liddell, F.D.K. (1960) The measurement of occupational mortality. *Br. J. ind. Med.*, **17**, 228–233

Little, A.S. (1952) Estimation of the T-year survival rate from follow-up studies over a limited period of time. *Human Biol.*, **24**, 87–116

Lubin, J.H. & Gail, M.H. (1984) Biased selection of controls for case-control analysis of cohort studies. *Biometrics*, **40**, 63–75

Lubin, J.H., Pottern, L.M., Blot, W.J., Tokudome, S., Stone, B.J. & Fraumeni, J.F., Jr (1981) Respiratory cancer among copper smelter workers: recent mortality statistics. *J. occup. Med.*, **23**, 779–784

Lubin, J.H., Blot, W.J., Berrino, F., Flamant, R., Gillis, C.R., Junze, M., Schmähl, D. & Viseo, G. (1984) Modifying risk of developing lung cancer by changing habits of cigarette smoking. *Br. med. J.*, **288**, 1953–1956

Lundin, F.E., Archer, V.E. & Wagoner, J.K. (1979) *An exposure–time–response model for lung cancer mortality in uranium miners.* In: Breslow, N.E. & Whittemore, A.S., eds., *Energy and Health*, Philadelphia, SIAM, pp. 243–264

MacMahon, B. (1962) Prenatal X-ray exposure and childhood cancer. *J. natl Cancer Inst.*, **28**, 1173–1191

Mancuso, T.F. & El-Attar, A.A. (1967) Mortality pattern in a cohort of asbestos workers. *J. occup. Med.*, **9**, 147–162

Mantel, N. (1973) Synthetic retrospective studies and related topics. *Biometrics*, **29**, 479–486

Mantel, N. & Stark, C.R. (1968) Computation of indirect adjusted rates in the presence of confounding. *Biometrics*, **24**, 997–1005

Mays, C.W. & Spiess, H. (1984) *Bone sarcomas in patients given radium-224.* In: Boice, J.D., Jr & Fraumeni, J.F., Jr, eds, *Radiation Carcinogenesis: Epidemiology and Biological Significance*, New York, Raven Press, pp. 241–252

McMichael, A.J., Jensen, O.M., Parkin, D.M. & Zaridze, D.G. (1984) Dietary and endogenous cholesterol and human cancer. *Epidemiol. Rev.*, **6**, 192–216

Mendelhall, W. & Lehman, E.H., Jr (1960) An approximation to the negative moments of the positive binomial useful in life testing. *Technometrics*, **2**, 227–242

Mendelsohn-Pottern, L., Stone, B.J., Day, N.E. & Fraumeni, J.F. (1980) Thyroid cancer in Connecticut 1935–1975: an analysis by cell type. *Am. J. Epidemiol.*, **112**, 764–774

Miettinen, O.S. (1972) Standardization of risk ratios. *Am. J. Epidemiol.*, **96**, 383–388

Miettinen, O.S. (1976) Estimability and estimation in case-referent studies. *Am. J. Epidemiol.*, **103**, 226–235

Miettinen, O.S. & Wang, J.D. (1981) An alternative to the proportionate mortality ratio. *Am. J. Epidemiol.*, **114**, 144–148

Miller, A.B., Howe, G.R., Sherman, G.J. & Lindsay, J. (1987) The Canadian study of cancer following multiple fluoroscopies. I: Mortality from breast cancer in women, 1950–1980. *J. natl Cancer Inst.* (in press)

Monson, R.R. (1974) Analysis of relative survival and proportional mortality. *Comp. biomed. Res.*, **7**, 325–332

Monson, R.R. (1980) *Occupational Epidemiology*, Boca Raton, Florida, CRC Press

Moolgavkar, S.H. (1978) The multistage theory of carcinogenesis and the age distribution of cancer in man. *J. natl Cancer Inst.*, **61**, 49–52

Moolgavkar, S.H., Day, N.E. & Stevens, R.G. (1980) Two-stage model for carcinogenesis: epidemiology of breast cancer in females. *J. natl Cancer Inst.*, **65**, 559–569

Moolgavkar, S.H., Lustbader, E.D. & Venzon, D.J. (1984) A geometric approach to nonlinear regression diagnostics with application to matched case-control studies. *Ann. Stat.*, **12**, 816–826

Mosteller, F. & Tukey, J.W. (1977) *Data Analysis and Regression: A Second Course in Statistics*, Reading, Mass., Addison & Wesley

MRC Environmental Epidemiology Unit (1984) *Expected Numbers in Cohort Studies (MRC Scientific Report No. 6)*, Southampton, Medical Research Council

Najarian, T. (1983) Comment. *Am. Stat.*, **37**, 455–457

Najarian, T. & Colton, T. (1978) Mortality from leukaemia and cancer in shipyard nuclear workers. *Lancet*, **i**, 1018–1020

Nelson, W. (1969) Hazard plotting for incomplete failure data. *J. Qual. Technol.*, **1**, 27–52

Newhouse, M.L. & Berry, G. (1976) Predictions of mortality from mesothelial tumours in asbestos factory workers. *Br. J. ind. Med.*, **33**, 147–151

Oakes, D. (1977) The asymptotic information in censored survival data. *Biometrika*, **64**, 441–448

Oakes, D. (1981) Survival times: aspects of partial likelihood. *Int. stat. Rev.*, **49**, 235–264

Office of Population Censuses and Surveys (1978) *Occupational Mortality: The Registrar General's Decennial Supplement for England and Wales 1970–1972*, London, Her Majesty's Stationery Office

Parkin, D.M., ed. (1986) *Cancer Occurrence in Developing Countries (IARC Scientific Publications No. 75)*, Lyon, International Agency for Research on Cancer

Pearson, E.S. & Hartley, H.O. (1966) *Biometrika Tables for Statisticians*, Vol. I (3rd Edition), Cambridge, Cambridge University Press

Persing, J.P. (1981) *Risk Factors for Breast Cancer in Women with BBD: Reproductive Factors and Exogenous Estrogens*, MS Thesis, Seattle, University of Washington

Peterson, A.V., Prentice, R.L. & Marek, P.M. (1983) *Implementation and computational considerations of the Cox partial likelihood analysis*. In: Heiner, K.W., Sacher, R.S. & Wilkinson, J.W., eds, *Computer Science and Statistics: Proceedings of the 14th Symposium on the Interface*, pp. 92–100

Peto, J. (1978) The hygiene standard for chrysotile asbestos. *Lancet*, **i**, 484–489

Peto, J. (1980) *Lung cancer mortality in relation to measured dust levels in an asbestos textile factory*. In: Wagner, J.C., ed., *Biological Effects of Mineral Fibres (IARC Scientific Publications No. 30)*, Lyon, International Agency for Research on Cancer, pp. 829–836

Peto, J. (1984) *Early- and late-stage carcinogenesis in mouse skin and in man*. In: Börzsönyi, M., Day, N.E., Lapis, K. & Yamasaki, H., eds, *Models, Mechanisms and Etiology of Tumour Promotion (IARC Scientific Publications No. 56)*, Lyon, International Agency for Research on Cancer, pp. 359–371

Peto, J., Henderson, B.E. & Pike, M.C. (1981) *Trends in mesothelioma incidence in the United States and the forecast epidemic due to asbestos exposure during World War II*. In: Peto, R. & Schneiderman, M., eds, *Quantification of Occupational Cancer (Banbury Report 9)*, Cold Spring Harbor, NY, CSH Press, pp. 51–69

Peto, J., Seidman, H. & Selikoff, I.J. (1982) Mesothelioma mortality in asbestos workers: implications for models of carcinogenesis and risk assessment. *Br. J. Cancer*, **45**, 124–135

Peto, J., Cuckle, H., Doll, R., Hermon, C. & Morgan, L.G. (1984) *Respiratory cancer mortality of Welsh nickel refinery workers*. In: Sunderman, F.W., ed., *Nickel in the Human Environment (IARC Scientific Publications No. 53)*, Lyon, International Agency for Research on Cancer, pp. 37–46

Peto, R. (1972) Contribution to discussion of paper by D.R. Cox. *J. R. stat. Soc. B*, **34**, 205–207

Peto, R. (1977) *Epidemiology, multi-stage models, and short term mutagenicity tests*. In: Hiatt, H.H., Watson, J.D. & Winsten, J.A., eds, *Origins of Human Cancer*, Cold Spring Harbor, NY, CSH Press, pp. 1403–1428

Peto, R. & Peto, J. (1972) Asymptotically efficient rank invariant test procedures (with discussion). *J. R. stat. Soc. A*, **135**, 185–206

Peto, R. & Pike, M. (1973) Conservatism of the approximation $\sum (O - E)^2/E$ in the logrank test for survival data or tumour incidence data. *Biometrics*, **29**, 579–584

Pierce, D.A. & Preston, D.L. (1984) *Hazard function modelling for dose-response analysis of cancer incidence in A-bomb survivor data*. In: Prentice, R.L. & Thompson, D.J., eds, *Atomic Bomb Survivor Data: Utilization and Analysis*, Philadelphia, SIAM, pp. 51–66

Pierce, D.A., Preston, D.L. & Ishimaru, T. (1985) *A Method for Analysis of Cancer Incidence in Japanese A-bomb Survivors, with Application to Acute Leukemia, (RERF Technical Report)*, Hiroshima, Radiation Effects Research Foundation

Pike, M.C., Krailo, M.D., Henderson, B.E., Casagrande, J.T. & Hoel, D.G. (1983) 'Hormonal' risk factors, 'breast tissue age' and the age-incidence of breast cancer. *Nature*, **303**, 767–770

Pike, M.C. (1985) Breast cancer and oral contraceptives (letter). *Lancet*, **ii**, 1180–1181

Pocock, S., Cook, D.G. & Beresford, S.A.A. (1981) Regression of area mortality rates on explanatory variables: what weighting is appropriate? *Appl. Stat.*, **30**, 286–295

Pregibon, D. (1979) *Data Analytic Methods for Generalized Linear Models*, Ph.D. Thesis, Toronto, University of Toronto

Pregibon, D. (1980) Goodness of link tests for generalized linear models. *Appl. Stat.*, **29**, 15–24

Pregibon, D. (1981) Logistic regression diagnostics. *Ann. Stat.*, **9**, 705–724

Pregibon, D. (1984) Data analytic methods for matched case-control studies. *Biometrics*, **40**, 639–651

Prentice, R.L. (1986) A case-cohort design for epidemiologic cohort studies and disease prevention trials. *Biometrika*, **73**, 1–12

Prentice, R.L. & Breslow, N.E. (1978) Retrospective studies and failure time models. *Biometrika*, **65**, 153–158

Prentice, R.L. & Mason, W.M. (1986) On the application of linear relative risk regression models. *Biometrics*, **42**, 109–120

Prentice, R.L. & Self, S.G. (1983) Asymptotic distribution theory for Cox-type regression models with general relative risk form. *Ann. Stat.*, **11**, 804–813

Prentice, R.L., Kalbfleisch, J.D., Peterson, A.V., Flournoy, N., Farewell, V.T. & Breslow, N.E. (1978) The analysis of failure times in the presence of competing risks. *Biometrics*, **34**, 541–554

Prentice, R.L., Yoshimoto, Y. & Mason, M.W. (1983) Relationship of cigarette smoking and radiation exposure to cancer mortality in Hiroshoma and Nagasaki. *J. natl Cancer Inst.*, **70**, 611–622

Prentice, R.L., Self, S.G. & Mason, M.W. (1986) *Design options for sampling within a cohort*. In: Moolgavkar, S.H. & Prentice, R.L., eds, *Modern Statistical Methods in Chronic Disease Epidemiology*, New York, Wiley, pp. 50–62

Quenouille, M. (1949) Approximate tests of correlation in time series. *J. R. stat. Soc. B*, **11**, 18–84

Ramlau-Hansen, H. (1983) Smoothing counting process intensities by means of kernel functions. *Ann. Stat.*, **11**, 453–466

Rao, C.R. (1965) *Linear Statistical Inference and its Applications*, New York, Wiley

Rinsky, R.A., Zumwalde, R.O., Waxweiler, R.J., Murray, W.E., Jr, Bierbaum, P.J., Landrigan, P.J., Terpilak, M. & Cox, C. (1981) Cancer mortality at a naval nuclear shipyard. *Lancet*, **i**, 231–235

Robins, J., Gail, M.H. & Lubin, J.H. (1986a) More on biased selection of controls. *Biometrics*, **42**, 293–299

Robins, J., Breslow, N. & Greenland, S. (1986b) A Mantel–Haenszel variance consistent under both large strata and sparse data limiting models. *Biometrics*, **42**, 311–323

Rose, G. & Shipley, M.J. (1980) Plasma lipids and mortality: a source of error. *Lancet*, **i**, 523–526

Rothman, K.J. (1976) Causes. *Am. J. Epidemiol.*, **104**, 587–592

Rothman, K.J. & Boice, J.D., Jr (1979) *Epidemiologic Analysis with a Programmable Calculator* (*NIH Publication 79-1649*), Washington DC, US Government Printing Office

Rowland, R.E. & Lucas, H.F. (1984) *Radium-dial workers*. In: Boice, J.D., Jr & Fraumeni, J.F., Jr, eds, *Radiation Carcinogenesis*: *Epidemiology and Biological Significance*, New York, Raven Press, pp. 231–240

Schlesselman, J.J. (1982) *Case-control Studies. Design, Conduct, Analysis*, Oxford, Oxford University Press

Schoenfeld, D. (1980) Chi-square goodness-of-fit tests for the proportional hazards regression model. *Biometrika*, **67**, 145–153

Schou, G. & Vaeth, M. (1980) A small sample study of occurrence/exposure rates for rare events. *Scand. actuarial J.*, **4**, 209–225

Segi, M. (1960) *Cancer Mortality for Selected Sites in 24 Countries* (*1950–1957*), Sendai, Tohoku University School of Medicine

Seidman, H., Selikoff, I.J. & Hammond, E.C. (1979) Short-term asbestos work exposure and long-term observation. *Ann. N.Y. Acad. Sci.*, **330**, 61–90

Selikoff, I.J., Hammond, E.C. & Seidman, H. (1973) *Cancer risk of insulation workers in the United States.* In: Bogovski, P., Gilson, J.C., Timbrell, V. & Wagner, J.C., eds, *Biological Effects of Asbestos (IARC Scientific Publications No. 8)*, Lyon, International Agency for Research on Cancer, pp. 209–216

Selikoff, I.J., Hammond, E.C. & Seidman, H. (1980) Latency of asbestos disease among insulation workers in the United States and Canada. *Cancer,* **46,** 2736–2740

Shapiro, S., Venet, W., Strax, P., Venet, L. & Roeser, R. (1982) Ten- to fourteen-year effect of screening on breast cancer mortality. *J. natl Cancer Inst.,* **69,** 349–355

Shore, R.E., Hempelmann, L.H., Kowaluk, E., Mansur, P.S., Pasternack, B.S., Albert, R.E. & Haughie, G.E. (1977) Breast neoplasms in women treated with X-rays for acute postpartum mastitis. *J. natl Cancer Inst.,* **59,** 813–822

Siemiatycki, J. & Thomas, D.C. (1981) Biological models and statistical interactions: an example from multi-stage carcinogenesis. *Int. J. Epidemiol.,* **10,** 383–387

Silcock, H. (1959) The comparison of occupational mortality rates. *Pop. Stud.,* **13,** 183–192

Smith, P.G. & Day, N.E. (1981) *Matching and confounding in the design and analysis of epidemiological case-control studies.* In: Bithell, J. & Coppi, R., eds. *Perspectives in Medical Statistics,* London, Academic Press, pp. 39–64

Smith, P.G. & Day, N.E. (1984) The design of case-control studies: the influence of confounding and interaction effects. *Int. J. Epidemiol.,* **13,** 356–365

Smith, P.G. & Doll, R. (1982) Mortality among patients with ankylosing spondylitis after a single treatment course with X rays. *Br. med. J.,* **284,** 449–460

Smith, P.G., Pike, M.C., Hill, A.P., Breslow, N.E. & Day, N.E. (1981) Multivariate conditional logistic analysis of stratum-matched case-control studies. *Appl. Stat.,* **30,** 190–197

Sprott, D.A. (1973) Normal likelihoods and their relation to large sample theory of estimation. *Biometrika,* **60,** 457–465

Stewart, A., Webb, J. & Hewitt, D. (1958) A survey of childhood malignancies. *Br. med. J.,* **ii,** 1495–1509

Stewart, W.H. & Pierce, D.A. (1982) Efficiency of Cox's model in estimating regression parameters with grouped survival data. *Biometrika,* **69,** 539–545

Storer, B.E. & Crowley, J. (1985) A diagnostic for Cox regression and general conditional likelihoods. *J. Am. stat. Assoc.,* **80,** 139–147

Storer, B.E., Wacholder, S. & Breslow, N.E. (1983) Maximum likelihood fitting of general risk models to stratified data. *Appl. Stat.,* **32,** 177–181

Suissa, S. & Shuster, J.J. (1985) Exact unconditional sample sizes for the 2×2 binomial trial. *J. R. stat. Soc. A,* **148,** 317–327

Szmuness, W. (1978) Hepatocellular carcinoma and the hepatitis B virus: evidence for a causal association. *Prog. med. Virol.,* **24,** 40–69

Tanner, M.A. & Wong, W.H. (1984) Data based nonparametric estimation of the hazard function with applications to model diagnostics and exploratory analysis. *J. Am. stat. Assoc.,* **79,** 174–182

Tarone, R.E. (1982) The use of historical control information in testing for a trend in Poisson means. *Biometrics,* **38,** 457–462

Tarone, R.E. (1985) On heterogeneity tests based on efficient scores. *Biometrika*, **72**, 91–95

Tarone, R.E. & Gart, J.J. (1980) On the robustness of combined tests for trends in proportions. *J. Am. stat. Assoc.*, **75**, 110–116

de-Thé, G.B., Geser, A., Day, N.E., Tukei, P.M., Williams, E.H., Beri, D., Smith, P.G., Bornkamm, G.W., Feorino, P. & Henle, W. (1978) Epidemiological evidence for causal relationship between Epstein-Barr virus and Burkitt's lymphoma from Ugandan prospective study. *Nature*, **274**, 756–761

Thomas, D.B., Persing, J.P. & Hutchinson, W.B. (1982) Exogenous estrogens and other risk factors for breast cancer in women with benign breast diseases. *J. natl Cancer Inst.*, **69**, 1017–1025

Thomas, D.C. (1977) Addendum to a paper by Liddell, F.D.K., McDonald, J.C. & Thomas, D.C. *J. R. stat. Soc. A*, **140**, 483–485

Thomas, D.C. (1981) General relative risk functions for survival time and matched case-control analysis. *Biometrics*, **37**, 673–686

Thomas, D.C. (1982) *Temporal effects and interactions in cancer: implications of carcinogenic models.* In: Prentice, R.L. & Whittemore, A.S., eds, *Environmental Epidemiology: Risk Assessment*, Philadelphia, SIAM, pp. 107–121

Thomas, D.C. (1983) Statistical methods for analysing effects of temporal patterns of exposure on cancer risks. *Scand. J. Work Environ. Health*, **9**, 353–366

Thomas, D.C. & McNeill, K.J. (1982) *Risk Estimates for the Health Effects of Alpha Radiation (Research Report INFU-0081)*, Ottawa, Atomic Energy Control Board

Thompson, R. & Baker, R. (1981) Composite link functions in generalized linear models. *Appl. Stat.*, **30**, 125–131

Thompson, W.D., Kelsey, J.L. & Walter, S.D. (1982) Cost and efficiency in the choice of matched and unmatched case-control designs. *Am. J. Epidemiol.*, **116**, 840–851

Titterington, D.M. (1985) Common structure of smoothing techniques in statistics. *Int. stat. Rev.*, **53**, 141–170

Tomatis, L., Turusov, V., Day, N. & Charles, R.T. (1972) The effect of long-term exposure to DDT on CF-1 mice. *Int. J. Cancer*, **10**, 489–506

Tsiatis, A.A. (1980) A note on a goodness-of-fit test for the logistic regression model. *Biometrika*, **67**, 250–251

Tsiatis, A.A. (1981) A large sample study of Cox's regression model. *Ann. Stat.*, **9**, 93–108

Tzonou, A., Kaldor, J., Day, N.E., Trichopoulos, D. & Smith, P.G. (1986) The effects of misclassification on case-control studies. *Rev. Epidemiol. Santé publ.*, **34**, 10–17

Ury, H. (1975) Efficiency of case-control studies with multiple controls per case: continuous or dichotomous data. *Biometrics*, **34**, 643–649

Ury, H.K. & Fleiss, J.L. (1980) On approximate sample sizes for comparing two independent proportions with the use of Yates' correction. *Biometrics*, **36**, 347–351

US Bureau of Censuses (1972) *Census of Population: 1970, General Population Characteristics (Final Report PC(1)-B)*, Washington DC, US Government Printing Office

Vaeth, M. (1985) On the use of Wald's test in exponential families. *Int. stat. Rev.*, **53**, 199–214

Vainio, H. (1985) Current trends in the biological monitoring of exposure to carcinogens. *Scand. J. Work Environ. Health*, **11**, 1–6

Wagoner, J.K., Infante, P.F. & Saracci, R. (1976) Vinyl chloride and mortality. *Lancet*, **ii**, 194–195

Wald, N.J. & Doll, R., eds (1985) *Interpretation of Negative Epidemiological Evidence for Carcinogenicity* (*IARC Scientific Publications No. 65*), Lyon, International Agency for Research on Cancer

Wald, N.J., Idle, M., Boreham, J. & Bailey, A. (1980) Low serum vitamin A and subsequent risk of cancer. Preliminary results of prospective study. *Lancet*, **ii**, 775–777

Walker, A.M. & Rothman, K.J. (1982) Models of varying parametric form in case-referent studies. *Am. J. Epidemiol.*, **115**, 129–137

Wall, W.D. & William, H.L. (1970) *Longitudinal Studies and the Social Sciences*, London, Heinemann

Walter, S.D. (1980) Matched case-control studies with a variable number of controls per case. *Appl. Stat.*, **29**, 172–179

Waterhouse, J., Muir, C., Correa, P. & Powell, J., eds (1976) *Cancer Incidence in Five Continents, Vol. III* (*IARC Scientific Publications No. 15*), Lyon, International Agency for Research on Cancer

Waxweiler, R.J., Roscoe, R.J., Archer, V.E., Thun, M.J., Wagoner, J.K. & Lundin, F.E. (1981) *Mortality follow-up through 1977 of the white underground uranium mines cohort examined by the US Public Health Service*. In: Gomez, M., ed., *Radiation Hazards in Mining: Control, Measurement, and Medical Aspects*, New York, New York Society of Mining Engineers of the American Institute of Mining, Metallurgical and Petroleum Engineers, Inc., pp.

Waxweiler, R.J., Beaumont, J.J., Henry, J.A., Brown, D.P., Robinson, C.F., Ness, G.O., Wagoner, J.K. & Lemen, R.A. (1983) A modified life table analysis system for cohort studies. *J. occup. Med.*, **25**, 115–124

Welsh, K., Higgins, I., Oh, M. & Burchfiel, C. (1982) Arsenic exposure, smoking, and respiratory cancer in copper smelter workers. *Arch. environ. Health*, **37**, 325–335

Wen, C.P., Tsai, M.S. & Gibson, R.L. (1983) Anatomy of the healthy worker effect: a critical review. *J. occup. Med.*, **25**, 283–289

Whittemore, A.S. (1981) Sample size for logistic regression with small response probabilities. *J. Am. stat. Assoc.* **76**, 27–32

Whittemore, A.S. & Keller, J.B. (1978) Quantitative theories of carcinogenesis. *SIAM Rev.*, **20**, 1–30

Whittemore, A.S. & McMillan, A. (1982) *Analysing occupational cohort data: application to US uranium miners*. In: Prentice, R.L. & Whittemore, A.S., eds, *Environmental Epidemiology: Risk Assessment*, Philadelphia, SIAM, pp. 65–81

Whittemore, A.S. & McMillan, A. (1983) Lung cancer mortality among US uranium miners: a reappraisal. *J. natl Cancer Inst.*, **71**, 489–499

Williams, D.A. (1976) Improved likelihood ratio tests for complete contingency tables. *Biometrika*, **63**, 33–37

Yandell, B.S. (1983) Nonparametric inference for rates with censored survival data. *Ann. Stat.*, **11**, 1119–1135

Yerushalmy, J. (1951) A mortality index for use in place of the age-adjusted death rate. *Am. J. publ. Health*, **41**, 907–922

Yule, G.U. (1934) On some points relating to vital statistics, more especially statistics of occupational mortality. *J. R. stat. Soc.*, **97**, 1–84

Zavon, M.R., Hoegg, U. & Bingham, E. (1973) Benzidine exposure as a cause of bladder tumors. *Arch. environ. Health*, **27**, 1–7

Zelen, M. & Dannemiller, M.C. (1961) The robustness of life testing procedures derived from the exponential distribution. *Technometrics*, **3**, 29–49

APPENDICES

APPENDIX I. DESIGN AND CONDUCT OF STUDIES CITED IN THE TEXT

APPENDIX IA

THE BRITISH DOCTORS STUDY

This prospective study of the health effects of smoking started in 1951. The first report appeared in 1954 (Doll & Hill, 1954) and was followed at regular intervals by the results of further follow-up (Doll & Hill, 1956, 1964; Doll & Peto, 1976, 1978; Doll et al., 1957, 1980). Members of the medical profession in the United Kingdom were asked to fill in a simple questionnaire, which was sent out on 31 October 1951 to 59 600 men and women on the Medical Register.

The questionnaire was intentionally kept short and simple to encourage a high proportion of replies. The doctors were asked to classify themselves into one of three groups – (1) whether they were, at the time, smoking; (2) whether they had smoked but had given up; or (3) whether they had never smoked regularly (that is, had never smoked as much as one cigarette a day, or its equivalent in pipe tobacco, for as long as one year). Present smokers and ex-smokers were asked additional questions. The former were asked the age at which they had started smoking and the amount of tobacco that they were currently smoking, and the method by which it was consumed. The ex-smokers were asked similar questions but relating to the time just before they had given up smoking.

In a covering letter, the doctors were invited to give any information on their smoking habits or history that might be of interest, but, apart from that, no information was sought on previous changes in habit (other than the amount smoked prior to last giving up, if smoking had been abandoned). The decision to restrict questions on amount smoked to current smoking habits was based mainly on the results of the earlier case-control study (Doll & Hill, 1950, 1952), based on interviews with nearly 5000 patients. This study had shown that the classification of smokers according to the amount that they had most recently smoked gave almost as sharp a differentiation between the groups of patients with and without lung cancer as the use of smoking histories over many years – theoretically more relevant statistics, but clearly based on less accurate data.

The results of ten years' follow-up were published in 1964 (Doll & Hill, 1964), in which a description of the cohort and its representativeness for all British doctors was described. The results of ten years' follow-up for men was published in 1976 (Doll & Peto, 1976) and of 22 years' follow-up for women in 1980 (Doll et al., 1980).

During the study, further questionnaires were sent out on three separate occasions to men (see Table IA.1) and on two occasions to women. The purpose was partly to obtain detailed information on smoking habits, in particular giving up smoking, and

Table IA.1. Response to questionnaires

	Second questionnaire	Third questionnaire	Fourth questionnaire
Survey period	November 1957– 31 Oct. 1958	March– 31 Oct. 1966	July– 31 Oct. 1972
Known to have died before end of survey period	3 122	7 310	10 634
Presumably alive at end of survey period	31 318	27 139	23 806
Replied by end of survey period (and % of men then alive)	30 810 (98.4)	26 163 (96.4)	23 299 (97.9)
Reasons for nonresponse:			
Too ill	31	65	21
Refused	36	63	102[a]
Address not found	72	403	22
Unknown and other reasons	369	445	362

[a] Includes all men who refused previously

also to ask additional questions, the relevance of which had emerged during the period of follow-up. Degree of inhalation was asked in these questionnaires, and the use of filter-tipped or plain cigarettes asked in the last questionnaire.

From the 59 600 individuals approached initially, 40 637 replies were received that were sufficiently complete to be used – 34 445 from men and 6192 from women. From a one-in-ten random sample of the register, it was estimated that this represented answers from 69% of the men and 60% of the women alive at the time of the inquiry. The degree of self-selection in those who replied was assessed in terms of the overall mortality using this one-in-ten sample. The standardized death rate of those who replied to the first questionnaire was only 63% of the death rate for all doctors in the second year of the inquiry, and 85% in the third year. In the fourth to tenth years the proportion varied about an average of 93%, and there was no evidence of any regular change with the further passage of years. Evidently the effect of selection did not entirely wear off, but after the third year it had become slight. One factor in this favourable mortality was the presence among those who replied of a relatively large number of nonsmokers and a relatively small number of heavy cigarette smokers, demonstrated by a small inquiry undertaken in 1961. Two small samples were drawn of (1) those who had replied in 1951 and (2) those who had not. Eliminating those who had died between 1951 and 1961, there were 267 previous 'answerers' and 213 previous 'nonanswerers'. They were asked about their smoking habits in 1961, and 261 (98%) of the answerers and 179 (84%) of the nonanswerers responded. Comparison of these two groups shows 21% (answerers) and 6% (nonanswerers) nonsmokers and 15% (answerers) and 28% (nonanswerers) as moderate or heavy cigarette smokers (15 or more daily).

The numbers of men replying to the subsequent questionnaires and the numbers not replying for different reasons are shown in Table IA.1. Further questionnaires were not

sent to doctors who had been struck off the Medical Register nor to those who had
refused to answer previously or had asked not to be written to again, although their
mortality was still monitored. The proportions of survivors who did not reply in 1957,
1966, and 1972 were, respectively, 1.6%, 3.6%, and 2.1%.

Information about the death of doctors was obtained at first directly from the
Registrars-General of the United Kingdom, who provided particulars of every death
identified as referring to a medical practitioner. Later, lists of deaths were obtained
from the General Medical Council, and these were complemented by reference to the
records of the British Medical Association and other sources at home and abroad.
Some deaths came to light in response to the questionnaires. Others were discovered in
the course of following up doctors who had not replied to or who had not been sent
subsequent questionnaires. Of the 34 440 men studied, 10 072 were known to have died
before 1 November 1971, 24 265 were known to have been alive at that date, and 103
(0.3%) were not yet traced.

Many of the 103 untraced doctors were not British, and 67 (65%) were known to
have gone abroad. It was felt unlikely that more than about a dozen deaths relevant to
the study could have been missed.

Information on the underlying cause of death in the 10 072 doctors known to have
died before 1 November 1971 was obtained for the vast majority from the official death
certificates. Except for deaths for which lung cancer was mentioned, the certified cause
was accepted and (unless otherwise stated) the deaths classified according to the
underlying cause. (In only four cases was no evidence of the cause obtainable.) The
underlying causes were classified according to the seventh revision of the *International
Classification of Diseases* (World Health Organization, 1957), except that a separate
category of 'pulmonary heart disease' was created.

Cancer of the lung, including trachea or pleura, was given as the underlying cause of
467 deaths and as a contributory cause in a further 20. For each of these 487 deaths,
confirmation of the diagnosis was sought from the doctor who had certified the death
and, when necessary, from the consultant to whom the patient had been referred.
Information about the nature of the evidence was thus obtained in all but two cases.
Doubtful reports were interpreted by an outside consultant, with no knowledge of the
patient's smoking history. As a result, carcinoma of the lung was accepted as the
underlying cause of 441 deaths and as a contributory cause of 17. Twenty-six deaths
were considered to be due to other underlying causes and three to other contributory
causes.

The results for female doctors were published later, in 1980, and for 22 rather than
20 years of follow-up. The methods of enquiry were similar to those used for male
doctors except that only three questionnaires were sent, in 1951, 1961 and 1973.

References

Doll, R. & Hill, A.B. (1950) Smoking and carcinoma of the lung. Preliminary report.
     Br. med. J., **iii**, 739–748
Doll, R. & Hill, A.B. (1952) A study of the aetiology of carcinoma of the lung. *Br.
     med. J.*, **iv**, 1271–1286

Doll, R. & Hill, A.B. (1954) The mortality of doctors in relation to their smoking habits. A preliminary report. *Br. med. J.,* **ii,** 1451–1455

Doll, R. & Hill, A.B. (1956) Lung cancer and other causes of death in relation to smoking; second report on mortality of British doctors. *Br. med. J.,* **ii,** 1071–1081.

Doll, R. & Hill, A.B. (1964) Mortality in relation to smoking: ten years' observations of British doctors. *Br. med. J.,* **i,** 1399–1410

Doll, R. & Peto, R. (1976) Mortality and relation to smoking: 20 years' observations on male British doctors. *Br. med. J.,* **ii,** 1525–1536

Doll, R. & Peto, R. (1978) Cigarette smoking and bronchial carcinoma: dose and time relationships among regular smokers and lifelong non-smokers. *J. Epidemiol. Community Health,* **32,** 303–313

Doll, R., Gray, R., Hafner, B. & Peto, R. (1980) Mortality in relation to smoking: 22 years' observations on female British doctors. *Br. med. J.,* **ii,** 967–971

World Health Organization (1957) *International Classification of Diseases,* Seventh Revision, Geneva

APPENDIX IB

THE ATOMIC BOMB SURVIVORS – THE LIFE-SPAN STUDY

A vast programme of studies has been conducted under the aegis of the Radiation Effects Research Foundation (RERF) and its predecessor, the Atomic Bomb Casualty Commission (ABCC), investigating both the short- and long-term effects of the radiation exposure suffered by the survivors of the atomic bomb explosions in Japan. These effects include:

Early somatic effects:
– acute radiation sickness
– abortion
– impaired fertility
– maldevelopment of the embryo and foetus

Late somatic effects:
– impairment of growth and stature
– cataract of the lens of the eye
– impairment of fertility
– cytogenetic abnormalities
– cancer
– other diseases
– effects on ageing
– effects on immunity

Genetic effects:
– stillbirths, changes in sex ratio, reduced birth weight, neonatal mortality, birth defects
– cytogenetic abnormalities
– protein polymorphisms

The main results on cancer mortality have come from the Life-span Study, the original description of which is given in a paper by Beebe *et al.* (1962). A feature of the Life-span Study has been the regular publication of technical reports by the RERF, with analyses of updated results.

The study was set up as a systematic search for any mortality differential associated with radiation, one aim being to ensure that effects would not be missed merely because they were not specifically looked for at the right time. It was intended that any new mortality differential uncovered by the Life-span Study could be pursued by pathologists and clinical investigators in a more definitive fashion. A portion of the mortality sample was the subject of a continuing clinical investigation embracing standard physical and laboratory investigations every two years, plus a wide variety of short-term, special studies.

The cohort for the Life-span Study was intended to include all survivors who had received appreciable radiation exposure, together with survivors more distant from the hypocentres of the explosions, who received lower doses. In the absence of suitable sampling frames established shortly after the bombs fell, the 1950 national census was used as a basis for cohort definition. In that census, 284 000 survivors were enumerated, of whom 195 000 lived in one of the bombed cities. The Japanese citizens among this latter group, with place of family registration in the city or nearby, constituted the sampling base. It was decided to include all individuals in this group who had received appreciable radiation, and a stratified sample of the remainder. At the time the sample was constructed, the air dose as a function of distance from the hypocentre of the bombs was estimated to be about 100 rads at 1500 metres, 15 rads at 2000 metres and 3 rads at 2500 metres. All eligible individuals who were within 2500 metres were therefore included. A comparison group was formed from among those more distally located at the time of the bomb, of the same size as the group exposed less than 2000 metres and of the same age and sex composition. Matching was done separately for people of each sex by single year of age.

A second control group was formed of people not resident in either of the two cities when the bombs fell, mainly to guard against the risk of missing effects that were not dose-dependent. Most of this group consisted of migrants to the two cities after the war, with considerable differences in background lifestyle. Doubts were raised early on as to the group's comparability, which were later confirmed (Beebe et al., 1971), and little reference is made to it in the more recent reports.

In the original 1950 census, there was an additional group (known as the 'reserve' group) of 9527 survivors exposed within 2500 metres, but whose place of family registration was too distant from the cities to satisfy the initial eligibility criterion. This criterion had been introduced to ensure uniformity in the follow-up procedures (see next section), but experience obtained during the conduct of the study indicated that the family registration system was highly effective for follow-up, and that this exclusion criterion was unnecessary. In the more recent reports, this group was included in the study cohort (Beebe et al., 1971).

Details of the full sample from the 1950 census are given in Table IB.1, which indicates those selected for the Life-span Study.

Follow-up procedures were based on the Japanese Family Registration System. Under the Family Registration Law of Japan (1947), a register is maintained by the mayor or equivalent authority for every family registered in his jurisdiction, and vital events are posted therein. The place of registration corresponds to a legal address for family purposes and is seldom changed even when physical residence changes. Officials responsible for the registration of births and deaths throughout Japan send copies of these vital documents to the places of family registration. Changes in the place of family registration and creation of registers for new families are so effected that knowledge of any one place of registration is a virtual guarantee that the present place of registration can be learned and survival status ascertained.

In connection with the present study, a test was made of the family registration

Table IB.1. The master sample, proper and reserve, by component, exposure category and city[a]

City and comparison group	Total	Proper part		Reserve
		Selected	Not selected	
Hiroshima				
Total	121 100	74 356	16 341	30 403
A 0–1999 m from hypocentre	26 174	21 329	—	4 845
B 2000–2499 m	14 543	11 524	—	3 019
C[b] 2500–9999 m	44 478	21 275	14 748	8 455
D[b] 10 000+ m or not in city	35 905	20 228	1 593	14 084
Nagasaki				
Total	42 620	25 037	10 458	7 125
A 0–1999 m from hypocentre	7 659	6 801	—	858
B 2000–2499 m	5 949	5 144	—	805
C[b] 2500–9999 m	18 151	6 742	8 900	2 510
D[b] 10 000+ m or not in city	10 860	6 350	1 558	2 952
Total				
Total	163 720	99 393	26 799	37 528
A 0–1999 m from hypocentre	33 833	28 130	—	5 703
B 2000–2499 m	20 492	16 668	—	3 824
C[b] 2500–9999 m	62 630	28 017	23 648	10 965
D[b] 10 000+ m or not in city	46 765	26 578	3 151	17 036

[a] From Kato (1984)
[b] Matched by age and sex to group A

system. For the Life-span Study, 20 000 individuals were checked against their family registers, and for only 17 could the register not be found. Investigation showed that nine of these were foreigners not eligible for family registration; for one person a register should have been made but had not been; and only seven, therefore, were really unknown. Since these individuals were being kept under active clinical surveillance, their mortality was known. The family registers returned mortality information on all but nine of the 1300 known deaths, or 99.3%, indicating that the family register approach provides information of nearly perfect completeness.

Information on cause of death was provided from vital statistics death schedules by the National Institutes of Health under official procedures specific to this joint NIH-ABCC study.

The cause of death as given on death certificates has been compared with that given by autopsy findings for those invididuals who came to autopsy – a small overall proportion – as shown in Table IB.2. To achieve comparability with official Japanese vital statistics, cause of death was coded according to the WHO *International Classification of Diseases, Injuries, and Causes of Death*. The 7th, 8th and 9th Revisions were used for the time periods 1950–1967, 1968–1978, and 1979 onwards, respectively

Table IB.2. Accuracy of causes of death – autopsy cases among Life-span Study sample, 1961–1975[a]

Cause of death	Death certificate	Autopsy report	Agreement	Confirmation rate	Detection rate
Tuberculosis	176	226	110	62.5	48.7
Malignant neoplasm of:					
buccal cavity & pharynx	19	17	13	68.4	76.5
oesophagus	50	53	36	72.0	67.9
stomach	444	495	374	84.2	75.6
large intestine	43	54	28	65.1	51.9
rectum	45	46	32	71.1	69.6
liver, gallbladder, bile ducts	42	169	26	61.9	15.4
pancreas	56	81	36	64.3	44.4
breast	40	49	38	95.0	77.6
uterus	70	83	57	81.4	68.7
prostate	13	24	5	38.5	20.8
urinary organs	38	60	30	78.9	50.0
malignant lymphomas	40	56	31	77.5	55.4
leukaemias	42	40	36	85.7	90.0
Benign neoplasms and neoplasms of unspecified nature	65	21	3	4.6	14.3
Disease of blood and blood-forming organs	30	14	12	40.0	85.7
Ischaemic heart disease	265	199	67	25.3	33.7
Gastric, duodenal & peptic ulcer	58	61	24	41.4	39.3
Cirrhosis of liver	153	149	80	52.3	53.7
Nephritis & nephrosis	62	29	11	17.7	37.9

[a] From Kato (1984)

Great efforts have been made to establish the dose received by each member of the Life-span Study group, and also the degree of accuracy of these dose estimates. In the early reports, the radiation dose estimates used were the so-called Tentative 1957 dose (T57D), which were considered to be accurate within a factor of 2. For each survivor included in the Life-span Study, information on location and shielding at the time of the bomb was obtained by interview and, in some cases, by mail questionnaire. These estimates were later revised, to give the T65 dose, which were used in reports on mortality experience up to 1974 (Beebe *et al.*, 1977). A minor change in the location of the hypocentre of the Nagasaki explosion led to some revision of the T65 dose, to give the T65DR estimates used in report number 7 (Kato & Schull, 1982). The average error in these estimates has been evaluated as 30% (Jablon, 1971). Further work has indicated that the T65DR estimates themselves may need major revision, based on a reassessment mainly of exposure to neutrons (Loewe & Mendelsohn, 1981).

Jablon (1984) and Fujita (1984) both discuss dosimetry revisions, in a monograph (Prentice & Thompson, 1984) of great value to those interested in the current status of the follow-up studies of the atomic bomb survivors.

References

Beebe, G.W., Ishida, M. & Jablon, S. (1962) Studies of the mortality of A-bomb survivors. I. Plan of study and mortality in the medical subsample (selection 1), 1950–1958. *Radiat. Res,* **16,** 253–280

Beebe, G.W., Kato, H. & Land, C.E. (1971) Studies of the mortality of A-bomb survivors. 4. Mortality and radiation dose, 1950–1966. *Radiat. Res.,* **48,** 613–649

Beebe, G.W., Kato, H. & Land, C.E. (1977) *Mortality Experience of Atomic Bomb Survivors 1950–74, Life Span Study Report 8* (*RERF Technical Report 1–77*), Hiroshima, Radiation Effects Research Foundation

Fujita, S. (1984) *Potential additional data sources for dosimetry and biological re-evaluation.* In: Prentice, R.L. & Thompson, D.J., eds, *Atomic Bomb Survivor Data: Utilization and Analysis,* Philadelphia, SIAM, pp. 183–194

Jablon, S. (1971) *Atomic Bomb Radiation Dose Estimation at ABCC* (*ABCC Technical Report 23–71*), Hiroshima, Atomic Bomb Casualty Commission

Jablon, S. (1984) *Dosimetry and dosimetry evaluation.* In: Prentice, R.L. & Thompson, D.J., eds, *Atomic Bomb Survivor Data: Utilization and Analysis,* Philadelphia, SIAM, pp. 143–152

Kato, H. (1984) *Data resources for the Life-span Study.* In: Prentice, R.L. & Thompson, D.J., eds, *Atomic Bomb Survivor Data: Utilization and Analysis,* Philadelphia, SIAM, pp. 3–17

Kato, H. & Schull, W.J. (1982) Studies of the mortality of A-bomb survivors. 7. Mortality, 1950–78. Part I. Cancer mortality. *Radiat. Res.,* **90,** 395–432

Loewe, W.E. & Mendelsohn, E. (1981) Revised dose estimates at Hiroshima and Nagasaki. *Health Phys.,* **41,** 663–666

Prentice, R.L. & Thompson, D.J., eds (1984) *Atomic Bomb Survivor Data: Utilization and Analysis,* Philadelphia, SIAM

HEPATITIS B AND LIVER CANCER

A large number of case-control studies and several cohort studies have been undertaken to investigate the association between the hepatitis B surface antigen (HBsAg) carrier state and the development of liver cancer. The first prospective study to report conclusive results was from Taiwan (Beasley *et al.*, 1981), in which male Chinese Government employees were enrolled through routine health care services. Since the term 'liver cancer' on a death certificate may imply secondary liver cancer, and hepatitis B virus (HBV) is related only to primary hepatocellular carcinoma (PHC), the causes of death of the study subjects were investigated in some detail. The study design and procedures were as follows (Beasley *et al.*, 1981).

The study was conducted among male Chinese Government employees (civil servants) in Taiwan whose life and health insurance system provides almost total ascertainment of the fact of death, with excellent determination of cause of death. The study was restricted to men, since the incidence of PHC is three to four times higher in men than in women, and male government employees are on average older and stay in government service longer. Initially, enrolment was restricted to men aged 40 to 59 years; later, because of the general popularity of the project, men of all ages were recruited. Study participants were recruited through two sources:

(1) at the Government Employees' Clinic Centre (GECC) during routine free physical examinations or at selected other clinics (e.g., dental, ear, nose and throat and ophthalmology), where no bias in liver disease status was considered likely (GECC group)

(2) among men recruited from the GECC ten years earlier, when they were 40–59 years old, for a prospective study of cardiovascular disease risk factors; they had been kept under active surveillance since then (CVDS group).

There were 1480 men in the CVDS group and 21 227 men in the GECC group. The CVDS and GECC groups were similar except that the CVDS group was older. It was stated that government employees and the general population were similar with respect to the frequency of HBV infections, the HBsAg carrier rate and the mortality rate from PHC and cirrhosis.

PHC was detected through health and life insurance, mandatory for all government employees and provided by a single large government bureau operating exclusively for this purpose. Insurance was usually retained after retirement and could be cancelled only at the request of the retired person. All deaths of active government employees and deaths of most retired government employees were thus known to the insurance bureau. Monthly lists of recent deaths and newly retiring employees who had cancelled their insurance were received from the bureau. In the 1981 report, only 643 men had cancelled their insurance (2.8% of study subjects), of whom 569 had been contacted by letter or telephone. Thus, only 74 (0.3%) of the original cohort might have died and the death not be known to the study.

To verify the completeness of the insurance system for the ascertainment of deaths, all HBsAg-positive men (3454) and controls matched for age and province of origin with each HBsAg-positive man were actively followed. This active surveillance involved annual completion of a health questionnaire and retesting for HBV markers. Adherence to follow-up averaged 95% annually. The state of health of those who failed to return for follow-up was determined by telephone or home visit. Contact was lost with only 74 men, whose vital status could not be ascertained. From this active surveillance we were able to verify that among men retaining their insurance all deaths are known to us.

The causes of death of all study subjects were investigated through the records of preceding periods in hospital. Among the 41 deaths due to PHC reported in 1981, 19 (46.3%) were confirmed histologically. Nineteen of the remaining patients had raised serum alpha fetoprotein (AFP) levels and changes on a liver scan, or angiography, or both, interpreted as PHC; one more patient had scans interpreted as PHC but AFP was not measured; and the remaining two patients had raised AFP levels and their clinical picture was interpreted as PHC. The clinical picture, liver scan and angiographic patterns did not differ between histologically confirmed and unconfirmed cases. Deaths attributed to cirrhosis all showed unequivocal clinical evidence of chronic hepatic failure in the presence of portal hypertension and other classical evidence of cirrhosis.

All recruitment and follow-up specimens were tested for HBsAg, alanine aminotransferase and AFP. Anti-HBs and anti-HBc (hepatitis B core antigen) testing were too expensive to undertake on all 19 253 HBsAg-negative subjects. All 1020 HBsAg-negative men from the CVDS group and controls matched for age and province of origin with each HBsAg-positive subject in the GECC group were selected from among the HBsAg-negative subjects for anti-HBs testing; 3661 men were tested for anti-HBs. Of these, all the 615 who were anti-HBs-negative were tested for anti-HBc. The anti-HBs and anti-HBc rates derived from the above sample were then used to project the frequency of these markers for the entire study population.

Reference

Beasley, R.P., Hwang, L.Y., Lin, C.C. & Chien, C.S. (1981) Hepatocellular carcinoma and hepatitis B virus. A prospective study of 22 707 men in Taiwan. *Lancet*, **ii**, 1129–1133

CANCER IN NICKEL WORKERS – THE SOUTH WALES COHORT

The risk of nasal sinus and lung cancer associated with nickel refining had been established in the late 1930s. In 1949, both diseases were prescribed as occupational diseases in the United Kingdom when they occurred in men 'working in a factory where nickel is produced by decomposition of a gaseous nickel compound'.

The principal cohort study of the South Wales cohort was first reported in 1970 (Doll *et al.*, 1970) and an extension of the study in 1977 (Doll *et al.*, 1977). Further analyses have been published since (Peto *et al.*, 1984; Kaldor *et al.*, 1986).

The aims of the study were succinctly described by Doll *et al.* (1970):

'Men employed in a nickel refinery in South Wales were investigated to determine whether the risk of developing carcinoma of the bronchi and nasal sinuses, which had been associated with the refining of nickel, are still present. The data obtained were also used to compare the effect of age at exposure on susceptibility to cancer induction and to determine the rate of change of mortality after exposure to a carcinogenic agent has ceased.'

The cohort was identified using the weekly paysheets of the company, on which all men receiving an hourly wage were listed by name and works' reference number. Initially, paysheets were inspected for the first week in April of the years 1934, 1939, 1944 and 1949, and all men were included whose names and numbers were recorded on any two of the sheets, unless they were noted on one of the two sheets as having been in the Armed Forces or transferred elsewhere for war work. By this means, the population was limited to men who were likely to have been employed for at least five years, and follow-up was facilitiated.

The names of all the men included in the study were identified in the company's register of new employees. This gave the year when they were first employed and much other information that helped in tracing them. From 1902 to 1933 the register of new employees also gave the men's ages; in later years this was sometimes omitted, in which case it had to be obtained from other sources, such as pension records or death certificates.

The study was later extended by examining the paysheets for the first week in April 1929. It is therefore effectively restricted to men employed for at least five years who were still employed in 1934 or later. The follow-up has been continued until 31 December 1981, by which time 788, or 81%, of the original cohort of 968 had died. Only 18 (2%) of the cohort were lost to follow-up.

Copies of the death certificates were obtained for all who were known to have died, and the cause of death was classified according to the Seventh Revision of the *International Classification of Diseases* (World Health Organization, 1957). The use of these rules for all periods rather than the ones that were current at the time of death has no effect on the estimated numbers of deaths attributed to cancers of the lung and nose.

Because of the method of selection, no one came under observation until 1934. The man-years at risk were, therefore, calculated for the period 1934–1981. Observed and expected deaths were calculated only up to age 85, at least in the last two reports (Peto *et al.*, 1984; Kaldor *et al.*, 1986), to minimize the effects of misclassification on the death certificates in old age. The numbers of deaths that would have been expected if the men had suffered the normal mortality in England and Wales as a whole were calculated by multiplying the man-years at risk in each five-year age group and each calendar period (1934–1938, 1939–1943, 1944–1948, 1949–1953, 1953–1958, 1959–1963 and 1964–1971) by the corresponding national mortality rates. Nasal cancer rates were not available before 1940, and the rates for 1940 were used for the earlier years.

References

Doll, R., Morgan, L.G. & Speizer, F.E. (1970) Cancers of the lung and nasal sinuses in nickel workers. *Br. J. Cancer,* **24,** 623–632

Doll, R., Mathews, J.D. & Morgan, L.G. (1977) Cancers of the lung and nasal sinuses in nickel workers: a reassessment of the period of risk. *Br. J. ind. Med.,* **34,** 102–105

Kaldor, J.M., Peto, J., Easton, D., Doll, R., Herman, C. & Morgan, L. (1986) Models for respiratory cancer in nickel refinery workers. *J. natl Cancer Inst.,* **77,** 841–848

Peto, J., Cuckle, H., Doll, R., Hermon, C. & Morgan, L.G. (1984) *Respiratory cancer mortality of Welsh nickel refinery workers.* In: Sunderman, F.W., ed., *Nickel in the Human Environment* (*IARC Scientific Publications No. 53*), Lyon, International Agency for Research on Cancer pp. 37–46

World Health Organization (1957) *International Classification of Diseases,* Seventh Revision, Geneva

APPENDIX IE

THE MONTANA STUDY OF SMELTER WORKERS

Earlier reports had indicated an excess risk of respiratory cancer among long-term metal miners. Among the agents possibly responsible for this increase were airborne radiation and arsenic compounds. The purpose of the Montana smelter study was to investigate the role of arsenic in the development of respiratory cancer, since smelters have negligible exposure to airborne radiation and higher exposure to arsenic. The original report was published in 1969 (Lee & Fraumeni, 1969) covering the mortality experience of the cohort in the period 1 January 1938 to 31 December 1963. The follow-up was later extended to 30 September 1977 (Lee–Feldstein, 1983). Further analyses of parts of the data have appeared (Lubin *et al.*, 1981; Brown & Chu, 1983), the latter structuring the analysis in terms of multistage models of carcinogenesis (see Chapter 6).

The study population comprised 8045 white men who had been employed as smelter workers for 12 or more months before 31 December 1956. Of this group, one-third was initially employed before 1938, one-third during 1938–1946, and one-third in 1947–1955.

Company records provided for each individual the date and place of birth, social security number, time and place of employment for each job held within a smelter before 1964, year last known alive, and the date and place of death for most decedents. In addition, follow-up information was obtained from death registers of state health departments, social security claims records of the Bureau of Old Age and Survivors Insurance, and other governmental agencies. The mortality experience of the group has been followed from 1 January 1938 to 30 September 1977 (Lee–Feldstein, 1983).

Death certificates were obtained for the smelter workers known to have died during the 26-year period, 1938–1963. Information on mortality and follow-up for the period 1964–1977 was obtained from company records, the Social Security Administration and death registers of various health departments. Underlying causes of death were classified according to the *International Classification of Diseases* appropriate for the calendar year of death and later, for convenience, were converted into the Seventh Revision code (World Health Organization 1957)

The follow-up status on 30 September 1977, together with the follow-up status given in the first report as of 31 December 1963, is shown in Table IE.1.

The study group was compared with the white male population of the same states through the use of expected deaths obtained by multiplying the age- and cause-specific mortality rates for the states by the person-years at risk for each cohort of smelter workers.

Table IE.1   Follow-up status of study group

Total study group, 1977		Follow-up status, 31 December 1963		
		Known to be living	Known to be deceased	Vital status not known
Known to be living	3707[a]	3342	0	365[b]
Known to be deceased	3522	1534	1877	111
Vital status not known	816	520	0	296
Total, 1963	8045[c]	5396	1877	772

[a] Includes 442 men still employed at the smelter on 30 September 1977
[b] Approximately half of the men reported lost to follow-up by Lee and Fraumeni (1969) were found to be alive on 30 September 1977.
[c] Two persons in the original study group of 8045 were women; they have been deleted from the present study.

The study group was categorized by exposure to varying levels of arsenic, sulfur dioxide and other chemicals. From measurements made in the smelters, each work area was rated on a scale from 1 to 10 with respect to the relative amount of arsenic trioxide in the atmosphere. Jobs in three areas, commonly known as the arsenic kitchen, cottrell, and arsenic roaster, afforded 'heavy' arsenic exposure (8–10 on the relative scale). 'Medium' arsenic exposure was associated with four work areas: converter, reverberatory furnace, ore roaster and acid plant, and casting (4–7 on the relative scale). Persons in all other areas had 'light' arsenic exposure (1–3 on the scale). Measurements in work areas may have varied over time, but it seems reasonable to assume that relative exposure in terms of these three broadly defined categories remained fixed. Most men had worked in several different areas, so, to be conservative, an individual was classified into one of the three arsenic groups based on his maximum (heaviest) exposure for the analyses reported by Lee and Fraumeni (1969).

The work areas were also categorized with respect to the level of sulfur dioxide, and study members were classified into one of the three exposure groups. 'Heavy' sulfur dioxide areas consisted of the reverberatory furnace and the converter, whereas 'medium' areas consisted of arsenic roaster, brickyard, ferromanganese plant, lead shop, cottrell, casting, ore roaster and acid plant, and phosphate plant. Finally, the work areas were rated by the levels of exposure to silicon dioxide (silica), lead fumes and ferromanganese.

References

Brown, C.C. & Chu, K.C. (1983) Implications of the multi-stage theory of carcinogenesis applied to occupational arsenic exposure. *J. natl Cancer Inst.*, **70**, 455–463

Lee, A.M. & Fraumeni, J.F., Jr (1969) Arsenic and respiratory cancer in man: an occupational study. *J. natl Cancer Inst.*, **42**, 1045–1052

Lee–Feldstein, A. (1983) Arsenic and respiratory cancer in humans: follow-up of copper smelter employees in Montana. *J. natl Cancer Inst.*, **70**, 601–610

Lubin, J.H., Pottern, L.M., Blot, W.J., Tokudome, S., Stone, B.J. & Fraumeni, J.F., Jr (1981) Respiratory cancer among copper smelter workers: recent mortality statistics. *J. occup. Med.*, **23**, 779–784

ASBESTOS EXPOSURE AND CIGARETTE SMOKING

Several cohorts of asbestos-exposed individuals have been studied in order to determine the joint effect of asbestos and cigarette smoking on the risk of lung cancer. The largest such study is that of the North American insulators, started in 1966. It has given rise to a number of publications, both on the effect of asbestos and on the combined effect of asbestos and smoking (Selikoff *et al.*, 1973; Hammond & Selikoff, 1973; Hammond *et al.*, 1979; Selikoff *et al.*, 1979, 1980). The study was based on the complete 1966 membership list of the International Association of Heat and Frost Insulators and Asbestos Workers, which has about 120 locals in the USA and Canada. Much of the material handled by these insulation workers contained asbestos, so that all of the members can be considered as asbestos workers. In 1966, each member was approached with a request to complete a questionnaire containing a number of questions, including those on his smoking habits and his use (or nonuse) of protective masks (11 656 completed the questionnaire). Date of birth and date of entry into the trade were ascertained from union records. All of these men were traced through 31 December 1976 and copies of the death certificates of those who died obtained. Some of the men on the 1966 membership list died before 1 January 1967, leaving 17 800 alive at that date. Altogether, 2271 died in the ten-year period 1 January 1967–31 December 1976; the number of man-years of observation totaled 166 853; and the average age of the men during the ten-year period was 44.4.

Since the aim of the study was to examine the joint effects of asbestos exposure and cigarette smoking and since the entire study group was taken to be exposed to asbestos, it was necessary to construct a special control group, not exposed to asbestos, for which the smoking history of the individuals was known. This group was obtained from the long-term prospective epidemiological study of the American Cancer Society (Hammond, 1966). Starting on 1 October 1959, 468 688 men and 610 206 women had been enrolled. All of them were over 30 years old at that time and most of them were over 40. Upon enrolment, each subject answered a detailed questionnaire; most of the survivors answered subsequent questionnaires distributed in 1961, 1963 and 1965. During that time, death certificates were obtained for those who died; and when cancer was mentioned on a death certificate, the doctor who signed the certificate was requested to supply additional information on the cause of death and the basis of the diagnosis. Follow-up was then discontinued for six years. Tracing of the subjects was resumed on 1 October 1971 and was continued through 30 September 1972. Because of the extremely large number of deaths after 1965, it was not feasible to request doctors to supply additional information on cause of death.

The socioeconomic distribution of the prospective study cohort differs markedly from that of the asbestos workers. To improve comparability, a selected subgroup of the overall cohort was taken as the control group, consisting of all male subjects who met the following criteria: white, not a farmer, no more than high-school education, a history of occupational exposure to dust, fumes, vapours, gases, chemicals or radiation and alive as of 1 January 1967 and traced thereafter. There were 73 763 such subjects. They were classified according to their smoking histories, and the age-specific death rates of each such class were computed.

There was a problem. Death rates in the control group were known for the period 1 January 1967 through 30 September 1972, while members of the asbestos insulation workers union were traced during the period 1 January 1967–31 December 1976. According to official mortality statistics, death rates of the general population of the USA changed somewhat during the second five-year period 1 January 1972–31 December 1976 compared with the first, 1 January 1967–31 December 1971, increasing for some diseases and declining for others. Under the assumption that these changes probably also applied to the control group, the death rates of the control group were extrapolated to take this into account. The principal effect of the extrapolation was to increase the death rates from lung cancer and decrease the death rates from heart disease during the last five years as compared with the first five years.

In this study, further information was obtained on the asbestos workers who died, including, in many instances, clinical data, histological sections and X-ray films. On the basis of this information, the cause of death as given on the death certificate could be reclassified, using the best available information. Table 1.11 gives a comparison between the cause of death as given on the death certificate and that based on the best available information. An equivalent review of the cause of death in the control group was not attempted, the number of deaths being too large. Care was taken to ensure that comparisons between the insulation workers and the control group were based on comparable information.

References

Hammond, E.C. (1966) Smoking in relation to the death rates of one million men and women. *Natl. Cancer Inst Monogr.*, **19**, 127–204

Hammond, E.C. & Selikoff, I.J. (1973) *Relation of cigarette smoking to risk of death of asbestos-associated disease among insulation workers in the United States.* In: Bogovski, P., Gilson, J.C., Timbrell, V. & Wagner, J.C., eds, *Biological Effects of Asbestos* (*IARC Scientific Publications No. 8*), Lyon, International Agency for Research on Cancer, pp. 312–317

Hammond, E.C., Selikoff, I.J. & Seidman, H. (1979) Asbestos exposure, cigarette smoking and death rates. *Ann. N.Y. Acad. Sci.*, **330**, 473–490

Selikoff, I.J., Hammond, E.C. & Seidman, H. (1973) *Cancer risk of insulation workers in the United States.* In: Bogovski, P., Gilson, J.C., Timbrell, V. & Wagner, J.C., eds, *Biological Effects of Asbestos* (*IARC Scientific Publications No. 8*), Lyon, International Agency for Research on Cancer, pp. 209–216

Selikoff, I.J., Hammond, E.C. & Seidman, H. (1979) Mortality experiences of insulation workers in the United States and Canada, 1943–1976. *Ann. N.Y. Acad. Sci.*, **330**, 517–519

Selikoff, I.J., Hammond, E.C. & Seidman, H. (1980) Latency of asbestos disease among insulation workers in the United States and Canada. *Cancer*, **46**, 2736–2740.

CORRESPONDENCE BETWEEN DIFFERENT REVISIONS OF THE INTERNATIONAL CLASSIFICATION OF DISEASES (ICD)

Comparison of the three digit codes used in the 7th , 8th and 9th Revisions of the International Classification of Diseases

Code	ICD7	ICD8	ICD9
140	Lip	Lip	Lip
141	Tongue	Tongue	Tongue
142	Salivary gland	Salivary gland	Salivary gland
143	Floor of mouth	Gum	Gum
144	Other parts of mouth; mouth unspecified	Floor of mouth	Floor of mouth
145	Oral mesopharynx	Other and unspecified parts of mouth	Other and unspecified parts of mouth
146	Nasopharynx	Oropharynx	Oropharynx
147	Hypopharynx	Nasopharynx	Nasopharynx
148	Pharynx unspecified	Hypopharynx	Hypopharynx
149	—	Pharynx unspecified	Pharynx unspecified
150	Oesophagus	Oesophagus	Oesophagus
151	Stomach	Stomach	Stomach
152	Small intestine	Small intestine	Small intestine
153	Large intestine, excl. rectum, incl. intestine NOS	Large intestine, excl. rectum, incl. intestine NOS	Colon (incl. large intestine NOS)
154	Rectum and rectosigmoid junction	Rectum and rectosigmoid junction	Rectum, rectosigmoid[1] and anus
155	Biliary passages incl. gallbladder and liver specified as primary	Liver and intrahepatic bile ducts specified as primary	Liver and intrahepatic bile ducts incl. liver not specified as primary or secondary
156	Liver secondary and unspecified	Gallbladder and extrahepatic bile duct	Gallbladder and extrahepatic bile duct
157	Pancreas	Pancreas	Pancreas
158	Peritoneum	Peritoneum and retroperitoneal tissue	Peritoneum and retroperitoneum
159	Unspecified digestive organs	Unspecified digestive organs	Other and ill-defined[2] sites within the digestive organs and peritoneum, incl. intestine NOS

[1] Skin of anus is coded to skin in all three Revisions, and the anal canal coded to rectum. Anus NOS, however, is coded to skin in the 7th and 8th Revisions, but to rectum in the 9th.

[2] Intestinal tract NOS is coded to 153 in ICD7 and ICD8, but to 159 in ICD9.

Code	ICD7	ICD8	ICD9
160	Nose, nasal cavities, middle ear and accessory sinuses (excl. skin and bone of nose in all three Revisions)	Nose, nasal cavities, middle ear and accessory sinuses	Nasal cavities, middle ear and accesscry sinuses
161	Larynx	Larynx	Larynx
162	Trachea, bronchus and lung (specified as primary)	Trachea, bronchus and lung	Trachea, bronchus, lung
163	Lung (unspecified whether primary or secondary)	Other and unspecified respiratory organs	Pleura
164	Mediastinum	—	Thymus, heart and mediastinum
165	Thoracic organs (secondary)	—	Other and ill-defined sites within the respiratory system and intrathoracic organs
170	Breast (male and female)	Bone and articular cartilage	Bone and articular cartilage
171	Cervix uteri	Connective and other soft tissues	Connective and other soft tissues
172	Corpus uteri	Melanoma of skin[3]	Melanoma of skin[3]
173	Other parts of uterus incl. chorionepithelioma	Other malignant[3] neoplasms of skin	Other malignant[3] neoplasms of skin
174	Uterus unspecified	Breast (male and female)	Breast – female
175	Ovary, fallopian tube and broad ligament	—	Breast – male
176	Other and unspecified female genital organs	—	—
177	Prostate	—	—
178	Testis	—	—
179	Other and unspecified male genital organs	—	Uterus, part unspecified
180	Kidney	Cervix uteri	Cervix uteri
181	Bladder and other urinary organs	Chorionepithelioma	Chorionepithelioma
182	—	Other malignant neoplasms of uterus, incl. uterus unspecified	Body of uterus
183	—	Ovary, fallopian tube and broad ligament	Ovary and other uterine adnexa
184	—	Other and unspecified female genital organs	Other and unspecified female genital organs
185	—	Prostate	Prostate
186	—	Testis	Testis
187	—	Other and unspecified male genital organs	Other and unspecified male genital organs
188	—	Bladder	Bladder
189	—	Other and unspecified urinary organs (incl. kidney)	Kidney and other and unspecified urinary organs
190	Melanoma of skin[3]	Eye	Eye

[3] Excludes skin of genital organs. ICD7 and ICD8 also exclude skin of breast (coded to breast).

Code	ICD7	ICD8	ICD9
191	Other malignant neoplasms of skin[3]	Brain	Brain
192	Eye	Other parts of nervous system	Other and unspecified parts of nervous system
193	Brain and other parts of nervous system	Thyroid	Thyroid
194	Thyroid	Other endocrine glands	Other endocrine glands
195	Other endocrine glands	Ill-defined sites	Other and ill-defined sites
196	Bone	Secondary and unspecified malignant neoplasms of lymph nodes	Secondary and unspecified malignant neoplasms of lymph nodes
197	Connective tissue	Secondary malignant neoplasm of respiratory and digestive system (incl. liver unspecified as primary or secondary)	Secondary malignant neoplasm of respiratory and digestive system
198	—	Other secondary malignant neoplasms of other specified sites	Secondary malignant neoplasms of other specified sites
199	Other and unspecified sites	Malignant neoplasm without specification of site	Malignant neoplasm without specification of site
200	Lymphosarcoma and reticulosarcoma	Lymphosarcoma and reticulum cell sarcoma	Lymphosarcoma and reticulosarcoma
201	Hodgkin's disease	Hodgkin's disease	Hodgkin's disease
202	Other forms of lymphoma	Other lymphoid tissue	Other lymphoid and histiocytic tissue
203	Multiple myeloma	Multiple myeloma	Multiple myeloma and immunoproliferative neoplasm
204	Leukaemia and aleukaemia	Lymphatic leukaemia	Lymphoid leukaemia
205	Mycosis fungoides[4]	Myeloid leukaemia	Myeloid leukaemia
206	—	Monocytic leukaemia	Monocytic leukaemia
207	—	Other and unspecified leukaemia	Other specified leukaemia
208	—	Polycythemia vera[5]	Leukaemia of unspecified cell type
209	—	Myelofibrosis[5]	—

[4] Mycosis fungoides is coded under 202 (as 202.1) in ICD8 and ICD9.
[5] Polycythemia vera and myelofibrosis are not coded as malignant neoplasms in ICD7 and ICD9.

Note
1. Uterus unspecified is coded with corpus uteri in ICD8, but given a separate 3-digit rubric in ICD7 and ICD9.
2. Other and unspecified urinary organs are coded with bladder in ICD7, but with kidney in ICD8 and ICD9.

U.S. NATIONAL DEATH RATES: WHITE MALES (DEATHS/PERSON-YEAR ×1000)

(a) All causes of death

Age group	1935-1939	1940-1944	1945-1949	1950-1954	1955-1959	1960-1964	1965-1969	1970-1974	1975-1979
0	15.090155	12.355103	9.633718	6.558825	6.537868	5.783995	4.944682	4.386003	3.683013
5	1.512075	1.123687	0.874162	0.640673	0.545455	0.490712	0.465096	0.435708	0.394271
10	1.354305	1.014955	0.828392	0.637076	0.549600	0.490108	0.482238	0.456612	0.433030
15	2.050257	1.735458	1.516066	1.347363	1.292953	1.215401	1.398888	1.472626	1.444567
20	2.725204	2.65871	2.151549	1.828221	1.787832	1.642321	1.837639	1.950797	1.894999
25	3.019979	2.541757	2.007412	1.684009	1.526650	1.486029	1.614999	1.694225	1.688568
30	3.606030	2.982105	2.398892	1.944711	1.767349	1.725782	1.800920	1.782359	1.694902
35	4.754416	4.039859	3.434303	2.782188	2.540642	2.498610	2.600209	2.484212	2.302031
40	6.878378	5.803823	5.172174	4.603532	4.221951	4.048614	4.135886	3.956904	3.635268
45	10.073833	8.836923	8.022261	7.493196	6.980722	6.833429	6.832890	6.501418	6.060059
50	14.405272	13.664108	12.908051	12.032722	11.623889	11.350258	11.280571	10.452522	9.713320
55	21.268906	20.694916	19.890091	18.537674	17.721161	17.542206	18.007660	16.720734	15.346365
60	30.761307	29.590622	28.714554	27.490128	27.061432	26.633423	27.203171	25.941437	24.437134
65	45.490067	42.773224	40.112122	40.288498	40.272156	40.383881	40.723648	38.572983	35.908997
70	65.333893	65.087128	60.756485	58.464386	57.640198	57.502396	59.767563	56.867615	54.622162
75	107.729950	98.246872	93.384598	87.799576	86.163193	84.236496	85.541626	85.420258	82.535858
80	163.118042	153.192078	134.480942	134.709656	133.321854	129.775757	125.819809	123.481873	118.320343
85	243.538437	238.410248	227.047104	204.860550	208.932007	230.693619	211.043625	186.255356	182.579224

Appendix III (cont'd)

(b) All malignant neoplasms

Age group	1935-1939	1940-1944	1945-1949	1950-1954	1955-1959	1960-1964	1965-1969	1970-1974	1975-1979
0	0.093430	0.110568	0.120175	0.125489	0.115679	0.084387	0.086541	0.072836	0.060039
5	0.057093	0.074363	0.081757	0.087156	0.091421	0.086692	0.082350	0.070881	0.060803
10	0.050084	0.057305	0.064863	0.057139	0.070663	0.067645	0.066173	0.055943	0.049658
15	0.071351	0.082535	0.095017	0.096333	0.095904	0.091542	0.091451	0.078406	0.071215
20	0.087208	0.110808	0.127404	0.124357	0.121628	0.112515	0.115589	0.111952	0.094780
25	0.118623	0.139066	0.153178	0.152257	0.147415	0.149026	0.143850	0.138268	0.125170
30	0.174696	0.193988	0.217294	0.207333	0.208630	0.210442	0.209528	0.194685	0.182164
35	0.290465	0.310748	0.335970	0.324324	0.326654	0.330676	0.350294	0.324935	0.293988
40	0.558559	0.553414	0.578648	0.594595	0.595899	0.599316	0.639675	0.634476	0.595643
45	1.020630	1.032964	1.062090	1.127988	1.127623	1.144600	1.193992	1.236712	1.243178
50	1.745554	1.849772	1.976320	2.017418	2.127339	2.137941	2.239856	2.257088	2.249419
55	2.832692	3.071470	3.323395	3.405025	3.478723	3.578072	3.837873	3.891954	3.782340
60	4.403046	4.542109	4.928676	5.149756	5.444480	5.528496	5.937672	6.154709	6.197082
65	6.509923	6.495900	6.750687	7.210414	7.692063	8.022576	8.574032	8.892487	8.872980
70	8.925286	9.278425	9.534017	9.638390	9.976719	10.286403	11.407393	11.981841	12.487869
75	12.638927	12.385037	13.181828	12.793587	12.871528	12.842813	12.337729	15.561729	16.167923
80	14.496526	15.194854	15.491899	16.084656	16.450943	15.862476	16.534668	18.353394	19.233383
85	15.146151	15.625639	17.797379	17.458130	17.702240	18.491318	18.790619	19.065338	20.466278

Appendix III (cont'd)

(c) Cancer of respiratory system

Age group	1935-1939	1940-1944	1945-1949	1950-1954	1955-1959	1960-1964	1965-1969	1970-1974	1975-1979
0	0.001746	0.001760	0.001251	0.001044	0.000942	0.000672	0.000646	0.000696	0.001040
5	0.001364	0.001501	0.001532	0.000917	0.000640	0.000467	0.000175	0.000382	0.000405
10	0.002420	0.001968	0.002505	0.000746	0.000906	0.000511	0.000368	0.000551	0.000228
15	0.004402	0.004043	0.005176	0.002604	0.001941	0.001082	0.001369	0.001561	0.001551
20	0.005787	0.007117	0.006789	0.004921	0.004115	0.003553	0.002832	0.002816	0.002190
25	0.008078	0.009520	0.008441	0.006886	0.007270	0.006986	0.005599	0.006204	0.006109
30	0.015083	0.016771	0.016744	0.017662	0.022139	0.023715	0.023521	0.021660	0.020351
35	0.032326	0.038453	0.045177	0.045509	0.054820	0.063577	0.075042	0.072661	0.065353
40	0.072322	0.089750	0.108127	0.126835	0.140732	0.161982	0.194655	0.215500	0.204149
45	0.148208	0.191795	0.232995	0.291139	0.332762	0.365263	0.420767	0.480238	0.502846
50	0.239424	0.331631	0.454028	0.564001	0.673495	0.741631	0.841064	0.913504	0.952510
55	0.331169	0.497759	0.727187	0.925482	1.137177	1.279813	1.456527	1.593035	1.597188
60	0.399714	0.594480	0.910775	1.258339	1.638880	1.895671	2.217393	2.485404	2.604812
65	0.433002	0.618815	0.930043	1.404181	1.960340	2.440346	2.971354	3.364429	3.477328
70	0.425743	0.613909	0.928421	1.383901	1.907932	2.490834	3.304993	3.992129	4.393531
75	0.453689	0.583911	0.886391	1.268537	1.736111	2.235025	3.158079	4.152960	4.643902
80	0.371528	0.525424	0.769048	1.116935	1.490533	1.872944	2.604069	3.678414	4.315789
85	0.323077	0.358974	0.643979	0.980080	1.194174	1.508670	1.945685	2.595173	2.981785

Appendix III (cont'd)

(d) All diseases of circulatory system

Age group	1935-1939	1940-1944	1945-1949	1950-1954	1955-1959	1960-1964	1965-1969	1970-1974	1975-1979
0	0.136651	0.089558	0.053331	0.051135	0.044999	0.037605	0.044222	0.060552	0.071630
5	0.077747	0.055734	0.035816	0.024465	0.017157	0.012852	0.012110	0.012789	0.012971
10	0.115249	0.084218	0.059499	0.037300	0.025064	0.019400	0.017336	0.015479	0.017198
15	0.157190	0.135348	0.103946	0.076806	0.054358	0.043296	0.036297	0.036922	0.037656
20	0.190581	0.181583	0.137757	0.109595	0.091907	0.071851	0.061590	0.061738	0.054995
25	0.262118	0.250540	0.197035	0.174063	0.150243	0.128281	0.110740	0.100867	0.094217
30	0.421207	0.425313	0.374947	0.357074	0.327580	0.300518	0.268933	0.225143	0.194408
35	0.779535	0.849473	0.848756	0.810016	0.773912	0.755144	0.715122	0.614382	0.528856
40	1.582577	1.670425	1.716481	1.837835	1.736228	1.673374	1.610294	1.443150	1.293776
45	2.938919	3.180255	3.307198	3.556956	3.369588	3.291026	3.173170	2.870263	2.591364
50	4.999078	5.617871	6.030265	6.318288	6.112041	5.898450	5.733212	5.115329	4.624130
55	8.361725	9.335401	9.850962	10.313844	9.847697	9.558846	9.591788	8.584021	7.741709
60	13.494988	14.318038	14.987144	15.914903	15.651752	15.182182	15.030571	13.840800	12.676222
65	21.380875	21.907501	21.995682	24.384079	24.282242	23.961594	23.530701	21.445801	19.344696
70	32.592224	34.847290	34.343796	37.063736	36.646530	35.840851	36.244812	33.286133	30.824768
75	55.897934	54.124817	54.808228	58.076111	57.631912	55.443085	54.658951	52.635254	49.210434
80	87.256897	86.440613	80.873764	92.443512	93.149704	89.922211	85.324646	81.058289	75.077774
85	128.546097	133.326874	136.821915	143.462128	151.346207	159.260071	150.262863	131.068344	125.710373

ALGORITHM FOR EXACT CALCULATION OF PERSON–YEARS[1]

We denote by t a multivariate time variable, for example, t_1 = age, t_2 = calendar time and t_3 = number of years since first exposure to a given risk factor. Entry into the study occurs at $t = e$ and exit at $t = e + f1$, where 1 is a vector of 1s and f is the total duration of follow-up. Thus, if a subject entered at age 26.3 years on 1 January 1950 having been initially exposed some 4.9 years earlier, and was followed for 23.7 years, we would have entry at $e = (26.3, 1950.0, 4.9)$ and exit at $(50.0, 1973.7, 28.6)$.

To start the algorithm, we set $t = e$ and determine the cell, denoted by a vector I of indices for each time variable, in which t lies. The designation $I = (3, 1, 2)$ in the example would mean that entry into the study occurred in the third age group, first calendar period, and second category of duration since initial exposure. The procedure is then as follows:

A   If u_I are the upper boundaries of the cell indexed by I (e.g., 30 years of age, calendar year 1955 and ten years since initial exposure), determine the contribution of the individual to this cell, C_I, as the smallest element of the vector $u_I - t$ *or* as the remaining follow-up time, if even smaller.

B   Set $t = t + C_I 1$.

C   Add C_I to cell I of the person-years cross-classification.

D   Check each element of t against the cell boundaries. For each element such that t_i is at the upper boundary, increase the corresponding element of I by 1.

E   Repeat until all follow-up is accounted for.

In the above example, the contributions to the first cell $I = (3, 1, 2)$ would be $3.7 = \min(30-26.3, 1955-1950.0, 10-4.9)$, t would change to $(30, 1953.7, 8.6)$ and the next cell to consider would be $I = (4, 1, 2)$.

---

[1] From Clayton (1984)

GROUPED DATA FROM THE MONTANA SMELTER WORKERS STUDY USED IN CHAPTERS 2–4

Age group	Calendar period	Period of hire	Arsenic exposure	Person-years	Numbers of deaths from:			
					All causes	Respiratory cancer	All cancer	Circulatory disease
1	1	1	1	3075.27	15	2	5	5
1	1	1	2	485.83	2	0	0	0
1	1	1	3	478.18	5	0	1	2
1	1	1	4	337.29	5	0	0	1
1	1	2	1	3981.61	27	2	2	10
1	1	2	2	656.06	5	1	2	1
1	1	2	3	190.34	2	0	0	1
1	1	2	4	12.46	1	0	0	1
1	2	1	1	936.75	4	0	1	2
1	2	1	2	194.58	1	1	1	0
1	2	1	3	164.87	2	1	1	0
1	2	1	4	121.00	0	0	0	0
1	2	2	1	10740.68	85	2	4	32
1	2	2	2	1696.77	9	1	2	4
1	2	2	3	870.52	14	0	1	6
1	2	2	4	224.00	0	0	0	0
1	3	2	1	12451.29	101	7	13	38
1	3	2	2	2511.97	15	0	2	5
1	3	2	3	868.35	12	0	2	5
1	3	2	4	291.78	4	0	1	2
1	4	2	1	7151.03	39	1	4	18
1	4	2	2	1341.63	18	3	3	8
1	4	2	3	419.81	6	0	1	2
1	4	2	4	160.61	2	0	0	1
2	1	1	1	2849.76	51	2	8	21
2	1	1	2	390.45	5	0	1	4
2	1	1	3	333.04	3	1	2	1
2	1	1	4	626.72	14	4	5	5
2	1	2	1	1912.89	30	4	7	15
2	1	2	2	202.69	4	0	0	1
2	1	2	3	90.50	3	0	0	3
2	1	2	4	14.96	1	0	0	1
2	2	1	1	2195.59	49	3	9	18
2	2	1	2	346.17	14	2	2	7
2	2	1	3	287.79	8	1	1	4
2	2	1	4	349.53	11	3	4	6
2	2	2	1	5624.50	109	5	15	48
2	2	2	2	933.45	26	7	9	9
2	2	2	3	410.94	8	1	4	0
2	2	2	4	75.41	6	2	2	1

Appendix V: Grouped Data from Montana Study (cont'd)

Age group	Calendar period	Period of hire	Arsenic exposure	Person-years	Numbers of deaths from:			
					All causes	Respiratory cancer	All cancer	Circulatory disease
2	3	1	1	747.77	24	3	4	8
2	3	1	2	142.13	3	0	0	1
2	3	1	3	127.51	2	1	1	0
2	3	1	4	142.33	5	1	1	2
2	3	2	1	9194.02	164	13	26	78
2	3	2	2	1919.44	42	5	6	18
2	3	2	3	902.38	20	2	2	8
2	3	2	4	487.17	12	3	4	2
2	4	2	1	8494.53	126	8	21	58
2	4	2	2	1896.43	39	6	8	21
2	4	2	3	688.03	12	3	4	4
2	4	2	4	425.13	9	0	0	7
3	1	1	1	2085.43	70	2	15	26
3	1	1	2	194.49	6	1	3	2
3	1	1	3	291.77	13	1	2	6
3	1	1	4	672.09	32	9	15	10
3	1	2	1	657.75	16	1	2	9
3	1	2	2	70.65	3	0	1	2
3	1	2	3	33.42	2	0	0	0
3	2	1	1	1675.91	63	7	12	28
3	2	1	2	225.40	14	2	5	3
3	2	1	3	209.68	13	1	4	6
3	2	1	4	441.10	20	7	7	7
3	2	2	1	1945.95	75	6	13	33
3	2	2	2	203.50	3	0	0	2
3	2	2	3	156.38	3	1	1	1
3	2	2	4	38.13	3	0	1	2
3	3	1	1	1501.73	68	10	16	33
3	3	1	2	234.83	10	4	4	5
3	3	1	3	190.86	8	3	5	3
3	3	1	4	244.82	13	3	5	7
3	3	2	1	4088.70	155	12	28	80
3	3	2	2	712.76	34	7	12	13
3	3	2	3	390.72	15	3	4	9
3	3	2	4	190.84	6	2	3	1
3	4	1	1	440.21	15	1	2	9
3	4	1	2	101.32	4	3	3	0
3	4	1	3	100.80	3	1	1	2
3	4	1	4	100.64	4	1	1	2
3	4	2	1	5100.05	184	19	40	93
3	4	2	2	1052.78	43	6	13	18
3	4	2	3	621.84	25	4	10	13
3	4	2	4	419.09	13	0	2	7
4	1	1	1	833.61	67	3	10	29
4	1	1	2	110.26	14	0	1	5

Appendix V: Grouped Data from Montana Study (cont'd)

Age group	Calendar period	Period of hire	Arsenic exposure	Person-years	Numbers of deaths from:			
					All causes	Respiratory cancer	All cancer	Circulatory disease
4	1	1	3	158.70	15	0	0	10
4	1	1	4	277.25	25	1	4	9
4	1	2	1	114.15	12	0	1	4
4	1	2	2	4.25	2	0	0	0
4	1	2	3	9.00	0	0	0	0
4	2	1	1	973.32	79	6	10	39
4	2	1	2	54.57	10	1	2	2
4	2	1	3	108.28	13	1	4	3
4	2	1	4	268.27	32	2	8	14
4	2	2	1	358.35	38	1	8	20
4	2	2	2	38.37	3	0	0	3
4	2	2	3	39.16	4	1	1	3
4	2	2	4	10.62	1	0	1	0
4	3	1	1	1027.12	77	6	13	47
4	3	1	2	105.58	7	2	2	2
4	3	1	3	54.74	5	0	0	3
4	3	1	4	197.20	24	1	5	13
4	3	2	1	1097.92	87	5	22	37
4	3	2	2	127.62	13	0	0	10
4	3	2	3	68.54	11	0	0	6
4	3	2	4	45.38	5	1	1	3
4	4	1	1	674.44	54	6	10	29
4	4	1	2	97.14	10	1	2	2
4	4	1	3	94.00	3	2	2	0
4	4	1	4	92.75	10	2	3	2
4	4	2	1	1763.50	141	14	22	86
4	4	2	2	324.74	15	2	5	7
4	4	2	3	180.22	6	0	1	4
4	4	2	4	114.36	5	0	1	4

GROUPED DATA ON NASAL CANCER DEATHS AMONG WELSH NICKEL WORKERS

Appendices VI and VII present grouped data derived from the Welsh nickel refinery cancer mortality study. Person-years (PY) and observed deaths were summed for all persons (N) with positive person-year contribution to each cell cross-classified by age first employed (AFE), year first employed (YFE), exposure index (EXP), and time since first employed (TFE). Expected deaths were based on national death rates for England and Wales in five-year age and calendar year strata (see Appendix IX). Of 400 possible cells in the four-way classification (Appendix VII), 242 had positive person-year contributions. The three-way classification (Appendix VI) was obtained by collapsing the four-way data over the EXP dimension. Of 80 possible cells in the three-way classification 72 had positive person-year contributions.

The categories of the four classification variables are:

AFE	YFE	EXP	TFE
1 = <20.0	1 = 1902–1910	1 = 0.0	1 = 0.0–19.9
2 = 20.0–27.4	2 = 1910–1914	2 = 0.5–4.0	2 = 20.0–29.9
3 = 27.5–34.9	3 = 1915–1919	3 = 4.5–8.0	3 = 30.0–39.9
4 = 35.0–54.4	4 = 1920–1924	4 = 8.5–12.0	4 = 40.0–49.9
		5 = 12.5 +	5 = 50.0 +

APPENDIX VI

NASAL SINUS CANCER MORTALITY IN WELSH NICKEL REFINERY WORKERS: SUMMARY DATA FOR THREE-WAY CLASSIFICATION

AFE	YFE	TFE	Nasal cancer deaths	Person-years	AFE	YFE	TFE	Nasal cancer deaths	Person-years
1	1	2	0	19.406	2	1	2	1	174.418
1	1	3	0	70.000	2	1	3	2	521.768
1	1	4	0	52.836	2	1	4	0	304.922
1	1	5	0	33.209	2	1	5	2	142.282
1	2	1	0	2.166	2	2	1	0	3.831
1	2	2	1	175.294	2	2	2	1	528.066
1	2	3	0	179.501	2	2	3	4	497.481
1	2	4	1	121.217	2	2	4	2	279.542
1	2	5	0	77.877	2	2	5	2	97.982
1	3	1	0	71.400	2	3	1	0	82.886
1	3	2	0	267.774	2	3	2	0	253.653
1	3	3	0	267.714	2	3	3	0	206.343
1	3	4	0	210.773	2	3	4	2	111.541
1	3	5	0	157.445	2	3	5	0	45.434
1	4	1	0	279.472	2	4	1	0	1021.139
1	4	2	0	344.109	2	4	2	1	1088.072
1	4	3	0	315.170	2	4	3	0	869.314
1	4	4	0	267.320	2	4	4	3	585.779
1	4	5	0	176.503	2	4	5	0	250.398

Appendix VI: Three-way Classification of Welsh Data (cont'd)

AFE	YFE	TFE	Nasal cancer deaths	Person-years	AFE	YFE	TFE	Nasal cancer deaths	Person-years
3	1	2	3	116.939	4	1	2	0	14.773
3	1	3	1	262.567	4	1	3	0	36.570
3	1	4	1	151.760	4	1	4	0	17.290
3	1	5	1	32.238	4	2	1	0	3.176
3	2	1	0	3.824	4	2	2	2	164.801
3	2	2	3	330.710	4	2	3	5	56.130
3	2	3	2	265.273	4	2	4	0	7.258
3	2	4	3	90.851	4	3	1	0	34.540
3	2	5	0	19.540	4	3	2	2	124.253
3	3	1	0	49.453	4	3	3	1	68.881
3	3	2	2	169.654	4	3	4	0	4.382
3	3	3	1	111.962	4	4	1	1	354.720
3	3	4	0	55.060	4	4	2	3	319.077
3	3	5	1	0.840	4	4	3	0	141.845
3	4	1	0	679.445	4	4	4	0	17.203
3	4	2	0	686.531					
3	4	3	1	458.838					
3	4	4	1	183.701					
3	4	5	0	42.665					

LUNG AND NASAL SINUS CANCER MORTALITY IN WELSH NICKEL REFINERY WORKERS: SUMMARY DATA FOR FOUR-WAY CLASSIFICATION

AFE	YFE	EXP	TFE	N	PY	Observed deaths			Expected deaths		
						Lung cancer	Nasal cancer	All causes	Lung cancer	Nasal cancer	All causes
1	1	2	2	1	1.8302	0	0	0	0.000501	0.000009	0.015749
1	1	2	3	1	10.0000	0	0	0	0.005548	0.000101	0.131953
1	1	2	4	1	0.8739	0	0	1	0.001180	0.000013	0.015226
1	1	3	2	3	7.1989	0	0	0	0.001972	0.000036	0.061946
1	1	3	3	3	30.0000	0	0	0	0.018695	0.000324	0.416487
1	1	3	4	3	26.0055	0	0	1	0.056554	0.000433	0.777975
1	1	3	5	2	21.9968	0	0	1	0.104245	0.000680	1.954394
1	1	4	2	3	7.6071	1	0	1	0.001647	0.000031	0.055648
1	1	4	3	2	20.0000	0	0	0	0.012367	0.000183	0.233173
1	1	4	4	2	15.9562	0	0	1	0.032319	0.000249	0.379826
1	1	4	5	1	7.2151	0	0	1	0.029605	0.000176	0.367500
1	1	5	2	1	2.7699	0	0	0	0.000759	0.000014	0.023835
1	1	5	3	1	10.0000	0	0	0	0.006666	0.000113	0.143022
1	1	5	4	1	10.0000	0	0	0	0.024173	0.000175	0.328920
1	1	5	5	1	3.9973	0	0	1	0.015579	0.000107	0.239810
1	2	1	1	2	0.9700	0	0	0	0.000066	0.000001	0.004107
1	2	1	2	6	49.0261	0	0	1	0.007615	0.000130	0.269025
1	2	1	3	5	50.0000	0	0	0	0.041582	0.000406	0.484250
1	2	1	4	5	50.0000	0	0	0	0.143042	0.000739	1.220072
1	2	1	5	5	35.8170	0	0	5	0.194630	0.000844	1.978039
1	2	2	1	2	0.9098	0	0	0	0.000056	0.000001	0.003699
1	2	2	2	10	80.7788	0	1	1	0.014266	0.000236	0.469375
1	2	2	3	9	81.6233	1	0	1	0.074494	0.000744	0.878157
1	2	2	4	8	46.0958	4	1	5	0.124914	0.000664	1.052235
1	2	2	5	3	27.1653	0	0	3	0.168732	0.000736	1.746187
1	2	3	1	1	0.2507	0	0	0	0.000017	0.000000	0.001062
1	2	3	2	4	35.4891	0	0	0	0.006504	0.000108	0.209898
1	2	3	3	4	37.8781	1	0	1	0.036124	0.000358	0.420860
1	2	3	4	3	22.3508	0	0	1	0.073292	0.000369	0.651239
1	2	3	5	2	14.8944	1	0	2	0.094093	0.000421	1.058619
1	2	4	1	1	0.0356	0	0	0	0.000002	0.000000	0.000151
1	2	4	2	1	10.0000	0	0	0	0.001438	0.000023	0.050957
1	2	4	3	1	10.0000	0	0	0	0.009036	0.000083	0.096519
1	2	4	4	1	2.7699	0	0	1	0.005879	0.000038	0.048107
1	3	1	1	17	50.1519	0	0	0	0.001557	0.000046	0.163907
1	3	1	2	20	181.0278	0	0	1	0.024588	0.000357	0.779594
1	3	1	3	21	190.5669	1	0	3	0.162638	0.001259	1.536345
1	3	1	4	17	146.8630	1	0	6	0.417245	0.001816	3.195433
1	3	1	5	11	107.9049	0	0	7	0.669160	0.002895	7.170720
1	3	2	1	7	17.0204	0	0	0	0.000706	0.000017	0.060004
1	3	2	2	7	66.7466	0	0	1	0.010052	0.000151	0.318440

Appendix VII: Four-way Classification of Welsh Data (cont'd)

AFE	YFE	EXP	TFE	N	PY	Observed deaths			Expected deaths		
						Lung cancer	Nasal cancer	All causes	Lung cancer	Nasal cancer	All causes
1	3	2	3	6	57.1471	0	0	1	0.053508	0.000438	0.515681
1	3	2	4	5	48.6658	0	0	1	0.150893	0.000654	1.195361
1	3	2	5	4	36.4930	0	0	3	0.226919	0.000998	2.619424
1	3	3	1	2	4.2274	0	0	0	0.000139	0.000004	0.013942
1	3	3	2	2	20.0000	0	0	0	0.002756	0.000041	0.092147
1	3	3	3	2	20.0000	0	0	0	0.018094	0.000149	0.173137
1	3	3	4	2	15.2439	0	0	1	0.042914	0.000196	0.324807
1	3	3	5	1	13.0465	0	0	1	0.085828	0.000377	0.859574
1	4	1	1	28	228.3376	0	0	1	0.007570	0.000157	0.747508
1	4	1	2	29	284.1088	0	0	2	0.063526	0.000719	1.132030
1	4	1	3	27	261.8770	0	0	3	0.297499	0.001698	2.385268
1	4	1	4	24	227.1940	2	0	4	0.762530	0.003367	5.741814
1	4	1	5	20	145.6633	1	0	9	0.878630	0.003459	8.045273
1	4	2	1	6	51.1345	0	0	0	0.001747	0.000038	0.166843
1	4	2	2	6	60.0000	0	0	0	0.013561	0.000153	0.239631
1	4	2	3	6	53.2930	0	0	1	0.056786	0.000323	0.458292
1	4	2	4	5	40.1261	0	0	1	0.133655	0.000590	0.992480
1	4	2	5	4	30.8396	0	0	2	0.189426	0.000740	1.730875
2	1	1	2	16	27.2839	0	1	1	0.011266	0.000258	0.363285
2	1	1	3	18	153.8885	2	0	5	0.116749	0.002275	3.592233
2	1	1	4	13	103.6338	1	0	5	0.207416	0.002433	5.494106
2	1	1	5	8	46.3060	0	0	6	0.157220	0.001916	5.416975
2	1	2	2	14	38.7660	0	0	0	0.015033	0.000335	0.477216
2	1	2	3	18	134.5756	3	0	8	0.111145	0.001899	2.727597
2	1	2	4	10	72.1631	1	0	6	0.183005	0.001500	3.319514
2	1	2	5	4	26.3951	0	1	3	0.115229	0.000944	2.855752
2	1	3	2	15	52.3291	0	0	1	0.021893	0.000503	0.703564
2	1	3	3	16	127.4445	2	1	5	0.109387	0.001829	2.714684
2	1	3	4	11	76.5519	2	0	5	0.172606	0.001661	3.731743
2	1	3	5	6	47.2267	0	1	3	0.189374	0.001729	5.178221
2	1	4	2	8	27.7354	1	0	1	0.011825	0.000274	0.378824
2	1	4	3	7	58.6919	1	0	2	0.055861	0.000864	1.298165
2	1	4	4	5	34.5167	2	0	2	0.093303	0.000770	1.757753
2	1	4	5	3	12.6444	0	0	2	0.049216	0.000461	1.422127
2	1	5	2	7	28.3033	0	0	0	0.011928	0.000275	0.380667
2	1	5	3	7	47.1670	2	1	4	0.042131	0.000702	1.073977
2	1	5	4	3	18.0565	1	0	2	0.044786	0.000420	1.003884
2	1	5	5	1	9.7096	0	0	0	0.033644	0.000408	1.270299
2	2	1	1	4	1.6687	0	0	0	0.000223	0.000004	0.009193
2	2	1	2	17	126.8835	0	0	1	0.047188	0.000908	1.305475
2	2	1	3	16	147.3439	2	0	4	0.210102	0.002145	3.088371
2	2	1	4	12	104.1298	0	1	4	0.386300	0.002357	5.133400
2	2	1	5	8	35.3401	1	0	7	0.204165	0.001159	3.459515
2	2	2	1	2	0.5453	0	0	0	0.000120	0.000002	0.004024
2	2	2	2	22	147.3027	3	0	4	0.054442	0.001098	1.595543
2	2	2	3	18	143.4004	0	0	5	0.183965	0.002064	2.944180

Appendix VII: Four-way Classification of Welsh Data (cont'd)

AFE	YFE	EXP	TFE	N	PY	Observed deaths			Expected deaths		
						Lung cancer	Nasal cancer	All causes	Lung cancer	Nasal cancer	All causes
2	2	2	4	13	86.5511	4	0	8	0.289411	0.001929	4.148711
2	2	2	5	5	38.0643	0	0	4	0.198582	0.001299	3.865778
2	2	3	1	2	0.7700	0	0	0	0.000167	0.000003	0.005635
2	2	3	2	21	155.1765	2	0	3	0.059191	0.001171	1.688422
2	2	3	3	18	134.5986	3	2	9	0.177506	0.001967	2.815660
2	2	3	4	9	51.4711	1	1	6	0.166513	0.001160	2.503561
2	2	3	5	3	18.5302	0	1	3	0.096347	0.000661	1.951160
2	2	4	1	1	0.4357	0	0	0	0.000101	0.000000	0.003334
2	2	4	2	10	74.6497	0	1	1	0.029773	0.000606	0.859406
2	2	4	3	9	59.6384	2	1	4	0.073933	0.000864	1.208902
2	2	4	4	5	37.3904	1	0	3	0.127317	0.000809	1.791119
2	2	4	5	2	6.0479	1	1	2	0.028994	0.000242	0.617074
2	2	5	1	1	0.4110	0	0	0	0.000113	0.000002	0.003537
2	2	5	2	3	24.0533	0	0	0	0.010351	0.000207	0.288814
2	2	5	3	3	12.4993	1	1	3	0.011295	0.000171	0.218863
2	3	1	1	10	32.7654	0	0	0	0.004667	0.000090	0.187169
2	3	1	2	12	105.3328	0	0	1	0.050795	0.000720	0.974806
2	3	1	3	11	88.2396	1	0	4	0.178689	0.001285	1.821627
2	3	1	4	7	54.1711	1	0	4	0.248082	0.001225	2.745999
2	3	1	5	3	12.5214	1	0	3	0.083994	0.000401	1.061039
2	3	2	1	13	39.9615	0	0	0	0.006060	0.000114	0.236859
2	3	2	2	13	130.0000	0	0	0	0.062156	0.000916	1.245923
2	3	2	3	14	108.1035	3	0	5	0.208017	0.001592	2.260874
2	3	2	4	9	47.3701	1	2	7	0.196524	0.000959	1.976272
2	3	2	5	2	28.4575	0	0	0	0.192905	0.000924	3.032250
2	3	3	1	2	10.1591	0	0	0	0.001217	0.000023	0.053197
2	3	3	2	2	18.3206	1	0	1	0.008768	0.000109	0.148577
2	3	3	3	1	10.0000	0	0	0	0.020875	0.000138	0.180384
2	3	3	4	1	10.0000	0	0	0	0.048323	0.000205	0.453334
2	3	3	5	1	4.4547	0	0	1	0.030170	0.000136	0.357358
2	4	1	1	75	636.6534	2	0	4	0.071267	0.001203	2.971809
2	4	1	2	72	677.4666	2	0	7	0.448932	0.004415	5.434327
2	4	1	3	65	568.3325	7	0	17	1.398524	0.007470	11.370510
2	4	1	4	48	379.5499	1	2	21	1.983351	0.008526	18.568737
2	4	1	5	27	167.9702	1	0	13	1.260037	0.005626	16.864193
2	4	2	1	41	335.2416	0	0	1	0.035677	0.000598	1.533288
2	4	2	2	41	369.7211	4	1	7	0.228690	0.002257	2.835229
2	4	2	3	32	289.4706	3	0	7	0.683183	0.003685	5.486624
2	4	2	4	25	196.2285	0	1	13	1.005349	0.004282	9.197350
2	4	2	5	12	78.6426	0	0	6	0.588204	0.002591	7.778345
2	4	3	1	7	49.2441	1	0	1	0.006178	0.000107	0.251981
2	4	3	2	6	40.8844	3	0	4	0.022000	0.000252	0.329680
2	4	3	3	2	11.5106	0	0	1	0.030754	0.000173	0.257286
2	4	3	4	1	10.0000	0	0	0	0.057345	0.000246	0.565400
2	4	3	5	1	3.7848	1	0	1	0.027976	0.000128	0.376292
3	1	1	2	8	30.9646	0	0	0	0.018602	0.000471	0.713553

Appendix VII: Four-way Classification of Welsh Data (cont'd)

AFE	YFE	EXP	TFE	N	PY	Observed deaths			Expected deaths		
						Lung cancer	Nasal cancer	All causes	Lung cancer	Nasal cancer	All causes
3	1	1	3	10	90.0610	0	0	1	0.085716	0.001714	3.700508
3	1	1	4	9	56.2800	1	0	6	0.099375	0.002043	5.033322
3	1	1	5	3	8.9761	0	0	1	0.023529	0.000424	1.434741
3	1	2	2	9	31.6553	0	0	1	0.018436	0.000466	0.673323
3	1	2	3	8	51.9076	1	0	5	0.047123	0.000913	1.805143
3	1	2	4	3	20.0629	0	0	1	0.044301	0.000682	1.609779
3	1	2	5	2	5.1459	0	0	1	0.014674	0.000236	0.813623
3	1	3	2	6	16.3969	0	0	1	0.010044	0.000253	0.406400
3	1	3	3	6	40.4081	0	0	4	0.032798	0.000709	1.420403
3	1	3	4	2	20.0000	0	0	0	0.039630	0.000762	1.912668
3	1	3	5	2	7.8320	0	0	1	0.021646	0.000365	1.142771
3	1	4	2	8	24.7081	0	2	2	0.013860	0.000347	0.503048
3	1	4	3	7	57.9165	0	0	1	0.055881	0.001028	2.061535
3	1	4	4	6	44.3951	1	1	3	0.097585	0.001371	3.243989
3	1	4	5	3	9.9196	0	0	3	0.027750	0.000459	1.264412
3	1	5	2	4	13.2140	0	1	1	0.006939	0.000172	0.236301
3	1	5	3	4	22.2736	0	1	2	0.025715	0.000367	0.662605
3	1	5	4	2	11.0219	1	0	1	0.030305	0.000317	0.764719
3	1	5	5	1	0.3643	0	1	1	0.001214	0.000016	0.037614
3	2	1	2	8	46.6960	0	0	2	0.025929	0.000617	0.880928
3	2	1	3	7	62.5234	0	0	2	0.088777	0.001137	2.325517
3	2	1	4	5	41.1809	0	1	1	0.130443	0.001382	3.439777
3	2	1	5	4	17.9314	1	0	1	0.069279	0.000702	2.589557
3	2	2	1	3	1.5001	0	0	0	0.000411	0.000008	0.012909
3	2	2	2	15	115.0914	1	1	3	0.066007	0.001451	2.027447
3	2	2	3	12	96.5497	0	2	8	0.149251	0.001705	3.341032
3	2	2	4	4	18.7769	0	1	4	0.060148	0.000552	1.348683
3	2	3	1	5	2.3235	0	0	0	0.001001	0.000023	0.031400
3	2	3	2	14	112.6292	2	1	4	0.071390	0.001567	2.278342
3	2	3	3	10	75.9399	2	0	8	0.115621	0.001421	2.970081
3	2	3	4	2	13.9891	0	0	1	0.044356	0.000496	1.395872
3	2	3	5	1	1.6083	0	0	0	0.005966	0.000063	0.248098
3	2	4	2	5	29.2269	0	0	3	0.016492	0.000379	0.509995
3	2	4	3	2	10.8987	1	0	1	0.020291	0.000195	0.401675
3	2	4	4	1	8.2767	0	0	1	0.029040	0.000284	0.693576
3	2	5	2	4	27.0659	0	1	1	0.015363	0.000358	0.503703
3	2	5	3	3	19.3617	1	0	2	0.029631	0.000342	0.690170
3	2	5	4	1	8.6274	0	1	1	0.031483	0.000278	0.679248
3	3	1	1	5	15.5463	0	0	0	0.004545	0.000091	0.144929
3	3	1	2	5	50.0000	0	0	0	0.038182	0.000619	0.815164
3	3	1	3	5	40.6248	0	0	1	0.105821	0.000753	1.476069
3	3	1	4	4	36.9518	0	0	2	0.167498	0.001175	3.079530
3	3	1	5	2	0.8402	0	1	2	0.003834	0.000026	0.120626
3	3	2	1	7	19.3579	1	0	1	0.005944	0.000119	0.187597
3	3	2	2	6	53.8741	0	0	1	0.039317	0.000662	0.857099
3	3	2	3	5	38.8685	0	0	2	0.097331	0.000709	1.372621

Appendix VII: Four-way Classification of Welsh Data (cont'd)

AFE	YFE	EXP	TFE	N	PY	Observed deaths			Expected deaths		
						Lung cancer	Nasal cancer	All causes	Lung cancer	Nasal cancer	All causes
3	3	2	4	3	16.5713	0	0	3	0.071583	0.000548	1.345318
3	3	3	1	7	12.8011	1	0	1	0.004282	0.000089	0.134381
3	3	3	2	6	50.7423	0	1	2	0.035059	0.000643	0.872330
3	3	3	3	4	28.0280	0	0	2	0.063334	0.000500	0.994420
3	3	3	4	2	1.5369	0	0	2	0.005663	0.000040	0.096456
3	3	4	1	2	1.7480	0	0	0	0.000711	0.000016	0.022298
3	3	4	2	2	15.0377	0	1	1	0.009166	0.000196	0.261667
3	3	4	3	1	4.4412	0	1	1	0.006977	0.000071	0.124634
3	4	1	1	46	366.4772	0	0	4	0.101905	0.001798	2.904719
3	4	1	2	40	362.2961	5	0	10	0.441966	0.004523	5.630685
3	4	1	3	30	258.8806	2	1	11	0.914011	0.005062	9.714138
3	4	1	4	19	127.8625	1	0	10	0.740171	0.003881	10.684372
3	4	1	5	9	34.1688	2	0	4	0.237515	0.001198	4.636051
3	4	2	1	36	302.5701	0	0	5	0.077265	0.001356	2.269936
3	4	2	2	33	304.8248	5	0	8	0.349723	0.003645	4.460165
3	4	2	3	25	189.9575	8	0	14	0.630007	0.003504	6.363993
3	4	2	4	11	52.2952	2	1	9	0.286616	0.001443	3.718540
3	4	2	5	2	8.4961	0	0	1	0.055865	0.000307	1.154069
3	4	3	1	2	10.3977	0	0	0	0.002449	0.000042	0.073716
3	4	3	2	2	19.4099	1	0	1	0.018544	0.000213	0.249869
3	4	3	3	1	10.0000	0	0	0	0.030400	0.000187	0.317061
3	4	3	4	1	3.5437	1	0	1	0.017331	0.000080	0.201905
4	1	1	2	1	3.2507	0	0	0	0.002090	0.000055	0.114900
4	1	1	3	1	10.0000	0	0	0	0.007862	0.000259	0.605049
4	1	1	4	1	8.7240	0	0	1	0.011710	0.000415	1.194058
4	1	2	2	2	8.3676	0	0	0	0.005357	0.000148	0.330412
4	1	2	3	2	20.0000	0	0	0	0.016183	0.000601	1.377671
4	1	2	4	2	8.5656	0	0	1	0.011862	0.000408	1.194423
4	1	3	2	1	3.1534	0	0	0	0.002028	0.000053	0.110443
4	1	3	3	1	6.5699	0	0	1	0.004622	0.000145	0.345160
4	2	1	2	5	31.7454	0	0	2	0.021618	0.000516	0.969634
4	2	1	3	3	2.1759	0	1	3	0.002073	0.000041	0.093540
4	2	2	1	1	0.7452	0	0	0	0.000466	0.000012	0.020219
4	2	2	2	5	45.2374	0	0	0	0.032784	0.000771	1.555950
4	2	2	3	5	20.6312	1	2	4	0.026131	0.000625	1.461149
4	2	2	4	1	4.4465	0	0	1	0.009194	0.000219	0.722761
4	2	3	1	6	2.4304	0	0	0	0.001428	0.000036	0.054792
4	2	3	2	9	78.5702	0	0	2	0.054769	0.001506	3.105979
4	2	3	3	7	33.3228	1	2	6	0.039947	0.001046	2.580065
4	2	3	4	1	2.8110	0	0	1	0.005305	0.000137	0.459733
4	2	4	2	3	9.2477	1	2	3	0.005915	0.000147	0.273481
4	3	1	1	10	17.8136	0	0	1	0.010409	0.000271	0.510801
4	3	1	2	9	73.3073	0	0	3	0.055422	0.001389	2.872154
4	3	1	3	6	58.3683	0	0	3	0.106349	0.001865	4.775894
4	3	1	4	3	3.5110	0	0	2	0.010589	0.000155	0.375698
4	3	2	1	6	14.6930	0	0	0	0.008516	0.000217	0.342941

Appendix VII: Four-way Classification of Welsh Data (cont'd)

AFE	YFE	EXP	TFE	N	PY	Observed deaths			Expected deaths		
						Lung cancer	Nasal cancer	All causes	Lung cancer	Nasal cancer	All causes
4	3	2	2	6	40.0914	0	2	5	0.034519	0.000665	1.238614
4	3	2	3	1	10.0000	0	0	0	0.018833	0.000281	0.658282
4	3	2	4	1	0.8709	0	0	1	0.001974	0.000041	0.093471
4	3	3	1	2	2.0330	0	0	0	0.001256	0.000032	0.052300
4	3	3	2	2	10.8544	1	0	1	0.008336	0.000186	0.381166
4	3	3	3	1	0.5123	0	1	1	0.000497	0.000010	0.021945
4	4	1	1	20	151.1498	0	0	3	0.081162	0.001719	2.551850
4	4	1	2	18	164.2301	0	2	4	0.265982	0.003007	5.759737
4	4	1	3	14	79.6339	2	0	10	0.260450	0.002350	5.923701
4	4	1	4	3	7.5938	1	0	3	0.033121	0.000282	0.955459
4	4	2	1	22	178.7898	1	1	3	0.102235	0.002249	3.350846
4	4	2	2	19	131.8055	2	0	10	0.199449	0.002261	4.225490
4	4	2	3	9	61.9921	1	0	6	0.207972	0.001873	4.734968
4	4	2	4	3	9.6090	0	0	2	0.042912	0.000345	1.267546
4	4	3	1	5	24.7805	0	0	1	0.013485	0.000329	0.596625
4	4	3	2	4	23.0416	0	1	3	0.026366	0.000417	0.796841
4	4	3	3	1	0.2190	0	0	1	0.000542	0.000004	0.009514

CONTINUOUS DATA (ORIGINAL RECORDS) FOR 679 WELSH NICKEL REFINERY WORKERS

ID	ICD code	Exposure level	Date of birth	Age at first employment	Age at start of follow-up	Age at death or withdrawal
3	0	5.0	1889.019	17.481	45.227	92.981
4	162	5.0	1885.978	23.186	48.268	63.271
6	163	10.0	1881.255	25.245	52.992	54.164
8	527	9.0	1886.340	24.721	47.907	69.679
9	150	0.	1879.500	29.958	54.746	76.844
10	163	2.0	1889.915	21.288	44.331	62.541
15	334	0.	1890.500	23.284	43.746	62.000
16	160	0.5	1874.332	50.357	59.915	65.583
17	420	0.	1909.500	15.462	34.746	50.514
18	12	0.	1892.500	24.139	51.746	57.593
19	160	10.0	1881.726	33.452	52.520	58.490
21	14	0.	1877.800	30.203	56.446	65.570
22	177	2.5	1879.500	28.669	54.746	67.481
23	162	0.	1900.500	22.648	33.746	52.703
26	999	0.	1887.474	28.197	46.772	77.056
27	420	0.	1893.849	28.962	40.397	68.521
28	420	0.	1905.849	14.052	28.397	61.529
29	434	0.	1873.500	36.744	60.746	63.008
30	420	1.0	1899.400	15.400	34.846	66.581
32	153	0.	1905.500	14.401	28.746	53.768
33	151	1.5	1883.500	27.796	50.746	61.810
34	154	4.0	1886.500	20.927	47.746	53.256
35	420	0.5	1886.395	23.523	47.852	82.827
37	162	0.	1889.093	34.490	45.153	63.043
40	162	1.0	1894.638	28.751	39.608	74.542
41	331	2.5	1886.967	27.819	47.279	65.109
42	420	0.	1899.499	24.194	34.748	83.049
44	998	0.	1889.500	34.959	44.746	56.478
47	160	1.0	1893.312	18.395	45.934	47.114
48	592	4.0	1884.500	26.834	49.746	63.634
49	162	2.5	1890.970	20.227	43.277	62.789
50	420	3.5	1896.500	26.360	37.746	54.969
51	151	1.0	1883.500	22.697	50.746	70.000
52	420	0.5	1894.748	20.752	39.499	86.688
53	160	1.0	1900.710	22.892	33.536	72.761
54	160	11.0	1889.397	25.288	44.849	77.808
55	0	0.	1900.986	22.726	33.260	81.014
56	502	2.0	1904.500	18.292	29.746	51.585
57	27	0.5	1882.500	34.560	51.746	58.434
58	241	0.	1872.500	45.640	61.746	66.768

Appendix VIII: Original Records from Welsh Study (cont'd)

ID	ICD code	Exposure level	Date of birth	Age at first employment	Age at start of follow-up	Age at death or withdrawal
59	420	0.	1901.225	22.164	33.022	81.019
60	422	5.0	1889.500	21.626	44.746	60.571
61	420	0.	1879.500	35.884	54.746	76.201
62	592	6.5	1879.500	34.152	54.746	73.432
63	160	14.0	1878.030	30.410	56.216	58.065
64	334	6.0	1888.500	18.807	45.746	64.812
65	502	6.0	1883.500	28.295	50.746	64.481
68	162	5.0	1897.849	16.651	36.397	79.830
70	162	0.	1901.274	21.570	32.973	54.748
71	163	0.5	1895.989	17.647	38.257	61.493
73	163	8.5	1887.293	25.188	46.953	78.715
75	0	0.	1905.408	16.880	28.838	76.592
76	332	7.5	1879.500	33.421	54.746	72.056
77	420	0.	1890.500	32.352	43.746	74.273
78	153	0.5	1894.915	28.099	39.331	72.389
79	334	1.0	1902.863	21.539	31.383	71.088
80	2	2.0	1889.500	33.311	44.746	64.138
82	527	3.0	1876.500	32.235	57.746	60.979
83	332	2.0	1880.500	30.777	53.746	76.022
84	0	0.	1895.479	27.542	38.767	86.521
85	151	6.5	1881.411	33.392	52.835	86.381
86	163	21.0	1885.500	22.267	48.746	59.612
87	163	4.0	1882.500	20.785	51.746	58.489
88	502	0.	1904.068	14.222	30.178	71.449
89	502	3.0	1875.500	43.432	58.746	68.505
90	491	0.	1900.953	19.596	33.293	76.882
91	154	3.5	1886.500	23.881	47.746	54.505
92	163	5.5	1895.175	24.156	39.071	52.477
93	443	0.	1888.303	20.451	45.943	81.089
94	420	5.5	1881.500	25.519	52.746	75.109
95	410	0.	1874.500	35.758	59.746	65.872
96	420	0.	1890.022	32.797	44.224	89.945
97	0	0.	1902.500	21.790	31.746	79.500
98	162	3.5	1894.159	28.808	40.088	61.822
99	420	0.	1883.500	31.768	50.746	62.393
100	331	5.0	1874.500	31.659	59.746	60.549
101	420	0.	1904.527	14.032	44.719	75.590
103	491	0.	1901.734	21.934	32.512	56.332
104	420	17.5	1883.500	26.021	50.746	73.555
106	160	11.0	1880.312	28.443	53.935	58.072
107	420	0.	1897.655	25.406	36.592	79.847
108	153	2.5	1880.500	35.653	53.746	65.445
109	592	5.5	1899.500	20.667	34.746	45.260
110	0	0.	1909.247	14.030	25.000	72.753
111	0	1.0	1905.222	17.425	29.025	76.778

Appendix VIII: Original Records from Welsh Study (cont'd)

ID	ICD code	Exposure level	Date of birth	Age at first employment	Age at start of follow-up	Age at death or withdrawal
112	491	0.	1897.452	25.573	36.794	78.578
113	998	7.5	1880.500	27.100	53.746	61.111
115	331	5.5	1888.500	25.152	45.746	66.656
116	162	1.5	1901.192	22.367	33.055	55.090
117	502	1.0	1891.652	24.364	42.594	66.337
118	493	7.0	1887.500	26.149	46.746	57.785
119	501	11.5	1881.500	26.336	52.746	58.284
120	502	7.0	1873.500	47.131	60.746	69.434
121	163	14.0	1882.011	27.556	52.235	68.578
122	162	0.	1893.238	30.301	41.008	82.805
124	331	0.	1871.500	36.000	62.746	84.724
126	162	18.0	1883.500	24.710	50.746	57.279
127	792	1.0	1900.500	22.319	33.746	62.000
128	163	0.	1886.500	20.925	47.746	53.637
129	450	2.0	1897.126	25.830	37.120	74.701
131	163	18.0	1881.959	26.675	52.288	67.197
132	332	0.	1900.929	22.088	33.318	69.745
135	491	0.	1892.109	31.208	42.137	84.893
137	465	0.	1905.386	19.081	28.860	74.279
138	181	3.5	1882.500	24.000	51.746	71.873
140	443	0.	1887.500	36.262	46.746	71.237
141	163	0.5	1891.500	18.503	42.746	62.253
142	160	7.5	1883.915	26.712	50.331	57.449
143	420	3.0	1887.500	32.951	46.746	77.303
144	160	1.5	1884.505	28.596	49.741	67.229
145	177	10.5	1882.729	27.038	51.518	91.827
147	420	4.0	1878.500	30.000	55.746	87.911
148	420	0.	1902.500	21.204	31.746	65.658
149	163	2.0	1889.997	33.307	44.249	69.036
150	160	9.5	1871.932	38.690	62.315	64.732
151	160	10.5	1875.364	32.830	58.882	77.745
152	420	4.5	1874.500	40.262	59.746	83.073
154	463	2.5	1900.150	22.655	44.096	70.000
155	434	0.	1880.500	32.719	53.746	58.237
156	196	12.5	1887.500	27.160	46.746	58.837
157	332	0.5	1905.751	16.331	28.496	74.752
158	163	5.5	1885.500	22.500	48.746	54.582
159	502	3.5	1886.500	23.747	47.746	55.612
161	162	2.5	1891.573	31.277	42.674	60.553
162	157	0.	1897.500	26.089	36.746	46.918
164	163	3.0	1896.500	24.413	37.746	52.610
165	502	2.0	1891.500	31.437	42.746	50.782
166	451	2.5	1901.063	21.641	33.183	67.511
170	420	0.	1893.619	29.433	40.627	78.741
172	163	3.0	1888.626	26.874	45.621	58.522

Appendix VIII: Original Records from Welsh Study (cont'd)

ID	ICD code	Exposure level	Date of birth	Age at first employment	Age at start of follow-up	Age at death or withdrawal
173	0	3.0	1895.929	26.921	38.318	86.071
175	332	0.	1887.500	26.000	46.746	76.295
176	198	4.5	1882.775	33.309	51.471	68.433
177	420	0.	1902.414	10.784	31.833	67.849
180	163	3.0	1892.500	21.311	41.746	48.117
181	526	2.0	1881.500	24.758	52.746	62.601
186	163	1.5	1897.929	25.652	36.318	61.096
187	999	0.	1906.500	18.098	27.746	34.500
190	163	5.0	1888.473	25.027	45.774	57.988
191	181	4.0	1886.500	35.092	47.746	69.814
194	446	1.0	1894.041	28.885	40.205	71.715
195	334	0.	1892.500	30.338	41.746	70.000
196	491	3.5	1892.563	27.937	41.684	81.832
197	356	2.5	1902.500	20.473	31.746	53.940
199	163	0.	1880.361	24.126	53.886	68.126
200	0	7.5	1885.866	20.548	48.381	96.134
202	541	0.5	1898.500	24.358	35.746	42.101
203	163	1.0	1886.649	36.471	47.597	71.880
204	502	6.5	1876.500	30.914	57.746	66.251
206	162	0.	1892.500	30.579	41.746	64.519
207	162	4.0	1895.690	18.074	38.556	60.312
208	163	1.5	1887.027	26.473	47.219	67.211
210	163	0.	1890.507	30.029	43.740	55.011
211	163	5.0	1886.500	31.922	47.746	50.030
212	163	1.5	1895.500	18.000	38.746	49.623
213	162	0.	1910.129	14.202	24.118	63.049
214	420	1.5	1886.655	29.142	47.592	78.559
215	434	0.	1885.500	25.111	48.746	54.366
216	420	0.	1881.500	23.464	52.746	66.669
218	491	10.0	1883.500	30.503	50.746	78.779
219	151	0.5	1884.391	38.730	49.856	83.182
221	163	11.0	1888.918	21.827	45.328	68.027
222	160	3.5	1876.085	37.737	58.162	70.910
223	162	0.	1889.500	33.867	44.746	63.758
224	434	0.	1903.500	13.774	30.746	37.645
225	177	0.	1883.849	25.608	50.397	83.770
226	260	0.	1883.500	21.000	50.746	67.999
227	0	0.	1904.344	12.585	29.902	77.656
228	502	0.	1906.912	15.671	27.334	71.660
229	420	0.	1901.500	23.363	32.746	62.735
230	0	0.	1903.500	13.063	30.746	78.500
231	162	3.0	1896.500	21.330	37.746	59.587
234	420	2.0	1882.500	27.651	51.746	71.456
236	161	0.	1892.500	21.889	41.746	68.281
237	163	5.0	1895.500	27.322	38.746	52.421

Appendix VIII: Original Records from Welsh Study (cont'd)

ID	ICD code	Exposure level	Date of birth	Age at first employment	Age at start of follow-up	Age at death or withdrawal
239	420	0.	1878.500	26.068	55.746	80.832
240	0	1.0	1902.500	20.533	31.746	79.500
243	998	2.0	1887.500	26.160	46.746	51.505
245	422	1.5	1886.500	23.930	47.746	73.587
246	163	0.	1894.500	20.788	39.746	55.642
248	420	1.0	1895.622	28.435	38.625	69.540
250	163	10.0	1885.500	24.842	48.746	59.897
251	153	3.5	1877.500	34.773	56.746	72.971
252	420	1.0	1888.500	17.579	45.746	58.453
255	0	0.	1899.162	23.943	35.085	82.838
256	223	2.0	1880.500	39.956	53.746	68.235
257	490	0.	1899.500	23.369	34.746	62.990
259	154	2.5	1885.500	37.426	48.746	76.489
261	0	0.	1901.384	21.929	32.863	80.616
265	999	0.	1902.500	13.495	31.746	55.892
266	331	0.	1887.500	34.514	46.746	61.060
267	2	3.0	1881.500	38.934	52.746	65.930
268	420	1.0	1894.500	20.790	39.746	88.412
270	163	2.0	1895.800	27.088	38.446	53.430
271	160	9.0	1884.519	30.549	49.727	64.990
272	420	5.5	1882.500	38.415	51.746	68.634
273	154	0.	1909.500	14.691	24.746	55.930
274	491	2.0	1883.438	36.977	50.808	75.066
275	331	0.	1880.500	44.112	53.746	54.155
276	153	1.0	1900.352	22.670	33.894	69.464
277	163	0.	1903.500	21.402	30.746	65.000
279	163	1.0	1880.500	27.653	53.746	63.308
281	420	0.	1893.285	26.939	40.962	76.531
282	162	6.0	1891.500	22.505	42.746	54.053
283	500	0.	1894.715	29.000	39.531	57.561
284	431	6.5	1880.500	26.451	53.746	56.377
285	420	0.	1899.063	15.721	35.183	68.334
286	421	5.0	1886.500	23.684	47.746	63.832
287	331	6.0	1878.500	28.000	55.746	84.064
289	162	0.	1884.951	35.771	49.296	76.942
291	502	8.0	1874.500	28.341	59.746	66.085
292	422	3.5	1871.500	37.137	62.746	86.223
293	610	8.5	1882.500	28.122	51.746	56.930
294	160	5.5	1885.299	35.270	48.948	62.096
295	196	0.	1889.019	35.448	45.227	74.937
297	420	5.0	1886.500	27.133	47.746	70.823
298	160	12.0	1885.822	25.230	48.425	54.700
299	160	0.	1898.500	23.432	35.746	68.653
300	163	5.0	1900.104	20.295	34.143	46.751
301	525	8.0	1889.500	22.582	44.746	51.322

Appendix VIII: Original Records from Welsh Study (cont'd)

ID	ICD code	Exposure level	Date of birth	Age at first employment	Age at start of follow-up	Age at death or withdrawal
302	593	0.	1900.508	15.232	33.738	75.421
303	422	7.5	1879.500	31.796	54.746	67.653
305	334	3.0	1899.871	16.629	34.375	73.907
306	999	0.	1897.500	25.322	36.746	37.300
307	422	0.	1877.500	27.352	56.746	85.215
309	331	3.5	1900.891	14.531	33.356	68.539
310	422	12.0	1878.500	27.601	55.746	76.434
313	0	0.5	1896.563	19.196	37.684	85.437
315	420	0.	1879.500	24.185	54.746	79.621
316	491	0.	1889.225	33.797	45.022	91.915
318	541	0.5	1899.500	17.000	34.746	43.747
319	160	0.	1900.738	22.123	33.509	66.320
321	0	0.	1897.433	25.584	36.814	84.567
322	592	0.	1900.500	22.675	33.746	55.059
324	332	0.	1885.249	37.586	48.997	83.869
325	434	0.	1910.500	14.074	23.746	43.034
326	502	3.0	1879.500	43.311	54.746	64.781
327	465	1.5	1903.962	13.655	30.285	73.057
328	331	1.5	1884.500	20.796	49.746	66.445
329	163	6.0	1888.500	23.790	45.746	51.344
330	160	0.	1881.578	28.899	52.668	70.079
332	420	0.	1884.328	38.560	49.919	69.310
334	162	6.0	1892.500	28.399	46.746	71.943
335	440	6.0	1884.500	26.678	54.746	78.467
336	420	12.0	1876.500	28.000	62.746	83.809
337	420	0.	1885.500	36.815	48.746	67.993
338	0	0.	1894.929	29.402	49.318	87.071
339	331	5.0	1882.500	28.459	51.746	72.448
340	502	0.	1894.285	28.726	39.962	66.568
341	154	0.	1888.500	31.686	45.746	51.481
344	420	1.0	1908.891	14.559	25.356	68.290
345	162	2.0	1900.828	22.027	33.419	54.350
346	163	4.5	1894.203	28.792	40.044	58.202
348	0	2.0	1901.329	21.792	32.918	80.671
349	332	0.	1899.249	23.967	34.997	75.414
351	331	6.0	1873.500	49.314	65.746	73.226
353	204	0.	1901.500	23.169	32.746	48.763
354	420	0.	1877.115	31.344	57.131	97.778
357	420	0.	1896.801	22.699	37.446	75.601
360	450	0.	1883.907	30.052	50.340	86.241
361	443	0.	1887.584	31.630	46.663	81.838
362	331	0.5	1889.181	21.433	45.066	88.258
363	160	10.0	1883.422	26.597	50.825	57.789
364	345	3.0	1886.500	21.697	47.746	60.664
365	420	0.	1900.202	22.669	34.044	60.415

Appendix VIII: Original Records from Welsh Study (cont'd)

ID	ICD code	Exposure level	Date of birth	Age at first employment	Age at start of follow-up	Age at death or withdrawal
368	420	2.0	1888.563	22.937	50.684	81.286
369	420	0.	1904.328	19.387	29.919	70.376
370	420	1.0	1899.619	14.595	34.627	76.963
371	600	8.0	1886.500	28.588	47.746	57.765
375	592	1.0	1885.500	26.790	48.746	60.226
376	332	0.	1907.047	15.036	27.200	68.838
377	153	9.5	1881.500	27.664	52.746	80.212
378	160	3.5	1893.500	19.911	40.746	63.974
380	411	0.	1907.153	14.740	27.093	53.663
381	160	13.0	1884.596	29.459	49.651	78.087
383	204	0.	1903.096	19.926	31.151	72.575
384	431	7.0	1877.500	37.462	56.746	64.533
385	0	0.	1903.534	16.600	30.712	78.466
386	451	5.0	1901.674	15.329	32.573	78.375
388	434	4.0	1892.500	30.316	41.746	49.547
389	420	0.5	1903.000	20.304	31.246	58.855
390	420	2.5	1886.504	22.996	52.742	85.791
391	162	13.0	1881.500	28.892	52.746	60.692
392	160	15.0	1891.019	21.505	43.227	57.585
394	237	0.	1904.571	14.004	29.675	65.829
395	160	3.0	1896.164	22.855	38.083	70.806
397	332	0.	1890.500	32.560	43.746	46.410
400	162	0.	1903.370	19.425	30.877	77.067
403	502	7.0	1887.500	35.330	46.746	48.596
404	155	0.	1902.904	20.578	31.342	77.555
406	163	5.5	1892.500	21.199	41.746	66.708
407	422	3.0	1883.500	39.360	50.746	66.566
408	443	1.0	1882.500	25.505	51.746	74.481
409	163	2.0	1874.500	38.404	59.746	70.807
410	162	0.	1900.500	22.525	33.746	51.661
412	420	0.	1880.500	35.182	53.746	78.215
416	162	0.	1893.811	29.770	40.436	61.685
417	162	7.0	1875.500	38.807	58.746	69.459
419	155	0.	1902.540	20.455	31.707	70.808
420	420	3.0	1894.500	24.823	39.746	71.338
421	160	1.0	1884.500	30.000	49.746	69.782
423	502	0.	1874.500	31.700	59.746	74.522
424	332	0.	1891.751	31.041	42.496	72.796
425	163	3.0	1897.500	13.316	36.746	55.514
427	422	3.5	1888.336	26.971	45.910	67.417
428	162	0.	1896.500	26.878	37.746	45.212
429	434	1.0	1897.562	25.249	36.685	79.154
432	0	0.	1904.112	18.852	40.134	77.888
433	146	3.0	1883.458	39.469	50.789	63.762
436	420	0.	1899.378	23.512	34.868	73.351

Appendix VIII: Original Records from Welsh Study (cont'd)

ID	ICD code	Exposure level	Date of birth	Age at first employment	Age at start of follow-up	Age at death or withdrawal
437	331	0.	1875.500	34.977	58.746	70.297
439	0	2.0	1901.178	21.786	33.068	48.970
440	162	0.	1892.500	26.000	41.746	66.716
442	590	0.	1873.500	34.116	60.746	75.705
443	420	0.	1905.326	14.556	28.920	65.762
444	0	0.	1908.036	14.778	36.211	73.964
446	160	0.	1888.071	35.050	46.175	65.017
447	432	0.	1890.463	21.849	43.783	74.989
449	153	0.	1885.500	20.579	48.746	65.577
452	500	0.	1891.260	28.677	42.986	76.770
453	160	0.	1892.503	31.308	41.744	64.183
455	332	5.5	1883.500	31.497	50.746	57.577
456	331	19.0	1888.500	21.253	45.746	54.796
457	181	2.0	1895.869	27.778	38.378	67.027
458	163	1.0	1878.500	27.338	55.746	58.996
459	610	7.0	1880.188	26.220	54.058	88.038
460	204	0.	1899.500	24.809	34.746	66.760
461	332	6.0	1896.992	22.334	37.255	76.789
462	421	4.5	1895.255	25.144	38.992	56.655
463	790	0.	1895.170	19.515	39.077	73.002
465	578	0.	1900.500	22.848	33.746	45.736
466	163	0.	1878.500	27.045	55.746	62.262
469	162	0.	1896.445	26.492	37.801	64.859
470	443	0.5	1892.500	26.000	41.746	57.541
473	162	7.0	1890.249	23.904	43.997	63.690
474	332	1.0	1886.792	38.011	47.455	83.137
475	550	0.	1891.500	30.421	42.746	50.122
476	162	0.	1894.992	28.186	39.255	81.134
477	502	0.	1896.503	26.451	37.744	86.056
478	204	0.	1895.337	28.720	38.909	73.926
484	151	0.	1888.500	22.648	50.746	68.372
485	162	5.0	1897.619	25.162	36.627	78.946
486	0	2.0	1901.500	21.621	32.746	44.821
488	936	0.	1899.762	23.940	34.485	75.227
490	162	2.0	1900.500	22.311	33.746	45.127
491	162	0.	1902.592	20.279	31.655	56.238
492	500	7.0	1883.500	31.262	50.746	68.719
495	420	0.	1873.500	29.881	60.746	77.779
496	181	2.0	1894.981	27.841	39.266	56.896
497	434	3.0	1875.500	30.295	58.746	62.640
499	331	9.0	1889.500	20.771	44.746	67.003
500	332	0.	1887.500	36.749	46.746	72.932
501	162	3.0	1883.477	26.871	50.770	73.335
502	733	0.5	1892.500	20.982	41.746	63.440
504	501	0.	1877.500	36.226	56.746	67.429

Appendix VIII: Original Records from Welsh Study (cont'd)

ID	ICD code	Exposure level	Date of birth	Age at first employment	Age at start of follow-up	Age at death or withdrawal
506	160	6.0	1889.460	21.605	44.786	67.523
507	163	5.0	1887.797	24.730	46.449	48.889
508	0	0.	1905.184	14.162	39.063	64.997
509	0	0.	1900.352	22.749	33.894	81.648
510	899	1.5	1899.126	15.482	35.120	79.099
511	146	0.	1881.500	23.782	52.746	75.049
512	163	1.5	1880.500	23.732	53.746	60.180
513	420	1.0	1886.500	29.953	47.746	61.385
514	162	6.5	1882.419	27.679	51.827	55.049
516	161	6.0	1887.723	30.510	46.523	71.734
518	160	5.5	1880.648	22.876	53.599	80.361
522	540	6.0	1885.500	21.489	48.746	63.276
523	0	1.0	1906.038	16.627	28.208	75.962
524	422	0.5	1880.500	32.651	53.746	72.851
525	420	0.	1899.312	21.600	34.934	65.439
526	525	8.0	1880.500	27.171	53.746	79.119
527	420	0.	1898.500	20.497	35.746	65.478
528	502	4.0	1896.445	26.335	37.801	75.467
529	160	1.0	1901.636	21.397	32.611	50.293
531	331	0.5	1892.432	30.398	51.815	85.946
533	434	0.	1902.041	21.008	32.205	75.636
535	422	3.0	1878.500	36.766	55.746	77.637
537	0	0.	1908.128	12.735	26.118	73.872
538	420	4.5	1895.247	16.778	39.000	59.129
540	157	2.5	1899.500	23.621	34.746	63.684
542	420	7.0	1875.500	33.232	58.746	87.919
544	420	8.5	1891.500	18.259	42.746	64.215
545	491	0.5	1900.251	20.631	33.995	71.436
546	0	0.	1909.500	14.495	24.746	72.500
547	420	1.0	1902.500	14.178	31.746	51.325
549	420	0.	1903.951	20.492	35.296	64.306
551	420	17.0	1888.260	18.760	45.987	72.757
553	420	0.	1896.609	26.566	37.637	70.495
554	163	0.	1892.500	28.279	41.746	54.210
556	0	0.	1908.555	14.823	25.692	73.445
559	422	1.0	1887.500	32.000	46.746	78.801
560	162	9.0	1881.500	30.262	52.746	61.160
561	162	16.0	1883.500	26.527	50.746	61.271
562	502	5.0	1875.500	32.555	58.746	65.049
563	163	0.	1894.148	20.844	40.099	56.978
565	163	0.	1882.500	28.842	51.746	81.382
566	160	2.5	1876.601	35.407	57.645	66.448
570	332	9.5	1890.500	15.000	43.746	72.215
572	420	5.0	1894.500	19.226	39.746	70.941
574	491	0.	1909.729	14.036	24.518	70.659

Appendix VIII: Original Records from Welsh Study (cont'd)

ID	ICD code	Exposure level	Date of birth	Age at first employment	Age at start of follow-up	Age at death or withdrawal
575	434	6.5	1871.500	35.903	62.746	72.473
577	163	9.0	1874.500	35.538	59.746	61.344
578	160	0.	1883.995	26.148	50.252	74.504
579	420	1.0	1881.500	25.193	52.746	78.820
582	502	0.	1892.623	30.232	41.624	79.557
584	163	8.0	1886.500	21.790	47.746	57.385
585	25	7.0	1878.500	27.642	55.746	63.884
586	493	0.	1902.500	21.863	31.746	40.752
587	153	6.5	1884.500	31.607	49.746	64.511
588	163	5.5	1871.500	43.829	62.746	64.683
590	610	2.0	1878.500	28.144	55.746	78.290
591	420	4.5	1884.500	25.023	49.746	67.240
592	163	8.0	1879.923	31.871	54.323	69.649
593	160	7.5	1882.438	31.885	51.808	61.821
595	160	8.0	1884.937	26.148	49.309	79.560
596	163	1.0	1892.948	31.650	41.298	69.871
597	491	7.0	1887.500	23.122	46.746	62.842
599	160	0.	1885.932	30.771	48.315	81.403
601	153	0.5	1880.500	29.818	53.746	67.155
603	162	0.	1899.318	24.479	34.929	57.622
605	420	0.	1896.303	18.804	52.943	83.568
606	181	5.5	1891.814	22.789	42.433	67.490
608	332	3.0	1900.503	22.281	33.744	72.634
609	160	3.0	1891.340	23.825	57.907	70.455
610	331	0.	1879.500	29.194	54.746	75.264
611	153	2.0	1875.500	47.292	58.746	68.888
612	422	0.	1892.500	30.495	41.746	60.755
615	420	0.	1897.879	14.079	36.367	78.203
616	420	0.5	1908.500	14.495	25.746	54.621
618	434	9.0	1882.500	30.574	51.746	53.735
620	177	0.	1903.222	16.025	31.025	63.425
621	434	0.	1871.500	44.051	62.746	83.692
622	422	4.5	1883.500	21.525	50.746	71.555
623	163	1.0	1877.500	44.434	56.746	61.922
625	420	0.5	1889.416	25.307	44.830	81.263
627	181	0.	1887.975	25.912	46.271	76.314
629	481	0.	1895.011	16.489	39.235	75.016
631	490	3.0	1886.500	29.000	47.746	66.437
632	501	0.	1889.789	23.534	44.457	74.979
633	422	0.	1894.500	26.068	39.746	69.628
635	420	9.0	1898.500	15.785	35.746	58.555
637	999	0.	1900.008	22.956	34.238	71.118
638	153	0.	1894.500	29.130	39.746	51.401
639	160	16.0	1881.912	27.781	52.334	78.145
640	163	8.5	1875.118	31.233	59.129	71.880

Appendix VIII: Original Records from Welsh Study (cont'd)

ID	ICD code	Exposure level	Date of birth	Age at first employment	Age at start of follow-up	Age at death or withdrawal
641	350	0.	1880.500	26.138	53.746	70.571
642	420	0.	1884.500	26.495	49.746	66.201
643	332	1.0	1874.500	33.932	59.746	73.995
645	999	1.5	1892.500	30.522	41.746	47.519
646	0	0.5	1896.131	26.891	43.115	85.869
647	420	0.	1900.295	23.899	33.951	74.513
648	420	2.0	1882.500	40.670	51.746	75.223
650	491	0.	1880.090	31.619	64.156	89.959
654	331	0.	1892.500	19.541	41.746	46.867
655	420	0.	1902.825	22.061	31.422	75.740
656	154	1.5	1879.500	45.098	54.746	63.388
658	160	1.0	1880.260	38.705	53.987	68.503
660	422	16.0	1881.373	25.290	52.874	85.726
662	491	0.	1877.773	29.904	56.474	93.493
663	521	0.	1876.500	45.108	57.746	73.111
664	454	0.	1900.232	20.546	34.014	68.645
665	420	0.	1879.500	26.774	54.746	77.434
667	422	4.5	1889.953	21.090	44.293	84.419
668	162	11.5	1888.137	21.817	46.110	65.551
669	420	0.	1882.500	27.664	51.746	57.242
674	160	12.5	1872.678	32.178	61.569	63.065
675	163	3.0	1898.500	24.322	35.746	53.831
676	163	1.0	1886.594	36.427	47.652	57.897
677	150	3.5	1889.353	27.365	44.893	69.490
679	490	3.0	1891.500	31.295	42.746	58.352
681	2	1.0	1894.500	28.333	39.746	46.508
682	154	0.5	1899.500	23.810	34.746	66.344
684	434	11.5	1886.500	27.341	47.746	58.637
685	151	0.5	1901.225	21.630	33.022	77.745
687	160	4.0	1885.170	28.907	49.077	78.433
688	541	0.	1885.500	20.777	48.746	56.522
689	443	0.	1893.500	25.116	40.746	64.232
690	420	0.	1906.500	17.221	27.746	55.122
694	0	0.	1900.500	15.000	33.746	46.347
696	191	0.	1877.500	46.105	56.746	73.648
697	162	0.	1906.145	14.120	28.101	63.373
698	422	8.0	1878.500	36.089	55.746	69.727
700	420	0.	1889.500	24.881	54.746	75.079
701	502	1.0	1898.956	25.235	35.290	82.186
702	522	10.0	1879.500	31.544	54.746	59.544
704	163	2.0	1894.500	28.358	49.746	69.423
705	420	3.0	1899.526	21.122	34.720	65.899
706	160	6.0	1874.441	38.636	59.805	74.937
707	163	0.	1881.337	42.225	52.909	76.005
710	0	0.5	1899.899	22.923	34.348	82.101

Appendix VIII: Original Records from Welsh Study (cont'd)

ID	ICD code	Exposure level	Date of birth	Age at first employment	Age at start of follow-up	Age at death or withdrawal
711	163	8.0	1880.563	34.122	53.684	69.711
712	422	0.	1870.500	44.840	63.746	85.653
713	810	2.0	1894.500	28.675	39.746	46.949
715	162	11.0	1891.049	22.562	43.197	54.658
716	491	0.	1894.699	25.430	39.548	84.334
717	160	11.5	1875.847	32.192	58.400	59.101
719	160	8.0	1880.738	34.465	53.509	56.030
721	334	6.5	1887.531	20.469	46.715	85.403
722	420	2.0	1896.355	26.516	37.891	74.017
723	502	0.	1889.500	33.640	49.746	77.021
724	163	1.0	1896.500	27.691	37.746	65.478
727	331	0.	1868.500	46.881	65.746	75.448
729	160	2.0	1892.500	29.804	41.746	70.333
730	163	0.	1888.475	27.314	45.771	79.341
731	163	4.5	1896.904	15.582	37.342	53.460
735	443	0.	1897.918	24.942	36.329	64.811
738	163	0.5	1894.668	28.167	39.578	64.027
742	527	3.0	1882.500	20.752	51.746	57.360
743	151	0.	1896.355	26.502	37.891	80.016
744	163	0.	1903.500	20.749	30.746	54.544
747	163	0.	1895.500	27.319	38.746	46.470
750	162	1.0	1886.500	32.708	47.746	49.256
751	420	3.0	1874.500	39.000	59.746	73.015
752	443	0.	1880.500	42.423	58.746	82.563
753	331	6.5	1875.500	36.300	58.746	69.533
754	163	2.5	1891.400	31.436	42.846	55.756
755	162	2.5	1891.500	30.522	42.746	53.445
756	998	3.5	1877.500	33.000	56.746	65.486
759	153	1.0	1901.500	21.823	32.746	62.533
760	0	0.	1893.500	29.284	40.746	88.500
763	450	0.	1877.704	32.773	61.542	72.512
764	163	3.0	1885.433	23.067	48.814	63.523
765	443	1.5	1891.452	32.192	42.794	69.753
766	420	0.	1900.333	23.811	33.913	66.456
768	160	13.0	1881.663	25.837	52.583	59.548
769	163	2.0	1886.500	27.114	47.746	51.141
772	420	0.	1895.500	27.369	38.746	55.275
773	0	0.	1891.500	32.100	42.746	44.626
774	163	1.0	1886.500	23.785	47.746	48.692
775	162	3.0	1892.008	28.721	42.238	61.066
776	160	0.	1876.500	36.022	57.746	66.881
777	451	0.	1897.638	21.540	46.608	79.132
778	163	5.5	1897.500	22.650	36.746	42.051
780	160	0.	1886.805	36.737	47.441	56.795
781	160	6.0	1875.789	39.414	58.457	69.926

Appendix VIII: Original Records from Welsh Study (cont'd)

ID	ICD code	Exposure level	Date of birth	Age at first employment	Age at start of follow-up	Age at death or withdrawal
782	792	1.0	1899.781	23.093	39.466	66.307
783	151	0.	1880.500	35.568	53.746	74.799
786	163	3.0	1891.932	26.970	42.315	68.700
787	163	0.	1892.500	32.074	41.746	56.670
788	0	0.	1901.890	22.722	32.356	80.110
789	332	2.0	1878.500	29.902	55.746	62.383
790	160	3.0	1884.626	29.456	49.621	59.341
792	0	0.	1908.500	13.549	25.746	73.500
794	205	0.5	1890.500	29.943	43.746	61.026
795	331	1.0	1885.500	37.390	48.746	67.547
796	334	1.0	1888.500	24.631	45.746	55.305
797	420	1.5	1870.500	37.729	63.746	78.432
798	420	5.0	1900.872	14.852	33.375	60.096
800	420	0.	1898.500	24.284	35.746	58.172
801	502	7.5	1884.500	25.834	49.746	58.432
802	332	0.	1876.500	27.267	57.746	86.094
803	540	1.0	1883.500	26.703	50.746	78.675
805	162	4.0	1880.500	30.275	53.746	58.393
806	163	0.	1891.819	22.504	42.427	55.290
808	431	10.0	1876.500	29.560	57.746	62.223
810	591	0.	1890.500	24.664	43.746	52.673
811	160	6.0	1882.411	27.386	51.835	63.367
812	0	0.5	1899.584	20.859	44.663	82.416
815	331	0.	1894.500	22.358	39.746	53.174
816	2	0.	1896.527	26.303	37.719	67.317
817	422	13.0	1877.500	32.930	56.746	70.492
818	160	4.0	1889.589	20.060	44.657	71.521
819	434	0.	1872.500	52.191	61.746	67.773
820	0	0.	1900.358	23.261	33.889	81.642
821	422	3.0	1893.104	29.751	41.142	55.800
822	332	14.5	1874.500	28.453	59.746	61.136
825	521	0.	1889.592	24.908	49.655	86.744
827	160	12.0	1874.978	36.726	59.268	64.510
828	0	0.	1908.667	14.380	25.580	73.333
829	156	3.0	1880.500	27.825	53.746	60.440
831	465	3.5	1890.173	32.622	44.074	71.016
832	163	8.5	1878.500	27.000	55.746	63.744
833	160	1.0	1876.609	38.999	57.637	62.443
834	163	0.5	1894.500	28.297	39.746	65.508
835	163	0.5	1897.321	21.819	36.926	54.868
836	998	6.5	1879.500	32.847	54.746	68.004
837	332	0.	1902.500	13.462	31.746	51.262
839	160	6.5	1889.000	25.666	45.246	62.334
840	334	0.	1874.545	48.362	69.701	93.613
841	422	3.0	1878.500	24.700	60.746	66.607

Appendix VIII: Original Records from Welsh Study (cont'd)

ID	ICD code	Exposure level	Date of birth	Age at first employment	Age at start of follow-up	Age at death or withdrawal
842	420	0.	1905.742	17.079	28.504	68.206
843	592	12.0	1881.500	28.000	52.746	79.563
845	163	9.0	1888.500	19.330	45.746	46.596
846	481	2.0	1895.926	27.699	38.320	77.066
847	610	0.5	1892.765	30.961	41.481	69.632
849	260	0.	1883.500	39.223	50.746	73.238
851	163	5.0	1897.500	25.371	36.746	50.108
852	350	0.	1892.156	32.093	42.091	73.392
853	181	6.0	1886.164	29.137	48.082	69.449
856	162	0.	1901.641	21.477	32.605	59.945
857	444	1.0	1890.175	28.860	44.071	69.214
858	502	0.	1902.945	20.159	46.301	63.367
859	2	5.0	1882.500	20.790	51.746	52.251
860	420	0.	1897.500	25.604	36.746	59.845
861	502	0.	1898.310	24.715	35.937	67.860
862	162	1.0	1894.586	28.277	39.660	58.102
863	332	0.	1898.767	24.104	35.479	73.547
864	420	0.	1895.531	27.589	38.715	80.444
866	332	0.	1870.500	34.309	68.746	84.533
868	177	0.	1900.609	14.418	33.637	63.292
871	420	1.0	1885.500	28.347	48.746	67.156
874	610	0.	1880.500	36.599	53.746	76.096
875	160	5.0	1873.967	40.737	60.279	76.501
876	541	0.	1906.500	15.429	27.746	43.292
879	163	2.0	1876.033	46.830	58.214	70.877
880	162	0.	1899.258	23.847	34.989	80.723
881	163	1.0	1889.036	34.134	45.211	63.257
883	304	0.	1894.085	28.767	40.161	66.440
884	0	0.	1904.380	18.456	29.867	77.620
885	0	0.	1899.500	24.042	34.746	82.500
886	163	0.5	1896.500	28.098	37.746	62.103
887	420	0.5	1874.500	40.495	59.746	84.941
888	331	2.0	1890.500	22.670	43.746	67.363
890	451	0.	1901.573	21.455	32.674	81.153
891	434	1.0	1901.500	22.270	32.746	42.484
892	163	6.0	1886.500	22.790	47.746	65.664
893	502	0.	1897.005	26.499	37.241	75.880
896	177	0.5	1891.500	22.821	42.746	71.547
898	420	8.5	1884.500	23.694	49.746	74.264
899	420	0.	1883.500	39.336	50.746	76.626
900	480	0.5	1890.800	21.000	43.446	79.219
901	421	0.	1902.500	21.719	31.746	52.853
903	451	0.	1903.203	14.005	41.044	77.297
904	420	8.5	1885.500	21.944	48.746	76.056
906	502	0.	1869.500	47.952	64.746	65.982

Appendix VIII: Original Records from Welsh Study (cont'd)

ID	ICD code	Exposure level	Date of birth	Age at first employment	Age at start of follow-up	Age at death or withdrawal
907	177	6.0	1887.500	18.640	46.746	73.117
908	420	0.	1889.710	33.074	44.537	69.997
909	177	2.0	1902.792	20.230	31.455	75.973
913	151	1.0	1904.142	14.148	30.104	62.814
914	331	2.0	1896.500	21.656	37.746	59.347
917	420	0.	1879.500	25.000	54.746	64.836
919	491	0.	1892.156	21.344	42.091	82.159
920	420	0.	1894.466	23.899	39.781	72.649
921	393	4.0	1879.500	25.774	54.746	56.817
923	334	0.	1893.230	27.368	46.016	81.770
924	420	0.	1896.101	27.288	38.145	85.570
925	502	2.0	1887.500	36.067	46.746	57.492
928	0	0.	1897.748	17.752	36.499	84.252
929	332	0.	1874.500	48.311	59.746	60.788
931	332	0.	1869.500	46.680	64.746	70.292
932	420	0.	1893.734	29.123	40.512	68.926
933	420	0.	1882.540	27.937	51.707	85.354
934	420	0.	1897.500	23.090	36.746	55.804
936	0	0.	1895.904	28.003	38.342	66.433
939	420	0.	1884.817	25.961	49.430	69.619
940	590	6.5	1879.500	35.103	54.746	61.418
941	0	3.5	1897.500	25.305	36.746	38.355
942	160	0.	1884.208	22.453	50.039	51.461
943	162	6.0	1883.500	30.000	50.746	59.125
944	502	0.5	1901.500	20.223	32.746	57.505
945	331	4.5	1863.500	49.555	70.746	83.289
946	999	0.	1894.500	28.273	39.746	46.096
947	0	0.	1896.940	26.230	37.307	69.030
949	162	0.	1902.500	13.245	31.746	50.126
950	0	0.	1902.500	22.342	31.746	33.735
952	153	0.	1887.063	35.806	47.183	70.510
953	177	2.0	1884.500	38.311	49.746	63.336
954	434	0.	1902.500	20.495	41.746	48.738
956	163	0.	1898.500	24.125	35.746	44.388
957	163	0.	1876.552	32.301	57.695	73.314
958	422	0.	1892.686	25.495	41.561	75.218
959	162	0.	1893.060	30.529	41.186	70.836
960	420	0.	1890.721	32.189	43.526	73.932
961	420	0.	1873.500	37.892	60.746	66.478
962	450	0.	1890.337	33.477	43.909	77.093
963	331	3.5	1886.500	28.462	47.746	51.695
964	502	3.0	1892.500	30.675	41.746	73.640
965	332	0.	1900.658	15.699	33.588	63.839
966	163	10.5	1883.904	23.712	50.342	64.495
967	162	0.	1886.005	36.885	48.241	67.515

Appendix VIII: Original Records from Welsh Study (cont'd)

ID	ICD code	Exposure level	Date of birth	Age at first employment	Age at start of follow-up	Age at death or withdrawal
968	420	0.5	1878.500	44.969	55.746	87.234
969	160	14.0	1881.500	28.799	52.746	57.686
971	154	0.	1894.500	28.358	39.746	57.803
972	162	0.	1903.589	14.753	35.657	57.329
973	162	0.	1894.562	20.400	39.685	79.353
0	490	0.	1880.500	22.938	53.746	55.174
0	177	3.5	1868.500	46.766	65.746	68.749
0	430	0.	1903.500	19.284	30.746	67.138
0	0	0.	1895.500	27.675	38.746	39.722

ENGLAND AND WALES: AGE- AND YEAR-SPECIFIC DEATH RATES FROM NASAL SINUS AND LUNG CANCER AND FROM ALL CAUSES

Calendar period	Age group (years)	Death rate (per 1 000 000 per year)		
		Lung cancer	Nasal cancer	All causes
1936 - 1940	10 - 14	1	0	1270
	15 - 19	2	0	2203
	20 - 24	6	0	3122
	25 - 29	14	0	3038
	30 - 34	30	1	3219
	35 - 39	68	1	4234
	40 - 44	149	3	5803
	45 - 49	274	5	8605
	50 - 54	431	10	13514
	55 - 59	586	15	20101
	60 - 64	646	16	30695
	65 - 69	636	19	45814
	70 - 74	533	27	73444
	75 - 79	464	48	120915
	80 - 84	324	47	183712
1941 - 1945	10 - 14	1	0	1195
	15 - 19	2	0	2223
	20 - 24	6	0	3703
	25 - 29	16	0	3191
	30 - 34	34	1	3123
	35 - 39	81	1	3631
	40 - 44	191	3	5035
	45 - 49	384	5	7664
	50 - 54	597	10	11860
	55 - 59	883	15	18522
	60 - 64	1021	16	28227
	65 - 69	970	19	42833
	70 - 74	748	27	64278
	75 - 79	631	48	104395
	80 - 84	385	47	161959

Appendix IX (cont'd)

Calendar period	Age group (years)	Death rate (per 1 000 000 per year)		
		Lung cancer	Nasal cancer	All causes
1946 - 1950	10 - 14	1	0	691
	15 - 19	3	0	1197
	20 - 24	8	0	1597
	25 - 29	18	0	1805
	30 - 34	36	1	2027
	35 - 39	94	1	2588
	40 - 44	236	3	3882
	45 - 49	544	5	6703
	50 - 54	954	10	10719
	55 - 59	1350	15	17423
	60 - 64	1717	16	28020
	65 - 69	1763	19	41767
	70 - 74	1400	27	64563
	75 - 79	1085	48	101751
	80 - 84	765	47	157771
1951 - 1955	10 - 14	0	0	480
	15 - 19	2	0	860
	20 - 24	7	0	1237
	25 - 29	13	0	1266
	30 - 34	35	1	1510
	35 - 39	98	1	2107
	40 - 44	248	3	3249
	45 - 49	579	5	5710
	50 - 54	1224	10	10456
	55 - 59	2003	15	17428
	60 - 64	2555	16	28435
	65 - 69	2926	19	44500
	70 - 74	2624	27	68059
	75 - 79	2069	48	108090
	80 - 84	1416	47	166158
1956 - 1960	10 - 14	0	0	403
	15 - 19	2	0	877
	20 - 24	4	0	1120
	25 - 29	12	0	1062
	30 - 34	35	1	1264
	35 - 39	93	1	1895
	40 - 44	251	3	3049
	45 - 49	590	3	5260
	50 - 54	1248	6	9550
	55 - 59	2317	12	17270
	60 - 64	3315	17	27884
	65 - 69	3926	24	43487
	70 - 74	3878	28	67418
	75 - 79	3332	43	103261
	80 - 84	2258	50	161489

Appendix IX (cont'd)

Calendar period	Age group (years)	Death rate (per 1 000 000 per year)		
		Lung cancer	Nasal cancer	All causes
1961 - 1965	10 - 14	0	0	407
	15 - 19	2	0	951
	20 - 24	5	0	1103
	25 - 29	11	0	1008
	30 - 34	34	0	1218
	35 - 39	90	1	1855
	40 - 44	223	3	3048
	45 - 49	563	4	5333
	50 - 54	1221	8	9327
	55 - 59	2284	9	16533
	60 - 64	3663	14	28089
	65 - 69	4844	18	44194
	70 - 74	4977	26	67547
	75 - 79	4513	41	102346
	80 - 84	3417	42	157935
1966 - 1970	10 - 14	0	0	389
	15 - 19	2	0	961
	20 - 24	4	0	975
	25 - 29	10	0	929
	30 - 34	25	0	1121
	35 - 39	76	1	1693
	40 - 44	216	2	3030
	45 - 49	531	5	5307
	50 - 54	1160	7	9255
	55 - 59	2201	11	15878
	60 - 64	3695	16	26829
	65 - 69	5273	23	43953
	70 - 74	6210	29	67717
	75 - 79	5914	36	100781
	80 - 84	4563	31	143567
1971 - 1975	10 - 14	0	0	346
	15 - 19	1	0	876
	20 - 24	4	0	987
	25 - 29	10	1	887
	30 - 34	24	1	1073
	35 - 39	58	1	1583
	40 - 44	177	4	2851
	45 - 49	503	4	5293
	50 - 54	1070	8	9096
	55 - 59	2077	11	15292
	60 - 64	3546	16	25132
	65 - 69	5174	26	41432
	70 - 74	6820	29	66018
	75 - 79	7273	33	99794
	80 - 84	6089	38	147939

Appendix IX (cont'd)

Calendar period	Age group (years)	Death rate (per 1 000 000 per year)		
		Lung cancer	Nasal cancer	All causes
1976 - 1980	10 - 14	0	0	293
	15 - 19	1	0	869
	20 - 24	2	0	932
	25 - 29	7	1	883
	30 - 34	17	1	994
	35 - 39	56	1	1511
	40 - 44	139	2	2535
	45 - 49	403	3	4717
	50 - 54	1003	9	8699
	55 - 59	1896	9	14449
	60 - 64	3342	15	24144
	65 - 69	4985	17	38731
	70 - 74	6718	20	62218
	75 - 79	8068	38	97305
	80 - 84	7744	33	145137

SUBJECT INDEX TO VOLUMES I AND II

PUBLICATIONS OF THE INTERNATIONAL AGENCY FOR RESEARCH ON CANCER
SCIENTIFIC PUBLICATIONS SERIES

(Available from Oxford University Press)
through local bookshops

No. 1 LIVER CANCER
1971; 176 pages; out of print

No. 2 ONCOGENESIS AND HERPESVIRUSES
Edited by P.M. Biggs, G. de-Thé & L.N. Payne
1972; 515 pages; out of print

No. 3 N-NITROSO COMPOUNDS: ANALYSIS
AND FORMATION
Edited by P. Bogovski, R. Preussmann & E. A. Walker
1972; 140 pages; out of print

No. 4 TRANSPLACENTAL CARCINOGENESIS
Edited by L. Tomatis & U. Mohr
1973; 181 pages; out of print

*No. 5 PATHOLOGY OF TUMOURS IN
LABORATORY ANIMALS. VOLUME 1.
TUMOURS OF THE RAT. PART 1
Editor-in-Chief V.S. Turusov
1973; 214 pages

*No. 6 PATHOLOGY OF TUMOURS IN
LABORATORY ANIMALS. VOLUME 1.
TUMOURS OF THE RAT. PART 2
Editor-in-Chief V.S. Turusov
1976; 319 pages
*reprinted in one volume, Price £50.00

No. 7 HOST ENVIRONMENT INTERACTIONS IN
THE ETIOLOGY OF CANCER IN MAN
Edited by R. Doll & I. Vodopija
1973; 464 pages; £32.50

No. 8 BIOLOGICAL EFFECTS OF ASBESTOS
Edited by P. Bogovski, J.C. Gilson, V. Timbrell
& J.C. Wagner
1973; 346 pages; out of print

No. 9 N-NITROSO COMPOUNDS IN THE
ENVIRONMENT
Edited by P. Bogovski & E. A. Walker
1974; 243 pages; £16.50

No. 10 CHEMICAL CARCINOGENESIS ESSAYS
Edited by R. Montesano & L. Tomatis
1974; 230 pages; out of print

No. 11 ONCOGENESIS AND HERPESVIRUSES II
Edited by G. de-Thé, M.A. Epstein & H. zur Hausen
1975; Part 1, 511 pages; Part 2, 403 pages; £65.-

No. 12 SCREENING TESTS IN CHEMICAL
CARCINOGENESIS
Edited by R. Montesano, H. Bartsch & L. Tomatis
1976; 666 pages; £12.-

No. 13 ENVIRONMENTAL POLLUTION AND
CARCINOGENIC RISKS
Edited by C. Rosenfeld & W. Davis
1976; 454 pages; out of print

No. 14 ENVIRONMENTAL N-NITROSO
COMPOUNDS: ANALYSIS AND FORMATION
Edited by E.A. Walker, P. Bogovski & L. Griciute
1976; 512 pages; £37.50

No. 15 CANCER INCIDENCE IN FIVE
CONTINENTS. VOLUME III
Edited by J. Waterhouse, C. Muir, P. Correa
& J. Powell
1976; 584 pages; £35.-

No. 16 AIR POLLUTION AND CANCER IN MAN
Edited by U. Mohr, D. Schmähl & L. Tomatis
1977; 311 pages; out of print

No. 17 DIRECTORY OF ON-GOING RESEARCH
IN CANCER EPIDEMIOLOGY 1977
Edited by C.S. Muir & G. Wagner
1977; 599 pages; out of print

No. 18 ENVIRONMENTAL CARCINOGENS:
SELECTED METHODS OF ANALYSIS
Edited-in-Chief H. Egan
VOLUME 1. ANALYSIS OF VOLATILE
NITROSAMINES IN FOOD
Edited by R. Preussmann, M. Castegnaro, E.A. Walker
& A.E. Wassermann
1978; 212 pages; out of print

No. 19 ENVIRONMENTAL ASPECTS OF
N-NITROSO COMPOUNDS
Edited by E.A. Walker, M. Castegnaro, L. Griciute
& R.E. Lyle
1978; 566 pages; out of print

No. 20 NASOPHARYNGEAL CARCINOMA:
ETIOLOGY AND CONTROL
Edited by G. de-Thé & Y. Ito
1978; 610 pages; out of print

No. 21 CANCER REGISTRATION AND ITS
TECHNIQUES
Edited by R. MacLennan, C. Muir, R. Steinitz
& A. Winkler
1978; 235 pages; £35.-

Prices, valid for October 1987, are subject to change without notice

No. 22 ENVIRONMENTAL CARCINOGENS:
SELECTED METHODS OF ANALYSIS
Editor-in-Chief H. Egan
VOLUME 2. METHODS FOR THE MEASUREMENT
OF VINYL CHLORIDE IN POLY(VINYL
CHLORIDE), AIR, WATER AND FOODSTUFFS
Edited by D.C.M. Squirrell & W. Thain
1978; 142 pages; out of print

No. 23 PATHOLOGY OF TUMOURS IN
LABORATORY ANIMALS. VOLUME II.
TUMOURS OF THE MOUSE
Editor-in-Chief V.S. Turusov
1979; 669 pages; £37.50

No. 24 ONCOGENESIS AND HERPESVIRUSES III
Edited by G. de-Thé, W. Henle & F. Rapp
1978; Part 1, 580 pages; Part 2, 522 pages; out of print

No. 25 CARCINOGENIC RISKS: STRATEGIES
FOR INTERVENTION
Edited by W. Davis & C. Rosenfeld
1979; 283 pages; out of print

No. 26 DIRECTORY OF ON-GOING RESEARCH
IN CANCER EPIDEMIOLOGY 1978
Edited by C.S. Muir & G. Wagner,
1978; 550 pages; out of print

No. 27 MOLECULAR AND CELLULAR ASPECTS
OF CARCINOGEN SCREENING TESTS
Edited by R. Montesano, H. Bartsch & L. Tomatis
1980; 371 pages; £22.50

No. 28 DIRECTORY OF ON-GOING RESEARCH
IN CANCER EPIDEMIOLOGY 1979
Edited by C.S. Muir & G. Wagner
1979; 672 pages; out of print

No. 29 ENVIRONMENTAL CARCINOGENS:
SELECTED METHODS OF ANALYSIS
Editor-in-Chief H. Egan
VOLUME 3. ANALYSIS OF POLYCYCLIC
AROMATIC HYDROCARBONS IN
ENVIRONMENTAL SAMPLES
Edited by M. Castegnaro, P. Bogovski, H. Kunte
& E.A. Walker
1979; 240 pages; out of print

No. 30 BIOLOGICAL EFFECTS OF MINERAL
FIBRES
Editor-in-Chief J.C. Wagner
1980; Volume 1, 494 pages; Volume 2, 513 pages;
£55.-

No. 31 N-NITROSO COMPOUNDS: ANALYSIS,
FORMATION AND OCCURRENCE
Edited by E.A. Walker, L. Griciute, M. Castegnaro
& M. Börzsönyi
1980; 841 pages; out of print

No. 32 STATISTICAL METHODS IN CANCER
RESEARCH. VOLUME 1. THE ANALYSIS OF
CASE-CONTROL STUDIES
By N.E. Breslow & N.E. Day
1980; 338 pages; £20.-

No. 33 HANDLING CHEMICAL CARCINOGENS IN
THE LABORATORY: PROBLEMS OF SAFETY
Edited by R. Montesano, H. Bartsch, E. Boyland,
G. Della Porta, L. Fishbein, R.A. Griesemer,
A.B. Swan & L. Tomatis
1979; 32 pages; out of print

No. 34 PATHOLOGY OF TUMOURS IN
LABORATORY ANIMALS. VOLUME III.
TUMOURS OF THE HAMSTER
Editor-in-Chief V.S. Turusov
1982; 461 pages; £32.50

No. 35 DIRECTORY OF ON-GOING RESEARCH
IN CANCER EPIDEMIOLOGY 1980
Edited by C.S. Muir & G. Wagner
1980; 660 pages; out of print

No. 36 CANCER MORTALITY BY OCCUPATION
AND SOCIAL CLASS 1851-1971
By W.P.D. Logan
1982; 253 pages; £22.50

No. 37 LABORATORY DECONTAMINATION
AND DESTRUCTION OF AFLATOXINS
B_1, B_2, G_1, G_2 IN LABORATORY WASTES
Edited by M. Castegnaro, D.C. Hunt, E.B. Sansone,
P.L. Schuller, M.G. Siriwardana, G.M. Telling,
H.P. Van Egmond & E.A. Walker
1980; 59 pages; £6.50

No. 38 DIRECTORY OF ON-GOING RESEARCH
IN CANCER EPIDEMIOLOGY 1981
Edited by C.S. Muir & G. Wagner
1981; 696 pages; out of print

No. 39 HOST FACTORS IN HUMAN
CARCINOGENESIS
Edited by H. Bartsch & B. Armstrong
1982; 583 pages; £37.50

No. 40 ENVIRONMENTAL CARCINOGENS:
SELECTED METHODS OF ANALYSIS
Edited-in-Chief H. Egan
VOLUME 4. SOME AROMATIC AMINES AND
AZO DYES IN THE GENERAL AND INDUSTRIAL
ENVIRONMENT
Edited by L. Fishbein, M. Castegnaro, I.K. O'Neill
& H. Bartsch
1981; 347 pages; £22.50

No. 41 N-NITROSO COMPOUNDS:
OCCURRENCE AND BIOLOGICAL EFFECTS
Edited by H. Bartsch, I.K. O'Neill, M. Castegnaro
& M. Okada
1982; 755 pages; £37.50

No. 42 CANCER INCIDENCE IN FIVE
CONTINENTS. VOLUME IV
Edited by J. Waterhouse, C. Muir,
K. Shanmugaratnam & J. Powell
1982; 811 pages; £37.50

SCIENTIFIC PUBLICATIONS SERIES

No. 43 LABORATORY DECONTAMINATION
AND DESTRUCTION OF CARCINOGENS IN
LABORATORY WASTES: SOME *N*-NITROSAMINES
Edited by M. Castegnaro, G. Eisenbrand, G. Ellen,
L. Keefer, D. Klein, E.B. Sansone, D. Spincer,
G. Telling & K. Webb
1982; 73 pages; £7.50

No. 44 ENVIRONMENTAL CARCINOGENS:.
SELECTED METHODS OF ANALYSIS
Editor-in-Chief H. Egan
VOLUME 5. SOME MYCOTOXINS
Edited by L. Stoloff, M. Castegnaro, P. Scott,
I.K. O'Neill & H. Bartsch
1983; 455 pages; £22.50

No. 45 ENVIRONMENTAL CARCINOGENS:
SELECTED METHODS OF ANALYSIS
Editor-in-Chief H. Egan
VOLUME 6. *N*-NITROSO COMPOUNDS
Edited by R. Preussmann, I.K. O'Neill, G. Eisenbrand,
B. Spiegelhalder & H. Bartsch
1983; 508 pages; £22.50

No. 46 DIRECTORY OF ON-GOING RESEARCH
IN CANCER EPIDEMIOLOGY 1982
Edited by C.S. Muir & G. Wagner
1982; 722 pages; out of print

No. 47 CANCER INCIDENCE IN SINGAPORE
1968-1977
Edited by K. Shanmugaratnam, H.P. Lee & N.E. Day
1982; 171 pages; out of print

No. 48 CANCER INCIDENCE IN THE USSR
Second Revised Edition
Edited by N.P. Napalkov, G.F. Tserkovny,
V.M. Merabishvili, D.M. Parkin, M. Smans & C.S. Muir,
1983; 75 pages; £12.-

No. 49 LABORATORY DECONTAMINATION AND
DESTRUCTION OF CARCINOGENS IN
LABORATORY WASTES: SOME POLYCYCLIC
AROMATIC HYDROCARBONS
Edited by M. Castegnaro, G. Grimmer, O. Hutzinger,
W. Karcher, H. Kunte, M. Lafontaine, E.B. Sansone,
G. Telling & S.P. Tucker
1983; 81 pages; £9.-

No. 50 DIRECTORY OF ON-GOING RESEARCH
IN CANCER EPIDEMIOLOGY 1983
Edited by C.S. Muir & G. Wagner
1983; 740 pages; out of print

No. 51 MODULATORS OF EXPERIMENTAL
CARCINOGENESIS
Edited by V. Turusov & R. Montesano
1983; 307 pages; £22.50

No. 52 SECOND CANCER IN RELATION TO
RADIATION TREATMENT FOR CERVICAL
CANCER
Edited by N.E. Day & J.D. Boice, Jr
1984; 207 pages; £20.-

No. 53 NICKEL IN THE HUMAN ENVIRONMENT
Editor-in-Chief F.W. Sunderman, Jr
1984: 530 pages; £32.50

No. 54 LABORATORY DECONTAMINATION
AND DESTRUCTION OF CARCINOGENS IN
LABORATORY WASTES: SOME HYDRAZINES
Edited by M. Castegnaro, G. Ellen, M. Lafontaine,
H.C. van der Plas, E.B. Sansone & S.P. Tucker
1983; 87 pages; £9.-

No. 55 LABORATORY DECONTAMINATION
AND DESTRUCTION OF CARCINOGENS IN
LABORATORY WASTES: SOME *N*-NITROSAMIDES
Edited by M. Castegnaro, M. Benard,
L.W. van Broekhoven, D. Fine, R. Massey,
E.B. Sansone, P.L.R. Smith, B. Spiegelhalder,
A. Stacchini, G. Telling & J.J. Vallon
1984; 65 pages; £7.50

No. 56 MODELS, MECHANISMS AND ETIOLOGY
OF TUMOUR PROMOTION
Edited by M. Börszönyi, N.E. Day, K. Lapis
& H. Yamasaki
1984; 532 pages; £32.50

No. 57 *N*-NITROSO COMPOUNDS:
OCCURRENCE, BIOLOGICAL EFFECTS
AND RELEVANCE TO HUMAN CANCER
Edited by I.K. O'Neill, R.C. von Borstel, C.T. Miller,
J. Long & H. Bartsch
1984; 1011 pages; £80.-

No. 58 AGE-RELATED FACTORS IN
CARCINOGENESIS
Edited by A. Likhachev, V. Anisimov & R. Montesano
1985; 288 pages; £20.-

No. 59 MONITORING HUMAN EXPOSURE TO
CARCINOGENIC AND MUTAGENIC AGENTS
Edited by A. Berlin, M. Draper, K. Hemminki
& H. Vainio
1984; 457 pages; £27.50

No. 60 BURKITT'S LYMPHOMA: A HUMAN
CANCER MODEL
Edited by G. Lenoir, G. O'Conor & C.L.M. Olweny
1985; 484 pages; £22.50

No. 61 LABORATORY DECONTAMINATION
AND DESTRUCTION OF CARCINOGENS IN
LABORATORY WASTES: SOME HALOETHERS
Edited by M. Castegnaro, M. Alvarez, M. Iovu,
E.B. Sansone, G.M. Telling & D.T. Williams
1984; 53 pages; £7.50

No. 62 DIRECTORY OF ON-GOING RESEARCH
IN CANCER EPIDEMIOLOGY 1984
Edited by C.S. Muir & G.Wagner
1984; 728 pages; £26.-

No. 63 VIRUS-ASSOCIATED CANCERS IN AFRICA
Edited by A.O. Williams, G.T. O'Conor, G.B. de-Thé
& C.A. Johnson
1984; 774 pages; £22.-

SCIENTIFIC PUBLICATIONS SERIES

No. 85 ENVIRONMENTAL CARCINOGENS:
METHODS OF ANALYSIS AND EXPOSURE
MEASUREMENT. VOLUME 10. BENZENE
AND ALKYLATED BENZENES
Edited by L. Fishbein & I.K. O'Neill
(in press)

No. 86 DIRECTORY OF ON-GOING RESEARCH
IN CANCER EPIDEMIOLOGY 1987
Edited by D.M. Parkin & J. Wahrendorf
1987; 685 pages; £22.-

No. 87 INTERNATIONAL INCIDENCE OF
CHILDHOOD CANCER
Edited by D.M. Parkin, C.A. Stiller, G.J. Draper, C.A.
Bieber, B. Terracini
& J.L. Young
(in preparation)

No. 88 CANCER INCIDENCE IN FIVE
CONTINENTS. VOLUME V
Edited by C. Muir, J. Waterhouse, T. Mack,
J. Powell & S. Whelan
(in press)

No. 89 METHODS FOR DETECTING DNA
DAMAGING AGENTS IN HUMANS:
APPLICATIONS IN CANCER EPIDEMIOLOGY
AND PREVENTION
Edited by H. Bartsch, K. Hemminki
& I.K. O'Neill
(in preparation)

No. 90 NON-OCCUPATIONAL EXPOSURE TO
MINERAL FIBRES
Edited by J. Bignon, J. Peto & R. Saracci
(in preparation)

No. 91 TRENDS IN CANCER INCIDENCE IN
SINGAPORE 1968-1982
Edited by H.P. Lee, N.E. Day &
K. Shanmugaratnam
(in press)

IARC MONOGRAPHS ON THE EVALUATION OF THE CARCINOGENIC RISK OF CHEMICALS TO HUMANS

(English editions only)

(Available from booksellers through the network of WHO Sales Agents*)

Volume 1
Some inorganic substances, chlorinated hydrocarbons, aromatic amines, N-nitroso compounds, and natural products
1972; 184 pages; out of print

Volume 2
Some inorganic and organometallic compounds
1973; 181 pages; out of print

Volume 3
Certain polycyclic aromatic hydrocarbons and heterocyclic compounds
1973; 271 pages; out of print

Volume 4
Some aromatic amines, hydrazine and related substances, N-nitroso compounds and miscellaneous alkylating agents
1974; 286 pages;
Sw. fr. 18.-

Volume 5
Some organochlorine pesticides
1974; 241 pages; out of print

Volume 6
Sex hormones
1974; 243 pages;
out of print

Volume 7
Some anti-thyroid and related substances, nitrofurans and industrial chemicals
1974; 326 pages; out of print

Volume 8
Some aromatic azo compounds
1975; 357 pages; Sw.fr. 36.-

Volume 9
Some aziridines, N-, S- and O-mustards and selenium
1975; 268 pages; Sw. fr. 27.-

Volume 10
Some naturally occurring substances
1976; 353 pages; out of print

Volume 11
Cadmium, nickel, some epoxides, miscellaneous industrial chemicals and general considerations on volatile anaesthetics
1976; 306 pages; out of print

Volume 12
Some carbamates, thiocarbamates and carbazides
1976; 282 pages; Sw. fr. 34.-

Volume 13
Some miscellaneous pharmaceutical substances
1977; 255 pages; Sw. fr. 30.-

Volume 14
Asbestos
1977; 106 pages; out of print

Volume 15
Some fumigants, the herbicides 2,4-D and 2,4,5-T, chlorinated dibenzodioxins and miscellaneous industrial chemicals
1977; 354 pages; Sw. fr. 50.-

Volume 16
Some aromatic amines and related nitro compounds — hair dyes, colouring agents and miscellaneous industrial chemicals
1978; 400 pages; Sw. fr. 50.-

Volume 17
Some N-nitroso compounds
1978; 365 pages; Sw. fr. 50.

Volume 18
Polychlorinated biphenyls and polybrominated biphenyls
1978; 140 pages; Sw. fr. 20.-

Volume 19
Some monomers, plastics and synthetic elastomers, and acrolein
1979; 513 pages; Sw. fr. 60.-

Volume 20
Some halogenated hydrocarbons
1979; 609 pages; Sw. fr. 60.-

Volume 21
Sex hormones (II)
1979; 583 pages; Sw. fr. 60.-

Volume 22
Some non-nutritive sweetening agents
1980; 208 pages; Sw. fr. 25.-

Volume 23
Some metals and metallic compounds
1980; 438 pages; Sw. fr. 50.-

Volume 24
Some pharmaceutical drugs
1980; 337 pages; Sw. fr. 40.-

Volume 25
Wood, leather and some associated industries
1981; 412 pages; Sw. fr. 60.-

Volume 26
Some antineoplastic and immunosuppressive agents
1981; 411 pages; Sw. fr. 62.-

IARC MONOGRAPHS SERIES

Volume 27
Some aromatic amines, anthraquinones and nitroso compounds, and inorganic fluorides used in drinking-water and dental preparations
1982; 341 pages; Sw. fr. 40.-

Volume 28
The rubber industry
1982; 486 pages; Sw. fr. 70.-

Volume 29
Some industrial chemicals and dyestuffs
1982; 416 pages; Sw. fr. 60.-

Volume 30
Miscellaneous pesticides
1983; 424 pages; Sw. fr. 60.-

Volume 31
Some food additives, feed additives and naturally occurring substances
1983; 14 pages; Sw. fr. 60.-

Volume 32
Polynuclear aromatic compounds, Part 1, Chemical, environmental and experimental data
1984; 477 pages; Sw. fr. 60.-

Volume 33
Polynuclear aromatic compounds, Part 2, Carbon blacks, mineral oils and some nitroarenes
1984, 245 pages; Sw. fr. 50.-

Volume 34
Polynuclear aromatic compounds, Part 3, Industrial exposures in aluminium production, coal gasification, coke production, and iron and steel founding
1984; 219 pages; Sw. fr. 48.-

Volume 35
Polynuclear aromatic compounds, Part 4, Bitumens, coal-tars and derived products, shale-oils and soots
1985; 271 pages; Sw. fr.70.-

Volume 36
Allyl compounds, aldehydes, epoxides and peroxides
1985; 369 pages; Sw. fr. 70.-

Volume 37
Tobacco habits other than smoking; betel-quid and areca-nut chewing; and some related nitrosamines
1985; 291 pages; Sw. fr. 70.-

Volume 38
Tobacco smoking
1986; 421 pages; Sw. fr. 75.-

Volume 39
Some chemicals used in plastics and elastomers
1986; 403 pages; Sw. fr. 60.-

Volume 40
Some naturally occurring and synthetic food components, furocoumarins and ultraviolet radiation
1986; 444 pages; Sw. fr. 65.-

Volume 41
Some halogenated hydrocarbons and pesticide exposures
1986; 434 pages; Sw. fr. 65.-

Volume 42
Silica and some silicates
1987; 289 pages; Sw. fr. 65.-

*Volume 43
Man-made mineral fibres and radon
(in press)

Volume 44
Alcohol and alcoholic beverages
(in preparation)

Supplement No. 1
Chemicals and industrial processes associated with cancer in humans (IARC Monographs, Volumes 1 to 20)
1979; 71 pages; out of print

Supplement No. 2
Long-term and short-term screening assays for carcinogens: a critical appraisal
1980; 426 pages; Sw. fr. 40.-

Supplement No. 3
Cross index of synonyms and trade names in Volumes 1 to 26
1982; 199 pages; Sw. fr. 60.-

Supplement No. 4
Chemicals, industrial processes and industries associated with cancer in h. *nans (IARC Monographs, Volumes 1 to 29)*
1982; 292 pages; Sw. fr. 60.-

Supplement No. 5
Cross index of synonyms and trade names in Volumes 1 to 36
1985; 259 pages; Sw. fr. 60.-

Supplement No. 6
Genetic and related effects: An update of selected IARC Monographs from Volumes 1-42
(in press)

Supplement No. 7
Overall evaluations of carcinogenicity: An update of IARC Monographs Volumes 1-42
(in press)

*From Volume 43 onwards, the series title has been changed to IARC MONOGRAPHS ON THE

INFORMATION BULLETINS ON THE
SURVEY OF CHEMICALS BEING
TESTED FOR CARCINOGENICITY

(Available from IARC and WHO Sales Agents)

No. 8 (1979)
Edited by M.-J. Ghess, H. Bartsch
& L. Tomatis
604 pages; Sw. fr. 40.-

No. 9 (1981)
Edited by M.-J. Ghess, J.D. Wilbourn,
H. Bartsch & L. Tomatis
294 pages; Sw. fr. 41.-

No. 10 (1982)
Edited by M.-J. Ghess, J.D. Wilbourn
& H. Bartsch
362 pages; Sw. fr. 42.-

No. 11 (1984)
Edited by M.-J. Ghess, J.D. Wilbourn,
H. Vainio & H. Bartsch
362 pages; Sw. fr. 50.-

No. 12 (1986)
Edited by M.-J. Ghess, J.D. Wilbourn,
A. Tossavainen & H. Vainio
385 pages; Sw. fr. 50.-

NON-SERIAL PUBLICATIONS

(Available from IARC)

ALCOOL ET CANCER
By A. Tuyns (in French only)
1978; 42 pages; Fr. fr. 35.-

CANCER MORBIDITY AND CAUSES OF
DEATH AMONG DANISH BREWERY
WORKERS
By O.M. Jensen
1980; 143 pages; Fr. fr. 75.-

DIRECTORY OF COMPUTER SYSTEMS
USED IN CANCER REGISTRIES
By H.R. Menck & D.M. Parkin
1986; 236 pages; Fr. fr. 50.-